Textbook of
Pharmaceutical
Packaging Technology

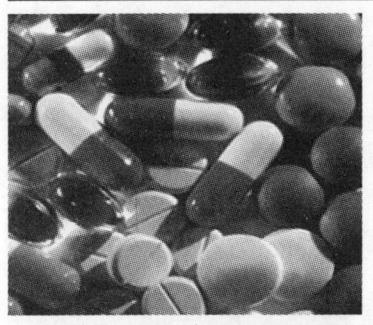
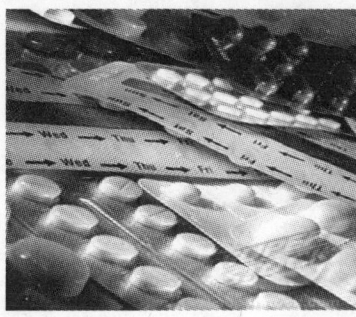
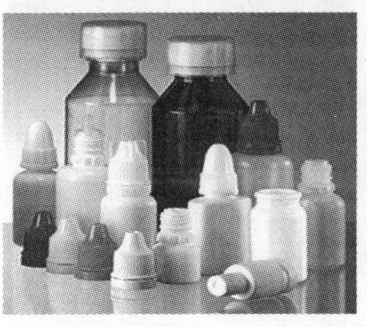
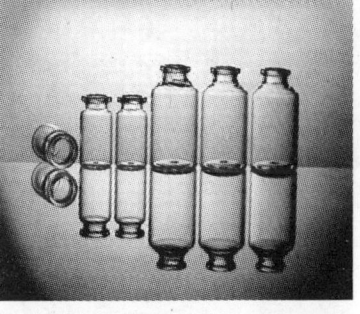
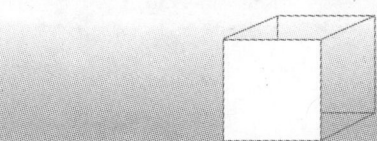

Textbook of
Pharmaceutical
Packaging Technology

Atul Kaushik M Pharm PhD
Professor, Department of Pharmaceutics, and
Principal, IPS College of Pharmacy
Gwalior

Bhaskar Chaurasia M Pharm
Assistant Professor
Shri RNS Institute of Pharmaceutical Sciences and Technology
Sitholi, Gwalior

Virendra Dhakar M Pharm
Assistant Professor
Shri RNS Institute of Pharmaceutical Sciences and Technology
Sitholi, Gwalior

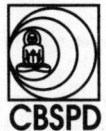

CBSPD

CBS Publishers & Distributors Pvt Ltd

New Delhi • Bengaluru • Chennai • Kochi • Kolkata • Lucknow • Mumbai
Hyderabad • Jharkhand • Nagpur • Patna • Pune • Uttarakhand

Textbook of
Pharmaceutical Packaging Technology

ISBN-13: 978-81-239-1987-4

First Edition: 2011

Reprint: 2015, 2017, 2019, **2024**

Published by **Satish Kumar Jain** and produced by **Varun Jain** for
CBS Publishers & Distributors Pvt Ltd
4819/XI Prahlad Street, 24 Ansari Road, Daryaganj, New Delhi 110 002, India
Ph: 011-23289259, 23266861   Website: www.cbspd.com
                                    e-mail: delhi@cbspd.com

Corporate Office: 204 FIE, Industrial Area, Patparganj, Delhi 110 092, India
Ph: 011-4934 4934   Fax: 011-4934 4935   e-mail: publishing@cbspd.com;
                                                 publicity@cbspd.com

Branches

- **Bengaluru:** Seema House 2975, 17th Cross, KR Road, Banasankari 2nd Stage, Bengaluru 560 070, Karnataka, India
  Ph: +91-80-26771678/79   Fax: +91-80-26771680   e-mail: bangalore@cbspd.com
- **Chennai:** 7, Subbaraya Street, Shenoy Nagar, Chennai 600 030, Tamil Nadu, India
  Ph: +91-44-26680620, 26681266   Fax: +91-44-42032115   e-mail: chennai@cbspd.com
- **Kochi:** 42/1325, 1326, Power House Road, Opp KSEB, Power House, Ernakulum Kochi 682 018, Kerala, India
  Ph: +91-484-4059061-65,67   Fax: +91-484-4059065   e-mail: kochi@cbspd.com
- **Kolkata:** 147, Hind Ceramics Compound, 1st Floor, Nilgunj Road, Belghoria, Kolkata-700056, West Bengal, India
  Ph: +033-25633055, 033-25633056   e-mail: kolkata@cbspd.com
- **Lucknow:** Basement, Khushnuma Complex, 7 Meerabai Marg (Behind Jawahar Bhawan), Lucknow-226001, UP, India
  Ph: +91-522-4000032   e-mail: tiwari.lucknow@cbspd.com
- **Mumbai:** PWD Shed, Gala no 25/26, Ramchandra Bhatt Marg, Next to JJ Hospital Gate no. 2, Opp. Union Bank of India Noorbaug, Mumbai-400009, Maharashtra, India
  Ph: 022-66661880/89   e-mail: mumbai@cbspd.com

Representatives

• Hyderabad	0-9885175004	• Jharkhand	0-9811541605	• Nagpur	0-8692091830
• Patna	0-9334159340	• Pune	0-9664372571	• Uttarakhand	0-9716462459

Printed at Neekunj Print Process, Haryana, India

to

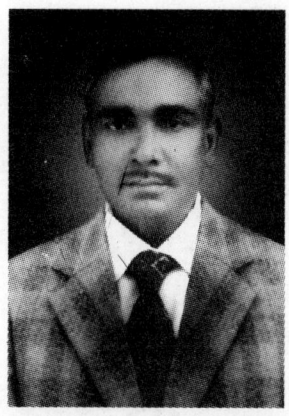

Late Dr BD Chaurasia
(Reader, Human Anatomy,
GR Medical College, Gwalior)

Preface

The pharmacy profession has made unlimited growth during the last 50 years and hence pharmaceutical education has also been promoted at the highest levels of standards. The present book will help readers in understanding the packaging technology, the different types of packaging, and the importance of packaging. It provides a very systematic and comprehensive coverage of the theory as well as the illustration of application thereof. This book is designed to serve as textbook for students who are studying packaging technology at both the undergraduate I postgraduate levels. It covers almost all types of packaging in industries.

The systematic structure of the book is assigned to cover the major syllabus of packaging technology over 19 chapters.

Chapters 1 to 6 describe what is packaging, future of packaging, packaging design research, different types of pharmaceutical containers, new trends in pharmaceutical packaging, different types of packaging materials and detailed study of glass, plastics and metal.

Chapter 7 describes the detailed study of blister and strip packaging. Chapters 8 and 9 explain ancillary materials and rubber.

Chapter 10 describes closures, different types of closures and liners. Chapter 11 explains corrugated fiberboard.

Chapters 12 and 13 describe sterilization methods of packaging materials and packaging of sterile pharmaceuticals.

Chapters 14 to 16 describe defects in packages, labelling of packages and package testing.

Chapters 17 and 18 describe stability of packages, packaging regulations and legal requirements.

Chapter 19 describes the detailed study of packaging functions.

We wish to acknowledge our indebtedness to our teachers and colleagues who have contributed towards this edition in one way or the other. However, our most sincere thanks are due to Dr Uma Shankar Nagayach (former Principal, Degree College, Mahoba), Dr Surendra Mohan Tiwari (former Reader, GR Medical College, Gwalior), Dr Prabhakar K Verma (Professor, Department of Pharmacy, MD University, Rohtak), Dr (Mrs) Suman Jain (Principal, Shri Ram College of Pharmacy, Banmore), Dr Ashutosh Kar (Director, Shri RNS College of Pharmacy, Gormi), and Dr Manoj Sharma (Principal, Shri RNS College of Pharmacy, Gormi).

We are thankful to Mr Ravindra S Dhakad and Mr Rajiv Chaurasia for their advise and constant encouragement in our endeavour.

We are also highly thankful to Mr Satish K Jain, Mr Vinod K Jain, and the editorial–production teams at CBSPD for their dynamic efforts in bringing out this publication.

We are also thankful to our family members and finally we are thankful to God.

Atul Kaushik
Bhaskar Chaurasia
Virendra Dhakar

Contents

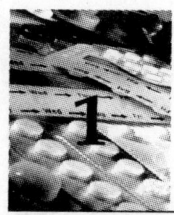# Pharmaceutical Packaging Technology

1.1 INTRODUCTION

Millions of years ago people hunted for food and ate it at once. Soon they realized they could keep their food longer if they protected it, so they made pockets from animal skin and large leaves, and kept water in containers made from coconut shells and dried vegetable skins. Gradually packaging came into existence to take care of food, medicine and consumer goods etc. Packaging was invented in 1875 by Henry J. Packaging. Packaging is heavily integrated into our daily lives; we see it all around us.

Packaging is the art, science and technology of protecting or enclosing products for distribution, storage, sale and use. Packaging also refers to the process of design, evaluation and production of packages.

It is used for several purposes:
- Contain products, defining the amount the consumer will purchase.
- Protects products from contamination, from environmental damages and from theft.
- Facilitate transportation and storing of products.
- Carry information and colourful design that make attractive displays.

Packaging makes a bridge between production and marketing. Virtually every product, whether grown or manufactured, must be packaged so that it reaches the consumer in an acceptable condition. Packaging is now generally regarded as an essential component of our modern lifestyle and the way business is organized. Packaging, today, is identified as a need for industrial growth and economic development of a country.

1.2 PACKAGING

The act, process, art, or style of packing is known as packaging. Or packaging is defined in the regulations as "all products made of any materials of any nature to be used for the containment, protection, handling, delivery and preservation of goods from the producer to the user or consumer." Or processes (such as cleaning, drying, preserving) and materials (such as glass, metal, paper or paperboard, plastic) employed to contain, handle, protect, and/or transport an article.

Role of packaging is broadening and may include functions such as to attract attention, assist in promotion, provide machine identification (barcodes, etc.), impart essential or additional information, and help in utilization. Pharmaceutical packaging is regarded as an whole conception of the modify pharmaceutical product. Packaging is more than just a product's pretty face. The package design may affect everything from breakage rates in shipment to whether stores will be willing to stock it. For example, "displayability" is an important concern. The original slanted-roof metal container used for Log Cabin Syrup was changed to a design that was easier to stack after grocers became reluctant to devote the necessary amounts of shelf space to the awkward packages. Other distribution-related packaging considerations include.

Labelling: Product may be required to include certain information on the label when it is distributed in specific ways. For example, labels of pharmaceutical and food products sold in retail outlets must contain information about their ingredients and nutritional value.

Opening: If the product is one that will be distributed in such a way that customers will want to – and should be able to – sample or examine it before buying, the packaging will have to be easy to open and to reclose. If, on the other hand, the product should not be opened by anyone other than the purchaser – an over – the-counter medication, for instance– then the packaging will have to be designed to resist and reveal tampering.

Size: If the product must be shipped a long distance to its distribution point, then bulky or heavy packaging may add too much to transportation costs.

Durability: Many products endure rough handling between their production point and their ultimate consumer. If distribution system can't be relied upon to protect the product, packaging will have to do the job.

Role of Packaging

The role of packaging is containment, protection, safety, and display.

1.3 CLASSIFICATION OF PACKAGING

Primary Packaging

Packaging material that is in direct contact with the product. It is generally composed of glass, or rigid or flexible plastics, and must keep the product stable until the expiration date. Or in other words product packaging such as the bottle, can, jar, tube, etc. that contains the item sold. It is the last packaging thrown by the consumer.

Choosing Appropriate Primary Pack

Product Characteristics/Sensitivity

- Hygroscopic
- Physical degradation
- Chemical degradation
- Drug release properties
- Mechanical properties
- Photosensitivity
- Gas liberation tendency
- Dimensional aspects.

Selection of Packaging Material

- Moisture barrier requirements
- Light barrier requirements
- Gas barrier requirements
- Chemical properties.

Secondary Packaging

That encloses the primary packaging, such as toothpaste tube in its box. Secondary packaging is outside the primary packaging–perhaps used to group primary packages together.
Examples: Boxes, cartons.

Tertiary Packaging

'Tertiary' or 'Transport' packaging is packaging that is used to group secondary packaging together to aid handling and transportation and prevent damage to the products, for example, the pallet and shrink wrap used to transport a number of cardboard outers containing boxes of soap powder. For the purposes of the Regulations, this does not include road, ship, rail or air containers.

1.4 PACKAGING ESSENTIAL REQUIREMENTS

(i) Requirements specific to the manufacturing and composition of packaging:

- The weight and volume of packaging must be the "Minimum Adequate Amount" to maintain the necessary level of safety, hygiene and acceptance for the packed product and the consumer.
- Noxious or hazardous substances in packaging must be minimised with regard to their presence in emissions, ash or leachate when packaging waste is incinerated or landfilled.
- Packaging must be reusable or recoverable including through recycling and its impact on the environment must be minimised when packaging waste is disposed of.

(ii) Requirements specific to the reusable nature of packaging:

- The physical properties of the packaging must enable a number of trips or rotations in normally predictable conditions.
- It must be possible to process the used packaging without compromising the health and safety requirements for the workforce.
- It must be possible to fulfil the requirements specific to recoverable packaging when the packaging becomes waste.

(iii) Requirements specific to the recoverable nature of packaging:

- **Recycling:** Packaging must enable the recycling of a certain percentage by weight of the materials used into the manufacture of marketable products.
- **Energy recovery:** Packaging shall have sufficient calorific value to allow optimisation of energy recovery.
- **Composting:** Packaging shall be of such a biodegradable nature that it should not hinder the separate collection and composting process into which it is introduced.
- **Biodegradable:** Packaging should be capable of undergoing Physical, Chemical, Thermal or Biological Decomposition, to such an extent that the final compost ultimately decomposes into carbon dioxide, biomass and water.

1.5 FUNCTIONS OF PACKAGING

Contaminant

- Not to leak, nor allow diffusion and permeation
- Strong enough to hold the contents during handling

Protection

- Light
- Moisture
- Oxygen
- Biological contamination
- Mechanical damage
- Counterfeiting

1.6 IMPORTANCE/SIGNIFICANCE OF PHARMACEUTICAL PACKAGING

Packaging has become a key driver for the protection of pharmaceutical dosage form physical and chemical factors.

- Derive suitable packaging on dosage form.
- Protection from moisture, gas, light and temperature
- Microbiological integrity.
- pH stability.
- Anti-counterfeit capability.
- Compliance – regulatory and patient.

Other Properties

- Package should be capable of easy opening, handling and storage.
- It should be easy to reclose
- Easy to inspect
- Easy to dispose of
- Also including the reusability and recyclability.

1.7 THE MAIN PACKAGING MATERIALS

- Plastic
- Glass
- Metal (Steel, aluminium, tin, lead)
- Paper/Fibreboard

Wood packaging and packaging made from other materials (for example hessian, jute, cork, ceramics and soon) are also included.

1.8 THE IDEAL PACKAGE

The perfect pharmaceutical package has all of the following criteria:
- Meets current legal requirements
- Compatible with product
- Protects against contamination from the environment
- Controls the product's environment
- Resists mechanical damage
- Sanitary
- Tamper-proof
- Attractive
- Convenient
- Inexpensive
- Lightweight
- Environmentally sound
- Functions as a preparation and/or serving vessel
- Sells itself
- Identifies the product and
- Supplies the required information.

Ideal Pack Requirements

- Product attributes, e.g. dosage form, physical and chemical robustness.

- Product protection needs, e.g. moisture and gas sensitivity, thermal stability, photostability, chemical compatibility, etc.
- Clinical requirements, e.g. dosing regimen, titration dosing, route of administration, need for dosing device.
- Patient requirements, e.g. specific handling requirements, patient handling studies.
- Commercial requirements, e.g. market presentation, pack sizes, market specific needs, patient handling needs.
- Manufacturing requirements, e.g. equipment capability, critical process parameters.
- Regulatory requirements, e.g. material compliance, pharmacopoeial monographs.

1.9 PROPERTIES OF IDEAL PACKAGING MATERIALS

Nevertheless, each and every function of the pack is meant to assume a certain degree of importance; however, protection predominantly occupies the most vital and ethical factor because it specifically controls the total shelf-life of the finished product.

Following are indeed some of the most important possible hazards that may require to be affording protection to the make finished secondary pharmaceutical product (i.e. dosage form), namely:

- Mechanical Factor
- Climatic Factor
- Biological Factor
- Chemical Factor

These four vital factors shall now be treating separately.

Mechanical Hazards

In fact, both physical/mechanical damage may incidentally take place because of the following reasons, such as:

1. **Impact or shock damage:** These are caused due to such factors as rough handling that includes sudden drops or impacts (deceleration). Importantly, shock may be minimized or overcome by various ways and means like proper cushioning, more careful handling, restriction of movement.

2. **Compression:** It has been duly observed that either loading or top pressure may crush or distort a pack and thereby damage the product packed inside.
   - Crushing of carton can render a product unusable even though no apparent damage has taken place to its contents.
   - Compression is most likely to take place in these three situations.
     - During stacking in the warehouse (or godown).
     - During transit when unavoidable vibration adds on to the further hazards and
     - Compression of pack may take place in certain other typical situations like:
       - Capping of tablet on production line.
       - Can occur while taking home the pack by its actual user.

3. **Vibration:** Vibration is the shaking comprises of two important variables such as: Frequency and Amplitude, e.g. extremely low amplitude + very high frequency. Thus, each extreme may effectively cause different types of damage to the product and/or pack. In other words, the various components of product may fall apart, e.g.
   - Screw caps may loosen to some extent
   - Labels may get disfigured, and
   - Decoration may abrade.

4. **Abrasion:** Abrasion may cause due to regular as well as irregular forms of vibration, e.g the visual appearance of product or pack may be affected, e.g.
   - A rectangular bottle in a carton shall move up and down and/or from side-to-side.
   - A round bottle under similar environment (condition) will experience from an additional chances of being undergoing rotation.

5. **Puncture or piercing:** A good number of packed materials do have the experience of suffering undergoing penetration from sharp objects. However, such events may eventually occur both in bulk drug and in finished pack. It may be avoided considerably by following two means:

- Avoiding fork lift trucks in handling of packed cartons or bulk – drug bags/drums.
- Provision of adequate cushioning and/or resistance to penetration.

Climatic or Environmental Hazards

In reality, the climatic or environmental hazards refer to the ever-present hazards that are specifically confined to a local environment. One may, however, come across such typical conditions usually covered by phrases, for instance: Arctic, Antarctic, Temperate, Subtropical, and Tropical, besides severe environmental conditions may take place in such adverse states as:

- Deep Freeze (–19 to –22°C)
- Bathroom or Kitchen
- Displayed under high wattage bulb in a shop (500W)
- Stored near hot – water pipes or heaters in a shop or warehouse.

Climatic hazards essentially include the following aspects detailed below:

1. **Moisture:** Moisture in the form of water vapour or liquid may eventually cause physical changes apparently, e.g. Softening, Hardening, Dulling, etc. whereas, chemical changes, e.g. effervescence, hydrolysis.
   - May also serve as a carrier for other contaminants.
   - There are some packaging materials are found to be permeable to moisture to a certain extent.
   - Screw type closure which ordinarily seem to render a good effective seal are prone to some passage of moisture that solely rests upon the sealing medium, the torque, the evenness, the shape, the sealing surface, the aperture size and circumferential area of container.
2. **Temperature:** It has been observed that extremes of temperature (either hot or cold) or cycling temperature may cause apparent deterioration product/or pack.
   - Higher temperature – emphatically designate a marked acceleration effect.
   - Low temperature – generally represent a marked deterioration effect, e.g. certain plastic packaging

materials (usually polymers) do have a tendency to become more brittle and undergo cracking.
- Importantly, both high temperature + High relative humidity shall cause shower effect if the temperature is lowered enough to reach the dew point.
- Contamination emenated from liquid moisture may progressively cause bacterial and mould growth.

3. Pressure: Air pressure differential are most commonly observed as a potential danger for materials that are dispatched by air employing un-pressurized aircraft.

Important points:
- Pressurized aircraft are usually pressurized to the equivalent to nearly 3000 m above sea-level, thereby affording a 0.25 bar differential in comparison to the take off status.
- Packed goods in manufacturing units are invariably at sea-level, and sent to high altitude location (i.e. mountainous areas like Ladakah, Srinagar, Leh, etc.) or vice-versa, will encounter similar patterns.
- *Example:* Goods Packed at Johannesburg (SA) located at 2000 m above sea-level, and subsequently dispatched to Durban located at sea level will be distinctively exposed to:
  - positive Pressure, and
  - variation in temperature as well.

4. Light: In fact, light rays comprises of wavelengths of various zones, such as:

UV Zone → Visible Zone → IR Zone.

Ultraviolet (UV) Zone-represents an extremely vital and potential source of photochemical change, which may or may not be visible apparently always.

It may cause:
- Decorated or printed materials may undergo appreciable discolouration, e.g.
  - White colour-change into yellow.
  - Deeper colour-change to fade.
- Product efficacy/strength may deteriorate considerably.

- UV-light may be barred by using selected material, e.g. aluminium foil, tin foil.
- Opacity and/or colour may reduce penetration or filter out selected wavelengths.
- Additional usage of UV-absorbers in plastics can also help in restricting light rays entering the pack.
- Several finished products are usually protected by a carton, outer, etc. significantly. In such cases, therefore, the actual protection zeroes down to only relatively short-display or usage duration when exposure to light takes place.

5. **Atmospheric gases:** Include essentially O_2, CO_2, N_2 and any other air borne gases.
   - *O_2:* Leads to oxidation accounts for more obvious hazard.
   - *CO_2:* May afford a shift of pH, e.g. unbuffered solution to plastic bottle (LDPE) which being more prone to CO_2 permeation, and/or lead to precipitation of certain products.
   - *Common gases:* Permeation through plastic is typically in ratio of 1:4:20 for N_2, O_2, and CO_2.
   - *CO_2:* Being most permeable in nature.
   - Odours gases/or volatile ingredients- intimately linked with perfumes, flavours and product formulations may either pass out of a pack or pass into a pack.
   - *Example:* In case of a volatile ingredient is ultimately escapes from a flavour, an unpleasant odour or taste may result.

6. **Solid airborne contamination (particulates):** Particulates may be incorporated/carried due to solid airborne contamination present in the atmosphere.

   Plastic contamination (particulates) may be enhanced by the electrostatic attraction preferably under dry conditions whereby the particulate matters are conspicuously taken up from the atmosphere by electrical charges.

   Consequently, the presence of particulates shall enhance the gross contamination due to various microorganisms (from the atmosphere) which may be minimized by installation of effective hepafilters in the production as well as "packing zone".

Biological Hazards

Biological hazards may be attributed due to the following three major factors, namely:

1. **Microbiological:** There exists an overall general tendency towards an improved microbial control for most of the secondary pharmaceutical products, i.e. dosage forms. In order to accomplish the aforesaid objective the following precautionary measures stringently:

   a. All packaging materials should be reasonably clean initially.

   b. Restrict any further contamination as far as possible.

   c. Specifically for sterile products (injectables, eye-drops, etc.) both the pack and the closure should maintain an absolute 100% effective seal against any possible ingress, i.e. infestation with microbes, moulds and yeasts.

2. **Other forms of infestation:** Quite common with food products, but other sources of infestation which may contaminate the pharmaceutical products profusely include attack particularly by: Insects, Termites, Vermin, Rodents, birds and animal contamination source.

   Such infestations do happen under extreme badly hygienic and house keeping parameters.

3. **Pilferage and adulteration risk factors:** Pilferage refers to the human failure aspect strictly, and may perhaps be legitimately categorized as another aspect of 'Biological Hazard', e.g. the spectacular example of Tylenol Poisoning of 1982 – has critically placed much greater practically feasible emphasis for the absolute need for Tamper-Resistant Packs.

   • Before this 'Shocking Episode' (in USA which shaken the world) various types of seals were used to imply/indicate whether any product had been removed or replaced – rather than as a means of causing protection against the deliberate adulteration.

   • *Security Seals:* Refers to a possibly preferred phrase so as to detect any tamper evidence, are now being widely employed across the globe for a variety of pharmaceutical products so as to serve as a means of definitely increasing and building up, and maintaining the consumer or patient confidence in the pack itself and hence the manufactured drug product.

Chemical Hazards

The chemical hazards usually come into being due to several factors, such as:

- Chemical interaction (in case, quite inherent to the basic formulation, cannot invariably be minimized or avoided by pack selection).
- Interaction or incompatibility between the product and the pack.
- Compatibility investigations should fundamentally cover any exchange, which can possibly take place between the product and the pack, and vice-versa.
- Compatibility studies may be intimately linked with other interaction or contamination, covering various aspects viz., migration, absorption, extraction, corrosion, erosion, etc. through which ingredients may be gained or lost.

Examples: These exchanges could be detectable easily due to:

- Degradation,
- Enhancement in toxicity/irritancy
- Organoleptic adulterations
- pH shift
- Haze and turbidity
- Colour change
- Loss/gain of microbial effectiveness

Obviously, there are some other external influences that may critically catalyze, induce or even nullify the chemical changes.

Examples of Chemical Interaction between a product and a pack and the overall outcome of contamination taking place are as enumerated under:

1. Adsorption of chemical entities upon the component surfaces occurs seldomly, e.g. losses of EDTA, some preservatives, such as:
   - Benzalkonium chloride, thiomersal, mercurials

2. Surface active ingredients, found in plastics can enter the product by dissolution and surface abrasion.
   Example: Antistatic additives, Slip additives, Mould Release agents, Antiblock agents, Lubricants.
3. Organoleptic adulterations can also take place due to permeation of volatile or odorous substances via plastic materials, e.g. solvent from printing inks.
4. Detachment of glass spicules can also occur when the alkaline solutions of citrales, tartrates, chlorides and salicylates are kept in cheap quality soda glass containers (bottles, jars).
5. More volatile preservatives such as chlorbutol, phenol, 2-phenyl ethanol. Usually exhibit rather fairly fast and rapid loss via low-density polyethene by absorption and surface evaporation. However, less than 10% losses may be prevented by an external over wrap that is not permeable to the preservative.

1.10 PACKAGING FORMATS IN PHARMA INDUSTRY

- Blister packs
- Strip packs
- Bottles for bulk packs
- Sachets or pouches
- Tubes for oral dosage
- Injectables
- Suppositories

1.11 PACKAGING RECYCLING SYMBOLS

Material	Symbol
Recyclable aluminium	(alu)
Recyclable steel	RECYCLABLE STEEL
Recyclable cardboard	or

Recyclable paper and cardboard (RESY)	Another symbol often displayed on paper and cardboard packaging is the RESY recycling symbol. This symbol guarantees that packaging with this symbol is recyclable and will be accepted by cardboard recyclers.
Recyclable glass	

Other Symbol

Material	Symbol
1. Biodegradable Plastic Packaging This is a relatively new symbol found on biodegradable plastic packaging. The symbol signifies that the packaging has been tested, and is suitable for putting into local authority compost collections.	
2. Recyclable Aerosols The main part of an aerosol is the can and 60% of these are made from tinplated steel. The remaining 40% are made from aluminium. Both of these metals are recyclable. Aerosols also contain some small plastic and rubber components including the lid, valve and dip tube.	**RECYCLE** **AEROSOLS**

1.12 FDA DEFINITIONS

All package types shall comply with any applicable 21 CFR regulations, CDER guidances, and compendial monographs. The container is that which holds the article and is or may be in direct contact with the article. The immediate container is that which is in direct contact with the article at all times. The closure is a part of the container.

Name	Definition	FDA Code
Ampoule	A container capable of being hermetically sealed, intended to hold sterile materials.	AMP
Applicator	A pre filled non injectable pipette, syringe or tube.	AP
Bag	A sac or pouch.	BAG
Blister Pack	A package that consists of molded plastic or laminate that has indentations (viewed as "blisters" when flipped) into which a dosage form, is placed. A covering, usually of laminated material, is then sealed to the molded part. A strip pack is a specialized type of blister pack where there are no pre-formed or molded parts; in this case there are two flexible layers that are sealed with the dosage form in between. Suppositories that are strip packed between two layers of foil are also considered a blister pack.	BLPK
Bottle	A vessel with a narrow neck designed to accept a specific closure.	BOT
Bottle, with Applicator	A bottle which includes a device for applying its contents.	BOTAP
Bottle, Dispensing	A bottle that is used by the pharmacist to dispense the prescribed medication. It includes preparations for which a dropper accompanies the bottle.	BOTDIS
Bottle, Dropper	A bottle that has a device specifically intended for the application of a liquid in a drop by drop manner, or a device intended for the delivery of an exact dose (e.g., calibrated dropper for oral medications).	BCTDR
Bottle, Glass	A glass vessel with a narrow neck designed to accept a specific closure.	BOTGL

Contd...

Contd...

Bottle, Plastic	A plastic vessel with a narrow neck designed to accept a specific closure.	BOTPL
Bottle, Pump	A bottle that is fitted with a pumping mechanism for the administration of drug product.	BOTPU
Bottle, Spray	A bottle that is fitted with an atomizer or a device which produces finely divided liquid carried by air.	BOTSPR
Bottle, Unit-Dose	A bottle that contains a single whole dose of a non-parenteral drug product.	BOTUD
Box	A square or rectangular vessel, usually made of cardboard or plastic.	BOX
Box, Unit-Dose	A box that contains a single dose of a non-parenteral drug product. [Note: Boxes that contain 100 unit dose blister packs should be classified under blister pack, since this is the immediate container into which the dosage form is placed.]	BOXUD
Can	A cylindrical vessel, usually made of metal.	CAN
Canister	A type of can for holding a drug product.	CSTR
Carton	A cardboard box or container which is usually considered a secondary packaging component.	CRTN
Cartridge	A container consisting of a cylinder with a septum at one end, and a seal at the other end, which is inserted into a device to form a syringe which contains a single dose of a parenteral drug product.	CTG
Case	A receptacle for holding something (e.g., that into which some oral contraceptive blister packs are placed).	CASE
Cello Pack	A plastic "clamshell" [thin plastic pre formed structure for a device].	CELLO
Container	A receptacle designed to hold a specific dosage form.	CTR
CUP	A bowl-shaped container.	CUP

Contd...

Contd...

CUP, Unit-Dose	A cup intended to hold a single dose of a non-parenteral drug product.	CUPUD
Cylinder	A container designed specifically to hold gases.	CYL
Dewar	A container, usually made of glass or metal, that has at least two walls with the space between each wall evacuated so as to prevent the transfer of heat. The inside of the container often has a coating (as silvering) on the inside to reduce heat transfer, and is used especially for storing liquified gases or for experiments at low temperatures. The size can vary from that of a small thermos bottle up to that which may be mounted upon a large truck (also known as a "cryogenic truck").	DEW
Dialpack	A dose pack container designed to assist with patient compliance. The patient turns a dial to the correct day and the correct dose is made available and the container indicates that the dose has been removed.	DLPK
Dose Pack	A container in which a preselected dose or dose regimen of the medication is placed.	DSPK
Drum	A straight sided cylindrical shipping container with flat ends; one of which can be opened/closed.	DRUM
Inhaler	A device by means of which a medicinal product can be administered by inspiration through the nose or the mouth.	INHL
Inhaler, Refill	A container of medication intended to refill an inhaler.	INHLRE
Jar	A rigid container having a wide mouth and often no neck which typically holds solid or semisolid drug products.	JAR
Jug	A large, deep container that has a narrow mouth, is typically fitted with a handle, and is used to hold liquids.	JUG

Contd...

Contd...

Kit	A package which includes a container of drug product(s) and the equipment and supplies used with it.	KIT
Not Stated	The package type is not stated or is unavailable.	NS
Package	The drug product container with any accompanying materials or components. This may include the protective packaging, labeling, administration devices, etc.	PKG
Package, Combination	A package in which two or more drug products that are normally available separately are now available together.	PKGCOM
Packet	An envelope into which only one dose of a drug product, usually in the form of granules or powder, has been directly placed. An example includes glassine powder paper containing aspirin. Other examples include aluminium foil packets into which alcohol swabs and pledgets are placed.	PKT
Pouch	A flexible container used to protect or hold one or more doses of a drug product (e.g. a pouch into which oral contraceptive blister packs are inserted, and an overwrap pouch for large volume parenterals).	POU
Supersack	A multilayer paper bag for shipping some solid bulk excipients, usually in the form of powder or granules.	SUPSACK
Syringe	A device for the administration of parenteral drug products that consists of a rigid barrel fitted with septum with a plunger at one end and a seal or needle at the other end. The needle assembly may be part of the device or separate.	SYR
Syringe, Glass	A device for the administration of parenteral drug products that consists of a rigid glass barrel fitted with septum with a plunger at one end and a seal or needle	SYRGL

Contd...

Contd...

Syringe, Plastic	at the other end. The needle assembly may be part of the device or separate. A device for the administration of parenteral drug products that consists of a rigid plastic barrel fitted with septum with a plunger at one end and a seal or needle at the other end. The needle assembly may be part of the device or separate.	SYRPL
Tamminder	A specialized package; it registers each time it is opened and is used for checking patient compliance to prescribed medication regimens.	TABMIND
Tank	A large receptacle used for holding, transporting, or storing liquids or gases, and often referred to as a reservoir.	TANK
Tray	A shallow flat receptacle, with a raised edge or rim, used for carrying, holding, or displaying finished drug product in its primary or market package. A tray and its contents may be encased in shrink-wrapped plastic for shipping, or with a cover or an overwrap as part of a unit of use package or kit.	TRAY
Tube	A flexible container for semisolid drug products which is flattened and crimped or sealed at one end and has a reclosable opening at the other.	TUBE
Tube, with Applicator	A tube which is provided with a device (the applicator) for administering the dosage form. The applicator may be part of the tube closure or be separate.	TUBEAP
Vial	A container designed for use with parenteral drug products.	VIAL
Vial, Dispensing	A vial that is used by the pharmacist to dispense the prescribed medication.	VIALDIS
Vial, Glass	A glass container designed for use with parenteral drug products.	VIALGL
Vial, Multi-dose	A vial intended to contain more than one dose of the drug product.	VIALMD

Contd...

Contd...

Vial, Patent Delivery System	A vial that has a patented delivery system.	VIALPAT
Vial, Pharmacy Bulk Package	A container of a sterile preparation whose contents are intended for use in a pharmacy admixture program and are restricted to the preparation of admixtures for infusion or, through a sterile transfer device, for the filling of empty sterile syringes.	VIALPHR
Vial, Piggyback	A vial that contains a parenteral preparation that can be attached directly to the tubing of a parenterally administered fluid.	VIALPIG
Vial, Plastic	A plastic container designed for use with parenteral 'rug products.	VIALPL
Vial, Single Dose	A vial containing a single unit of a parenteral drug product.	VIALSD
Vial, Single-Use	A vial where a single dose of a parenteral drug product can be removed, and then the vial and its remaining contents can be disposed.	VIALSU

1.13 NEW CONCEPT AND FUTURE OF PACKAGING

In the recent past there has been a growing demand for novel packaging methods for the fast growing pharmaceutical industry. Pharmaceutical packaging demands high standards such as, user safety, preservation, hygiene, packaging differentiation and efficiency. There is a strong and increasing demand for innovative packaging in the retail sector for pharmaceuticals. Chemical resistance, transparency and toughness of packaging enhance safety and efficiency of the drugs. Pharmaceutical packaging adds value to the product by preserving quality and lengthening shelf life. It also plays a major role in creating brand awareness and expanding consumer preferences. Products are packaged to meet the criteria of safety, convenience and attractiveness. In essence, packaging boosts consumption of products, and thereby economic growth.

Features of Good Packaging Systems

The pharmaceutical packaging industry is constantly advancing, and as with most other packaged goods, they need reliable and speedy packaging solutions that deliver a combination of product protection, quality, tamper evidence, patient comfort and security needs. Constant innovation in drug making and advance drug delivery systems such as prefilled syringes, blow fill seal vials, powder applications, etc. have direct impact on packaging. Oral drugs such as tablets, capsules, soft gels, syrups, etc. are the most widely consumed. They are packed in blister packs, plastic containers, glass containers, sachets, etc. Need for easy handling of drugs has made a huge impact on the packaging industry to deliver innovative packaging solutions. This has led to the importance of providing tailored packaging solutions, which assures the effectiveness of the drug.

Qualities of Effective Packaging Systems

- Easy dispensing of oral drugs.
- Child resistance and senior-friendliness.
- Quickly identifiable, functional and hermetically sealed packs.
- Convenience and hygiene.

Packing and Filling Machinery

Once the drug is ready to be introduced in the market, fast and efficient packing system is of principle importance. Efficiency of the packing and filling machinery plays a major role in delivering a perfectly packaged drug to the consumer. Precise filling mechanisms is essential to avoid filling wrong dosage of a medicine and proper packing systems to provide hermetically sealed packs for higher product safety. Proper packing increases the shelf life of the product and ensures fullproof packaging. The whole drug manufacturing process is driven by cost as drug makers face increased cost pressures right through the entire production and packaging process. This requires efficient packaging lines that offer user friendly, flexible and easily operable packaging systems.

New and Upcoming Forms of Packaging

In a fast paced lifestyle there is heightened need for easy usage and efficient packing of drugs. There is a steady shift towards packaging of prescription drugs in unit dose packages. This in turn leads to the growth of blister packs to house solid oral drugs. Blister packs provide easy dispensing of drugs and also make it easy to consume the right dosage at the right time. On the other hand, there is an increased shift towards more accurate dosage of drugs and home use of parenteral drugs. Prefilled syringes, with their single-use, disposable format; eliminate the many steps involved in using a vial and is the fastest growing packaging format.

Unit-of-use formats of consuming drugs can be relied upon to:
- Provide tamper evidence.
- Increase shelf life.
- Facilitate distribution.
- Increase brand awareness.
- Facilitate compliance with pharmaceutical regimens.
- Check counterfeiting and diversion.
- Protect each dosage unit from the time it is manufactured until the time it is ingested.

Potential for RFID in Pharmaceutical Packaging

The World Health Organization estimates that counterfeit drugs cost the pharmaceutical industry nearly $40 billion per annum. Innumerable anti-counterfeiting initiatives are underway in the pharmaceutical sector, where not just brand protection is at risk, but also the very lives of the people who consume these packaged drugs. Newer methods are required in order to tackle the counterfeited drugs scattered in the market. Smart packaging solutions add value to the product and also protect them from counterfeiting. For example, ensuring that people take the correct pill at the correct time and also safeguarding the pill container from being duplicated. Radiofrequency Identification Device (RFID) can improve the lives of patients and at the same time keep track of drug counterfeit. In addition to combating non-compliance, RFID-enabled packaging offers the following benefits that are expected to improve the overall quality of the healthcare system:

- Engaging the patient as a participant in their own treatment.
- Simplifying administration of drugs through automation.
- Providing interaction with the patient so that the course of therapy is continuously reinforced.
- Identifying tampered pharmaceutical packages the moment they enter the market.

Packaging has become a marketing tool for the product, along with important features like child resistance, tamper evidence, protection against counterfeiting and increased patient convenience. Hence new packaging designs would in turn protect the brand identity of the product and become an essential part of drug manufacturing.

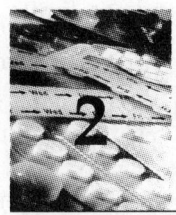

Package Design Research and New Trends in the Pharmaceutical Packaging

2.1 INTRODUCTION

Packaging can be define as an economical means of providing presentation, protection, identification/information, containment, convenience and compliance for a product during storage, carriage, display and use until such time is as the product used or administered.

Following examples satisfy the above definition:

1. Used of solid dosage form (especially sustained release dosage form). It offers patient convenience a selected number of units can be readily detached and improve patient compliance.
2. Use of blister or strip package need relatively little space compares to bottle.
3. Examples of packs offering patient convenience include a range of unit dose presentations that permit immediate disposal offer use, metered dose aerosols, nasal sprays. Which combine convenience with dosage control, squeeze eye drop packs compared to earlier bottle, dropper.

2.2 PHARMACEUTICAL CONTAINER

A container for pharmaceutical use is an article which contains or is intended to contain a product and is, or may be, in direct contact with it. The closure is a part of the container.

The container is so designed that the contents may be removed in a manner appropriate to the intended use of the preparation. It provides a varying degree of protection depending on the nature of the product and the hazards of the environment, and minimizes the loss of constituents. The container does not interact physically or chemically with the contents in a way that alters their quality beyond the limits tolerated by official requirements.

1. Primary containers: Immediate container in direct contact with pharmaceutical article. This container protects the drug from environment, e.g. gas, moisture and light. The primary container must satisfy all requirements specified by both USP and FDA.

2. Secondary container: It encloses the primary container. It may contain one or more primary containers and provides protection and labeling for the primary container. These containers may be combined with other additional packaging to constitute the unit of sale package. Many units of sale are usually packaged together during shipping and surrounded by a final exterior package on which a shipping label and identification bar code should be affixed.

Desirable Characteristics of Pharmaceutical Containers

They should have the following characteristics:

1. They should be capable of affording protection to the medicaments against environmental conditions like air, light, and moisture and biological intruders like bacteria, moulds and insects.
2. They should not permit loss of contents due to leakage, spillage or permeation.
3. The container should not interact with the preparation in any manner during storage.
4. The constituents of containers should neither absorb or adsorb the ingredients from the preparation nor should they themselves leach out into the preparation.
5. They should not impart any taste or odour to the preparation.
6. They should be rigid and strong enough to withstand normal handling and transport.
7. They should be able to withstand sterilization temperature and pressure, if so required.
8. Container meant for sterile products should remain sterile until the contents have been used up.
9. They must be adaptable to commonly employed high-speed packaging equipment.

10. They should be economical, easy to clean, and have good appearance.

Selection of Containers

Selection of container depends upon the following properties:

1. **Sterility of the product:** If the product is to be supplied in sterile form, it is necessary to use hermetic or airtight containers. For injectables, hermetic containers are used and for other preparations, airtight containers are used. The main purpose is product remain sterile.

2. **Light sensitivity of medicaments:** For light sensitive drugs, light resistance containers such as amber glass container or black thermoplastic container should be used. Sometimes, ordinary containers completely wrapped in black papers may also be used for light sensitive substances.

3. **Volatility of medicament and other ingredients:** If the product contains a volatile substance or if preparation is volatile in nature, an airtight container should be used to prevent the evaporation of the preparation.

4. **Pressure inside the container:** If there are chances of increasing internal pressure or if the pressure inside the container remains higher than the atmospheric pressure as in case of aerosols, a mechanically strong container should be used.

5. **Incompatibility between the constituents of the product and the container:** Some medicaments like alkaline liquids have the capacity to extract out alkali from glass containers. The extracted alkali can deteriorate the product and it can be incompatible with the constituents of the product. So, for these types of preparations, only those containers which comply with the limit test of alkalinity of glass should be used. Some medicaments can extract out lead or arsenic from glass containers. For these preparations lead or arsenic free glass containers should be used. Before the final selection of a container, it should be confirmed that there is no incompatibility between the constituents of the container and the constituents of the preparation.

6. **Hygroscopic properties of the preparation or medicament:** If the product contains a hygroscopic substance or if the preparation is hygroscopic in nature, an airtight container should be used so that during storage the preparation should not absorb atmospheric moisture.

7. **Utility of the product:** The container should be selected depending upon the use of the product and the mode of administration. For eye and ear drops, dropping bottles are used. For ointments and creams, collapsible tubes or wide mouth bottles are used. For ointments to be applied in the return or other body cavities like nose, collapsible tubes with nozzles are used. Capsules and tablets can be supplied in strips or in bottles. For injectables, vials and ampoules are used. For IV fluid bottles or thermoplastic bags are used. Similarly, for other products, proper container should be selected and used.

Types of Containers

1. According to the Number of Dosage form Packed in it:

1. **Single unit container:** It contain the drug product for a single dose for use immediately after it is opened.

2. **Single dose container:** A single-dose container for substances that can be taken orally, particularly pharmaceutical products, comprises a hollow body for containing the substance, which is provided with a dispensing opening, and has external curvatures formed on its lateral surface, which are adapted to constitute means for gripping the container. It contains the drug quantity for the single dose.

3. **Unit dose container:** A unit dose container is for articles intended for other than parenterals. A unit dose is the amount of a medication administered to a patient in a single dose.

   Unit-dose packaging is the packaging of a single dose in a nonreusable container. It is increasingly used in hospitals, nursing homes, etc. Medications in unit-dose packaging are easily identifiable and can be returned to the pharmacy if the medication is discontinued.

A liquid containing thermoplastic unit dose container which comprises a body portion, a neck portion and an outlet opening at the end of the neck portion which is sealed by a non-resealable cap. The outside wall of the neck portion comprises a thread engagement portion, which is located at, or proximate the outermost edge of the neck portion so that after removal of cap thread engagement portion is adapted to engage within an inwardly facing screw thread channel at the end of a syringe. This enables sealing connection of the container to the syringe so that liquid within container may be directly transferred from the container to the syringe.

4. **Multiple unit container:** A multiple dose container is a container that permits withdrawal of successive portion of the contents without changing the strength, quality or purity of the remaining portion.
   - Economic in comparison to single unit container, e.g. plastic bottles.
   - Both OTC and prescription medicine, Tablets, Capsules, etc. are packaged in plastic bottles.
   - Plastic bottles provides adequate barrier to moisture, light, etc.
   - The bottle can be made opaque (using HDPE), transparent (PET bottle) or amber coloured (PP bottle)
   - Child resistant and temper evident wrap can be applied if necessary.
   - Desiccant materials can be entered in the container to decrease the relative humidity of local atmosphere.
   - Medications packaged for tropical use should be tropicalized in this way to prevent excessive water absorption by the preparation itself.
   - Plastic container may also be used for oral powders, granules or oral liquids (if oral liquid do not extract leachant from the bottles).
   - Drawback of plastic container–heat intolerance is measure drawback so, these are not suited for sterile application otherwise they will melt.

- For parenteral products, generally glass is used. In glass container elastomer closure is used. The closure is formed by plastic membrane plug that can be penetrated by syringe needle. This closure style allow for sterile withdrawal of pharmaceutical preparation.
- Additional multiple unit containers are in wide spread use such as collapsible tubes (for ointments and pastes), metered dose inhalers and aerosol containers.
- Collapsible tube container.

Multi-unit Container Package

A multi-unit container package comprising in combination an outer one piece sleeve-form open end wrapper and a plurality of container units therein each consisting of a plurality of containers detachably bonded together by adhesive means applied to each container on a side wall contacting a side wall of another container, each unit being free of any holder, strap, tray or space consuming means, said outer wrapper having a flat top overlying in direct contact the tops of the containers, a flat bottom supporting in direct contact the bottoms of the containers, opposite side walls directly contacting the side walls of a plurality of containers in a plurality of units, and a tear strip located midway between and parallel to the open ends of the outer wrapper extending around the outer wrapper said tear strip having a pull tab cut out of the outer wrapper material at one end of the strip, whereby the outer wrapper and contents may be divided into two parts each consisting of an outer wrapper and a plurality of units each consisting of a plurality of adhering containers.

   5. **Multiple dose container:** It is for articles intended for parenterals.

2. According to the Protection Offered or Permeability

  i. **Well-closed container:** A well-closed container protects the contents from extraneous solids and from loss of the articles under normal conditions of handling, shipment, storage and distribution.

 ii. **Tightly-closed container:** A tightly closed container protects the contents from contamination by extraneous liquids, solids or vapours. From loss of deterioration of the article from effervescence, deliquescence or evaporation under normal conditions of handling, shipment, storage and distribution. A tightly-closed container must be capable of being tightly reclosed after use.

iii. **Hermetically sealed container:** A hermetically sealed container is impervious to air or any other gas under normal conditions of handling, shipment, storage and distribution.

iv. **Light resistant container:** A light-resistant container protects the contents from the effects of light by virtue of the specific properties of the material of which it is made. Alternatively, a clear and colourless or a translucent container may be made light-resistant by means of an opaque (light-resistant) covering and/or stored in a dark place.

v. **Tamper-evident container:** A temper evident container is a closed container fitted with a device or mechanism that reveals irreversibly whether the container has been opened.

vi. **Tamper resistant packaging:** Drugs marked for ophthalmic use or for OTC.

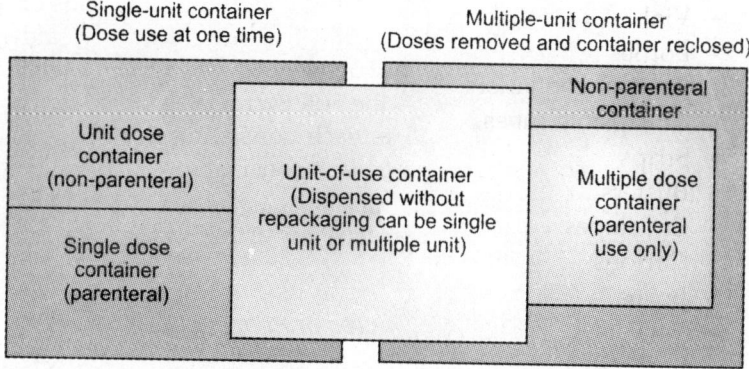

Fig. 2.1: Containers based on their dosage capacity

3. According to the Type of Material Construction

1. Paper container
2. Glass container

3. Plastic container
4. Metal container

Metal containers used in pharmaceutical packaging:

- Hard metal containers
- Soft metal containers

These metal containers are made up of aluminium, stainless steel, lead, tin, etc.

Hard metal containers are mainly used for packing of solid dosage forms such as tablets, powders, capsules, etc. It is also used for packaging of aerosols. Big metallic drums are also used for the supply and storage of solid drugs, powders, liquid paraffin, turpentine oil, etc.

Soft metal containers are used for pharmaceutical and cosmetic products. In pharmaceutical preparations, collapsible tubes made from tin are preferred because tin is unreactive with most of the products. Aluminium tubes are used for toothpaste and creams. Tin coated tubes are used for water based ointments and creams. Lead tubes are not used because of toxicity of lead.

4. According to the Shape and Intended use:

- Ampoules
- Vials
- Bottles
- Aerosol containers
- Collapsible tubes
- Strips
- Blisters
- Envelopes
- Cartons
- Boxes
- Packets
- Sachets

2.3 APPROACH TO PACKAGE DESIGN

As no two products are precisely identical pack requirement of and two products may differ fundamental however, approach to design of a package will be irrespective to the products.

1. What is Packaging?

- Multi-dimension/multi-disciplinary/Dynamic.
- Link between production and consumption.
- Part of physical distribution.
- Means of ensuring the safe delivery of a product to the ultimate consumer in sound condition at a minimum overall cost.
- What it protects. it must sell, and what it sells, it must protect.
- Represents the last output of manufacturing, but the first input in marketing.
- A tool of marketing.
- Technique of preparing goods for transport and marketing.
- An integral part of production.
- An art, science and technology to protect, preserve and present the products effectively to satisfy the consumers
- A critical part of companies marketing activity modes expenditure and improve productivity marketing share and compatibility.

2. Functions of a Package

Primary

    i To contain
    ii To protect
  iii To preserve
  iv. To represent/communicate
    v. To dispense

Secondary

    i. Easy to handle
    ii. Easy to store
  iii. Easy to open
  iv. Easy to inspect
    v. Easy to reclose
  vi. Easy to dispose of
  vii. Reusability
 viii. Recyclability, etc.

3. Types of Packages

- Retail pack/consumer pack/unit pack/primary pack.
- Shipping container/bulk pack/transport pack.
- Intermediate pack.

4. Guidelines for Retail Packages

- Packages should adequately contain, protect and preserve product.
- Package material should not have adverse effect on the content (Compatibility).
- Package must comply with all relevant legal requirements.
- Package for hazardous products must contain them safely. Incorporate suitable warnings and be fitted with appropriate closures.
- Package must not mislead about the nature quality or quantity of the contents.
- Package should be convenient for consumer and safe in normal use including dispensing.
- Package should properly identify the product and provide instruction for use.
- Package should provide safeguard from pilferage or contamination.
- Package should be attractive or presentable with appropriate graphics/printing.
- Package should be designed with regard to its reuse, recycling and ultimate disposal.

5. Guidelines for Shipping Containers

- Must contain the product efficiently and effectively.
- Must provide protection against external climatic conditions and contaminants.
- Must be easily and efficiently filled and closed.
- Must be compatible with the products.
- Must be easily handled by appropriate means (mechanical/manual).
- Must remain securely closed in transit but open easily and when required (e.g. Customs Inspection) be capable of efficient and secure reclose.

- Must communicate necessary information (e.g. product, destination, how to handle and open the pack).
- Must be virtually unbreakable of products which are dangerous or potentially harmful, e.g. chemicals, acids, bases.
- Must be reasonable cost.
- Must be readily disposable, reusable or have an after use for some other purposes package design.

6. Factors Influencing Design/Selection of Package

- Product (Nature of content) factor
- Distribution factor
- Marketing factor
- Statute and regulation factor
- Packaging operation factor
- Cost factor

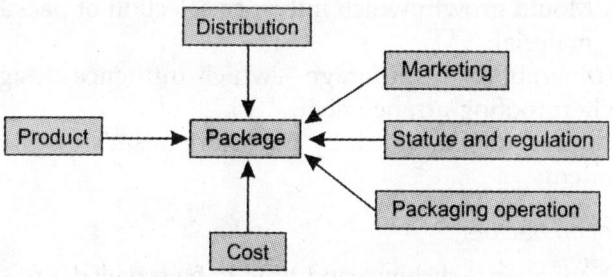

Fig. 2.2: Factors influencing design

Product Factor

Kind of products
- Consumer/industrial
- High-value/low value
- Standard/gift/seasonal

Physical properties/characteristics
- Physical state (solid/liquid/semisolid/powder)
- Single item/composite or assembly
- Weight/density
- Volume/size

- Surface finish (smooth/rough)
- Shape/form
- Stability and CG
- Fragility
- Rigidity
- Flammability/volatility

Vulnerabilities of contents

i. Compatibility of product with package.
ii. Vulnerability to environmental atmospheric conditions leading to:
   - Change of state (e.g. crisp to soggy)
   - Accumulation of dirt
   - Discolouration
   - Loss of taste or flavour
   - Acquisition of undesirable odour
   - Corrosion
   - Mould growth which influence selection of packaging material.
iii. Vulnerability to pilferage—which influence design of pilferproofing arrangement.
iv. Vulnerability to attack by micro-organism's insects and rodents.

Distribution Factors

- Destination – distance and time to be traveled.
- Handling – manual/mechanical
- Transport – road/rail/sea/air (single or in combination)
- Number of Transshipments
- Warehouses/storage – stacking pattern/Stack Height.
- Hazards – drop (height), Horizontal impact intensity, Compression (stack load with size), vibration (frequency/amplitude), puncture, etc.
- Atmospheric conditions – temperature/RH/Pressure (max. and min. values with time of exposure).
- Other environmental condition – rodents insects/water/ contamination from contents of other pack (degree of protection needed – matter of judgment).

- Limitations – carrying capacity of human being for manual handling; capacity of lifting equipment/conveyors etc.
- Marking – general/special (for dangerous goods).
- Unit load systems – palletisation/containerisation.

Marketing Factors

- Merchandising system – over the counter/super market
- The customer – sex/age/income group/social level.
- Customer buying habit (quantity).
- Location of market – local/regional/national/export.
- Consumers convenience – inspection before purchase, easy opening, reclosability, measured dose, dispensing aid, easy grip, easy dispensability.
- Appearance of package to convey impression, luxury/hygiene/economy/odernity, etc.
- Average marketing time
- Display shelves space/positioning, size/form/shapes of package.

Statute and Regulation

- Obligatory requirements.
- Standards of weights and measures act (to prevent deception).
- Weight and quantity to be packed.
- Marking of retail price.
- FDA regulation.
- Regulations of the carriers.
- International air transport association.
- Inter government maritime consultative organization.
- Legislation of importing countries controlling entry of certain packaging materials.

Packaging Operation Factor

Matching of packaging systems with production:
1. Time factor
2. Convenience factor
3. Versatility factor
4. Growth factor

- Consideration for seasonal products demand higher at one time.
- Either packaging system should be adaptable to demand or package product.

Cost Factor

- Materials and containers depend on functions of package and size of order.
- Contents require special/complex, design cost more reusability/returnable (from one unit to another) handling, transportation and storage of empty packages, e.g. glass bottles *vs* flexible pouches. Setup vs Folding boxes (some packaging material, e.g. cellophane need conditioned storage space; economic advantage of cheaper rate for bulk buying vs Storage cost).
- Package operation cost.
- Labour and overhead .
- Maintenance and depreciation.
- Storage of filled package type.
- Transportation of filled package.
- Freight by weight/volume.
- Loss and damage cost
- Replacement/repairing defective items.
- Loss of goodwill cost.
- Insurance cost.
- Package development cost.

2.4 NEW TRENDS IN THE PHARMACEUTICAL PACKAGING

Using DNA Labels to Protect Against Product Piracy

Some bio-technology companies are using the building blocks of the human genetic material DNA for forgery-proof identification.

Foils

VAW Flexible Packaging has developed a new blister material with the name Polybar (Polybar®). This is a co-extruded flat foil, the middle layer of which is made up of the barrier-forming polymer COC. The middle layer is embedded on both sides in two PP layers, which gives the packaging material good forming properties, according to the company. According to the manufacturer, the blister material developed by VAW, in contrast to the PVC/PVDC normally used, is more friendly for the environment, lighter and therefore also of greater economic advantage for the customer.

Packaging Suitable for Seniors

Wishes of elderly customers and their requests of the packaging industry and the designers:

Seniors Want

- A clearer sell-by date
- More legible writing
- Not so much shiny material
- Smaller packages and
- Packages which can be opened easier.

Wallet – The Package with a Future

The multi-phase contraceptive pill can be named here as a typical example of this product solution. In this case the important thing is to pack the tablets so that the sequence for taking the pills is clearly defined for the consumer. The wallet, having disappeared from view for a while, has regained a lot of significance in recent years on account of its specific merits. Some of the advantages are:

That the insert with its important administering information is firmly connected to the medication package (product liability). That the package is attractive and therefore can be readily taken everywhere by the consumer. That several product components can be packaged in a consumer-friendly way, e.g. integration of diagnostic strips, monthly or weekly preparations. That the outer envelope of the wallet can also be used as an attractive display surface; and That the packages can be economically produced in large quantities using high-performance machines.

Design of Package Inserts for Pharmaceuticals

The content and design of package inserts for pharmaceuticals has been criticized for years. Initiatives by the pharmaceutical industry as well as on the part of the responsible authorities have already brought about improvements, but not yet satisfactory results. At a chemist's shop in Jena, patients have now been polled about their wishes regarding ranking of information on package inserts.

Blister Foil with Flexible Printed Circuits (FPC)

The "electronic blister" is a further development of ordinary blisters, consisting of a standard blister pack which is sealed with a new kind of FPC film. The whole system consists of the blister with printed circuits, a monitor and a docking station. The FPC film has integrated FPC's that are stretched over the dragée indentations of a blister. The blister is placed into a shell, the so-called monitor, which supplies a voltage through certain contact surfaces of the blister to the opposite contact point. Inside the monitor, an electronic system is at work, which reacts to a dragée being taken out: When pushing out a dragée, a printed circuit, and therefore current flow, is irreversibly interrupted. The electronics of the monitor register this changed state. The first time a dragée is taken out of the blister, a regimen program is started for the patient. The patient is guided from the first time to the next time for taking the medication and is reminded of taking it via the optical display and acoustically via a sound generator, should he exceed this period. The times for taking the medication are stored in the monitor. These times can be transferred to the docking station via an interface. At the doctor's office, the docking station takes over the monitor's data and graphically shows the history of when a dragée has been taken out of the monitor on a display. This is how the physician in charge can recognize compliance with the medication regimen, i.e. the patient's behavior, at a single glance.

Fake Pharmaceuticals/Counterfeit Drugs

Basically counterfeit drugs are homemade fake drugs that are being sold under the product name without proper endorsement. These also include products without the active ingredient or with the active ingredient, but not enough of it, or they could include the wrong active ingredient, or have fake packaging. These are the different characteristics of counterfeit drugs. There is a big difference between non-registered drugs and those that are registered and the classification of whether they are "counterfeit" or not. A medicine that is not registered, but available in a particular country is not a counterfeit, but just simply an unregistered product. Counterfeit drugs were initially noticed in 1968 in Nigeria.

Identifying counterfeits: I was searching the internet in more depth on the process of identifying counterfeit drugs. Between the years 2000 and 2006 the WHO have witnessed an 800% increase of new counterfeit drug cases. The growth of these cases can be attributed to organized crime groups such as; the "Russian mafia", Chinese triads, Mexican gangs, Colombian drug cartels, and also some terrorist groups. 60% of the cases being found are in developing countries. Counterfeit drugs are such a big problem because when the medicine, thought to be the correct one, has incorrect levels of the active ingredient which causes the weaker strains of the agent to be destroyed. Furthermore, it allows the drug-resistant strains to adapt to the active ingredient and multiply. This has been attributed to the doubling of malaria deaths in the past 20 years. The disease has become resistant to the real drugs because of the fake drugs.

India prevalence: In India counterfeit drugs account for about one-third of the drugs that are produced world-wide. In 2008 it was said by the Organization for Economic Co-operation and Development (OECD) that 75% of fake drugs in the whole world had originated from India. Nigeria is also receiving drugs from India. India is another source, besides China, for the creation of forged drugs and is responsible for the numerous killings of innocent Nigerians. In 2003 there were three fatal open heart surgeries performed on little children who died immediately after surgery. Later it was found that the adrenaline and suxamethonium, which induces muscle relaxation, were fake. Nigeria has recently threatened to ban all drugs from India, to help combat the problem of counterfeit drugs in their country.

Drug resistant: It is said that most of the data of epidemiology of counterfeited drugs are kept secret through the pharmaceutical industries and governmental agencies. Drug companies will hire investigators to find counterfeiters and will shut them down. Usually this occurs in private. According to the WHO the types of drugs that are most commonly forged include antibiotics, antimalarials, hormones, antiviral, anticancer, and steroids. The counterfeiters typically take chalk, various chemicals, or anything they can put their hands on and package these up to look like real drugs and then sell them to consumers. Most of these drugs do not help at all and sometimes can be toxic; even lethal. These drugs are becoming a leading cause in people being disease resistant and not healing.

E-prescriptions

Today there seems to be a big push towards doctors filing e-prescriptions.

Benefits of e-prescriptions: Looking at the Government's Health and Human Services website they give some reasons electronic prescriptions are beneficial. Here are a few reasons why it is beneficial (The Benefits on Electronic Prescribing).

1. Improve quality and proficiency.
2. Reduce costs (co-payments).
3. Work-flow efficiencies.
4. Eliminate ineligibility problems of hand-written prescriptions.
5. Reduce incidence of drug diversion by alerting health care providers (i.e. duplicating prescriptions).

When dealing with counterfeit drugs electronic prescriptions may or may not help. It seems to be very beneficial. The consequences though, may be that people are more apt to purchase their drugs online since the prescriptions are electronic. This could pose as a huge problem and a better way to get fake pharmaceuticals to more people. Consumers are still going to have to be smart.

Innovations Made of Aluminium

The job was to develop new potential for aluminium in pharma-packaging. After much preliminary reflection and talks with aluminium-foil specialists, four solutions were developed and followed through to the production of mock-ups:

The blister box: A folded solution consisting of two opposing blister cards. The blisters are on the outside of the package, so that the lidding foil is covered.

Sliding blister: The backs of two blister cards are placed against each other so that they can be shifted.

Fold-away blister with horizontal cavities: Of interest are blister packages with internally staggered blisters, where the cavities fit into each other like push buttons.

The "snapdragon": The capsule, made of an aluminium-plastic composite, can be pushed open from the side, so that single tablets can be taken out.

New pharma-sticker in Italy: The Italian government has introduced a new accounting label containing a sequential serial number besides the already existing product number. The designated supply of sequentially numbered rolls of labels for an intended use to individual manufacturers as well as the accounting through every stage of the trade channel enable seamless tracing of all pharmaceutical products and monitoring of the flow of pharmaceuticals.

Multiple-component Packages with Extraordinary Convenience Functions

Pharma industry has designed a multiple-component package with extraordinary convenience functions for the idea was to offer the anti-coagulant Clivarin Pen in a form which makes it easier for the patient to treat himself. The package was supposed to contain all components necessary for medication: the pen with ten single doses, the injection needle, the alcohol swab, directions for use and administration and a possibility for the disposal of used needles. The patient activates the tensioning device, places the pen and pulls the trigger. The needles are disposed of cleanly and without risk of injury in the integrated collection compartment. If the pen is empty, the package can be closed again and disposed of together with the household waste.

For this, in pharma industry has designed a mono-material cardboard package. The special feature of this one-piece package is that the pen and the ten injection needles with protective cap are securely fixed in an integrated insert. Furthermore, the package is fitted with a turned-over mirror on the lid which is turned over during the gluing process and glued on. That means costly backside printing can be eliminated.

The package is delivered in a pre-glued and flat-lying state it is manually set up and filled. For a complex product with 18 individual parts, this would not be possible any other way.

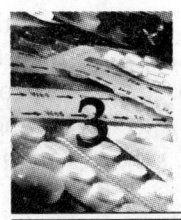

Packaging Materials

3.1 INTRODUCTION

Packaging provides physical protection from forces such as shock, vibration, compression, temperature, in addition to offering barrier protection from external influences including water vapour, dust, oxygen, etc. The information function of packaging ensures communications on product use, transport, recycle, or disposal. Some information about pharmaceuticals, medical, and chemical products is required by governments under the law. Moreover, packaging is also instrumental in controlling shipment of counterfeit pharmaceutical and medical products. For instance, pharmaceutical products often include tamper resistance packaging to prevent or to uncover any attempts at tampering. Convenience of handling, display, stacking, and distribution.

Unit dose packing was first started in 1927 for an Aspirin based product (ASPRO). Blister packaging was first introduced in American Hospitals. Visibility in Blister to recognize the product easily.

Packaging materials such as glass are often made in developing countries but materials such as plastic film are more commonly imported from multinational packaging manufacturers. Most multinationals have a retail agent situated in developing countries and contact addresses can be found in local business directories. Further information regarding suppliers and local costs of materials can be obtained from local packaging institutes; again these can be located through business directories.

Functions of Packaging

A good package should therefore perform the following functions:
- It should provide a barrier against dirt and other contaminants thus keeping the product clean.
- It should prevent losses. For example, packages should be securely closed to prevent leakage.
- It should protect dosage form against physical and chemical damage. For example, the harmful effects of air, light, insects, and rodents. Each product will have its own needs.
- The package design should provide protection and convenience in handling and transport during distribution and marketing.
- It should help the customers to identify the dosage form and instruct them how to use it correctly.
- It should persuade the consumer to purchase the dosage form.

3.2 PACKAGING MATERIALS

Any material intended to protect an intermediate (tablet, capsules, syrups, aerosols, opthalmics, parenterals, etc.) during storage and transport. An economical means of providing protection, presentation, identification, information and convenience for pharmaceuticals product from the moment of production until it is used or administered.

Developments in materials technology depend to some extent on the importance of the intrinsic value of each, and the proportion of total cost, which is accounted for by raw materials. At the two extremes are the traditional inorganic materials glass and metals. While only about 25% of a glass container's cost is for its raw material content, for metals the proportion is 70–80%. For the organically derived materials, paper and plastics, the comparable figure is something like 50%.

Materials reduction is usually achieved through work on the geometry of the pack, the mechanical properties of the material, and the forming technology. The elements of this triple-pronged attack are used to different degrees in individual situations.

Importance of Packaging Material in Pharma Industry

- Protection of product.
- Protection from physical damage
- Protection from chemical deterioration.
- Protection from mechanical and climatic hazards.
- Protection from microorganisms.
- Compatibility of product and packaging material.
- Child resistant.
- Temper evident.
- Drugs need more care in their packaging than do most other product, because any failure in their packing could result in changes in the drug that lead either to a failure to cure, to illness, to injury or even cause death of patient.

Type of Packaging Materials used by Pharma Industry

Primary Packaging Material

(Also known as Critical Packaging Component).

Secondary Packaging Material

(Also known as Non-critical Packaging Component).

Tertiary Packaging Material

(Also known as Non-critical Packaging Component).

Table 3.1: Packaging material/base material used in pharma industry for packaging

Base material	Packaging material
Paper	Labels, Leaflets.
Board	Cartons, Display Units.
Glass	Ampoules, Vials, Syringes, Bottles, etc.
Metals (Aluminium, Tin Plate)	Collapsible Tubes, Foils, etc.
Plastics (e.g. Polyethylene, Polypropylene)	Closures, Tubes, PET Bottles, etc.
Metal/Plastic	Flip Off Aluminium Seals

3.3 CLASSIFICATION OF PACKAGING MATERIALS

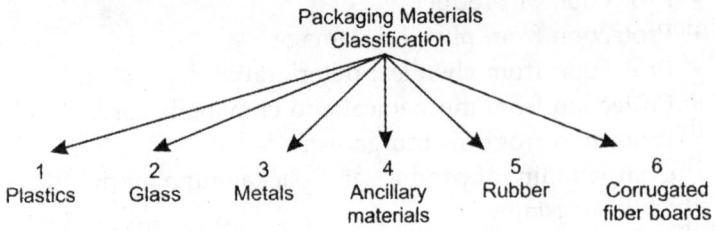

Fig. 3.1: Classification of packaging materials

1. Plastic Packaging

In the plastics sector opportunities continue to be identified in the basic materials, processing developments, and even in container geometry. A better understanding of relationships between molecular structure and physical properties is being combined with improved ability to tailor molecules in the polymerization process to produce enhanced performance.

Linear low-density polyethylene was the first such material to be commercialized on a large scale, and new 'super' polyolefins are becoming available which will ensure that this group, by far the largest sector of all plastics, will maintain its pre-eminence. Polyethylene terephthalate (PET), developed initially as an engineering and textile polymer, found packaging applications relatively recently. In 20 years or so, it has become the industry standard for large containers for carbonated soft drinks due to its light weight, clarity, extreme strength and good gas retention characteristics.

Its low intrinsic viscosity made it unsuitable for blow moulding, but ideal for the newest technique of injection-stretch blow moulding. Recently new grades with higher intrinsic viscosity have become available, and can now be expected to challenge PVC for such applications as bottles for pharmaceutical product, edible oil, wine, and mineral waters.

After years of research, higher temperature-tolerant formulations have appeared, based on a new polymer, polyethylene naphthalate (PEN), which is used in combination with PET. This offers improved strength, UV barrier and gas barrier properties, in addition to being hot-fillable at temperatures from 85°C to over 100°C.

Interest in environmental aspects of packaging has resulted in the wider use of refillable multi-trip containers. For this application polycarbonate, PET and the new PET/PEN grades are the main contenders.

The use of various plastics for containing and wrapping dosage form depends on what is available in a particular country. Plastics are extremely useful as they can be made in either soft or hard forms, as sheets or containers, and with different thickness, light resistance, and flexibility. The filling and sealing of plastic containers is similar to glass containers.

Plastic Container (Bottles): Materials

High, Medium, and Low Density Polyethylene (PE) Bottles

Plastic bottles are most commonly made from Polyethylene (PE) in high, medium and low density (HDPE, MDPE, and LDPE). The higher the density the more rigid the container is. Bottles that are made from PE that have no colourant added are called Natural as they are not clear like glass, but are transparent. A good example of a natural container is most one gallon plastic milk jugs.

Polyethylene Terephthalate (PET) Bottles

Polyethylene terephthalate (PET), bottles are growing in popularity faster that any other material. PET is a plastic resin and a form of polyester. PET bottles and PET jars are becoming so popular because of its strength, thermostability and it incredible transparency since Natural PET can be as clear as glass. PET bottles are most commonly used in the food and beverage industry to package soda, water, juice, vegetable oils, salad dressings, peanut butter, and hundreds of other food and beverage products.

The personal care and cosmetic industry have switched much of what was previously packaged in glass to PET as it is inexpensive, lightweight making it easier to handle and cheaper to ship than glass as well as it being shatter-resistant and recyclable. It is less reactive and permeable to gas than its closest plastic counterpart Polyvinylchloride (PVC) so soda, beer, and water can be filled in PET bottles and what is inside does not get the plastic taste or lose the carbonation that would happen with other plastics bottles.

When Glycol modifiers are added to minimize brittleness and premature aging, the material is becomes PETG. It offers the most transparency of any type of PET, however PETGs water and gas transmission rates are not as good as PETE or even PVC. While PETE offers better transmission rates, its clarity is not as good as PETG.

Polypropylene (PP) Bottles

Polypropylene (PP) bottles are very similar to HDPE bottles. The only major exception is that polypropylene can be processed (clarified) in its natural uncoloured state is more transparent or cleared than HDPE can be however it will never have the clarity that PET or PVC will have.

Polyvinylchloride (PVC) Bottles

Plastic bottles made from Polyvinylchloride (PVC) have dwindled somewhat in the past few years in popularity but are still an excellent choice for many personal care, cosmetic, and household chemicals due to the strength and transparency PVC has to offer. PVC recycling unfortunately is not nearly as popular as PET, PP and HDPE recycling, so some environment concerns do exist.

Properties and Advantages

Flexible films are the most common form of plastic. Generally, flexible films have the following properties:

- Their cost is relatively low.
- They have good barrier properties against moisture and gases.
- They are heat sealable to prevent leakage of contents.
- They have wet and dry strength.
- They are easy to handle and convenient for the manufacturer, retailer and consumer.
- They add little weight to the product.
- Lighter than glass or metal.

- They fit closely to the shape of the product, thereby wasting little space during storage and distribution.
- Less prone to breakage and in case breakage occurs, fragments are less hazardous.

Disadvantages

- Low chemical inertness compared to glass.
- More permeable than glass.
- Low resistance to high temperature compared to glass.
- For topical ointments, vaccines and transfusion bottles, flexible plastic called polyolefins are used.

Plastic Collapsible Tubes

Plastic tubes are available in different sizes with different specification such as Latex Lining, Shoulder Coating, Sealed Nozzle, Elongated Nozzle, Plastic Nozzle, etc. Plastic Collapsible tubes provide a cost effective, attractive and durable plastic packaging solution for a wide range of consumer products. In addition they are increasingly being used to package products for the pharmaceutical, food and DIY market sectors. Designs can be reproduced in up to six colours using dry-offset litho printing or foiled using the hot-stamping process.

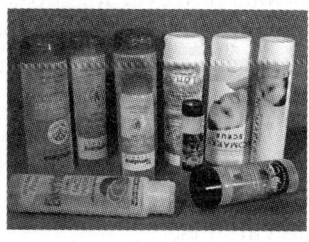
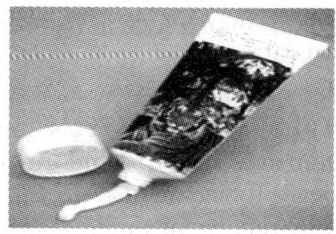

a   b

Figs 3.2a and b: Collapsible tubes

Protection: Plastic tubes offer effective protection for the majority of products which in turn safeguards the shelf life of the product.

UV inhibitors can be added to single layer tubes for increased protection for products susceptible to light degradation.

Sunscreens will turn a LDPE grade tube yellow in colour, in these instances, HDPE can be used to manufacture the tubes and therefore protect the tube from the product.

Durability: Plastic tubes do not require a protective outer carton, the material has "memory" which means it retains its shape well and can withstand the rigours of transportation and handling.

User Friendly: Plastic tubes stand upright on the tube cap and allow the product to be easily and hygienically dispensed.

The durable nature of plastic tubes means they are suitable for use in many different environments from the bathroom to the beach to the workshop.

Point of sale appeal: The wide range of colours, finishes and decorative effects are on offer. This adds up to an attractive packaging solution which has a strong impact on the shelf and allows plenty of opportunity for product differentiation.

Tube caps and closures: A wide range of caps are available including smooth sided, ribbed, rounded profile, disc top and flip top screw-on available in colours that can be matched to the artwork design, if preferred to white or clear.

Tube Decoration

Hot stamping: Foil adds a final touch to the design of a tube and improves the appearance for premium products.

Mold offers a range of standard foils however it is possible to colour match foils to meet customer requirements but these would be subject to development lead times and minimum order quantities.

Tube labelling: Labels can be used when complexity of design exceeds the boundaries of offset and silk screen printing. Labeled tubes are also useful when producing small runs for test marketing or foreign language variants.

Lacquer/Varnish: The finish of the tube can be enhanced with a final coating of gloss or matt lacquer. This process provides additional protection for the offset inks and tube.

Offset printing: The most intricate designs can be produced in up to six colours using offset printing. Tubes are printed in-line using the rotary dry-offset process, designs range from line and text to more complex illustrations and vignettes.

Tube colour: Tube colour can be matched to meet specific customer requirements, a wide range of colours, tints and pearlescent finishes can be achieved. However, if the colour of the product is itself a feature then the tube can be produced in a clear polyethylene.

Application

Plastic tubes are used to package the following products: Cosmetic Creams, Shampoo, Shower Gel, Sunscreens, Inks, Paints, Eatable Sauces, Motor Greases, Glues, Tile Grout, etc.

2. Glass Packaging

Glass Container (Bottles): Glass Types and Materials

Types I, Type II and Type III glass containers are all suitable for parenteral (injection or intravenous) preparations as specified by the US Pharmacopoeia on the basis of chemical durability tests.

Type I Glass: Type I glass bottles are made from borosilicate, which have has a highly resistant composition and releases the least amount of alkali. It is commonly used for pharmaceutical or fine chemical products that are sensitive to pH changes.

Type II Glass: Type II glass containers are made from commercial soda lime glass that has been de-alkalized to obtain a great improvement in chemical resistance by treating the interior surfaces at a high temperature to heat away the alkali on or near the glass surfaces. The undesirable characteristic of Type II Glass is that the treating etches the surface, causing a frosted appearance.

Type III Glass: Type III glass bottles and containers are made of untreated commercial soda-lime glass and has average or somewhat above average chemical resistance. It is the most common in use and is compatible with most items such as: food; beverages; common chemicals, etc.

Type NP Glass: Untreated glass containers made of ordinary soda-lime glass. This glass cannot be used for parenteral preparations.

Properties

Glass has many properties which make it a popular choice as a packaging material:

- Glass is able to withstand heat treatments such as pasteurization and sterilization.
- It does not react with drug.
- It is rigid and protects the dosage form from crushing and bruising.
- It is impervious to moisture, gases, odours and microorganisms.
- It is re-usable, re-sealable and recyclable.
- It is transparent, allowing products to be displayed. Coloured glass may be used either to protect the dosage form from light or to attract customers.

Advantages

1. Is chemically inert.
2. Is impermeable and nonporous.
3. Is resealable.
4. Is microwavable.
5. Is stackable on shelves.
6. Is retortable.
7. Is transparent.
8. Is made from abundant raw materials.
9. Can achieve a hermetic seal, prolong shelf life.
10. In amber or green, can filter out harmful UV rays.
11. Is autoclavable.
12. Has almost a zero rate of transmission.
13. Is great for carbonated beverages.
14. Can be irradiated.
15. Combined with foil, can make an effective tamper-evident container.
16. Does not deteriorate, corrode, stain or fade.
17. Needs no protective coating inside.
18. Is economical.
19. A proven package for strong chemicals and solvents.
20. Has FDA acceptance.
21. Is attractive, connotes richness and substance.
22. Is compatible with child resistant closures.

Disadvantages

Despite its many advantages, glass does have certain disadvantages:

- Glass is heavier than many other packaging materials and this may lead to higher transport costs.
- It is easy to fracture, scratch and break if heated or cooled too quickly.
- Potentially serious hazards may arise from glass splinters or fragments in the dosage form.

Preparation of Glass Containers

A good product packaged in a dirty container will soon deteriorate and therefore the following stages are recommended:

Inspection: This stage applies equally to both new and reused containers. Any chipped, cracked, or heavily soiled containers must be rejected. Containers which have been used to store strong smelling substances such as kerosene should be rejected.

Washing: It is preferable that detergent and bleach are used for cleaning. However, if these are not available, soap or ashes may be used. Simple hand-held brushes can be used to aid the cleaning process on a small scale. For higher rates of production, powered washers are available.

Rinsing: Thorough rinsing of containers is essential. A simple rinsing system, illustrated below, involves a series of spigots set into a length of pipe which act as rinse sprays.

Sterilization: It is strongly recommended that prior to filling, glass containers are heat sterilized. Sterilization can be achieved very simply by holding the open neck of the container over the spout of a kettle containing boiling water. Containers can be inverted over a steam pipe, which is supplied from a water boiler. The vertical pipe is vital as it acts as a safety valve. Alternatively, glass containers can be boiled in water for ten minutes to sterilize them.

Sealing and capping: Bottles suitable machines for sealing bottles can be produced locally. There are two types of cap commonly used: those that thread onto the bottle neck, and crown caps which are pushed on under pressure. Simple low cost crown capping machines are available.

Jars: The sealer shown below is an efficient method for sealing jam jars with push-on lids (compared to domestic methods of using plastic and rubber bands). If bottle or jar necks are not always regular in size, a flexible plastic material allows the sealer to be fitted on different sizes of container.

Cooling: Many products are filled into glass containers while they are hot and then need to be cooled quickly. To achieve the containers can be stacked and cooled by circulating air.

The Advantage of Glass Bottles over the Plastic Ones

The environmental concerns of the world we are living in have determined the replacement of glass with other recyclable materials. The most relevant case is the replacement of glass bottles with plastic pets; the latter have the advantage of being a lot lighter, easier to manufacture and to recycle, not to mention that the costs of plastic are infinitely lower than those of glass. Hence, little by little the use of glass bottles has entered a descending path; nevertheless, they cannot be eliminated from the storing or packaging process of many types of goods. Coke-Cola or Pepsi can be bottled in pets, milk can be sold in cartons, and beer in tin cans, but a good Bordeaux wine will never be stored in plastic.

The advantage of glass bottles over the plastic ones is the quality of the material. Despite the long-use tradition, glass has the purity of structure that makes any interaction with the stored liquid impossible. Plastic on the other hand is known to alter the properties of certain beverages because of the chemical reactions that appear in time between the artificial structure and the possible acids in the beverage.

Glass bottles also have the great advantage of preserving a certain temperature for a longer period of time. They do not dilate when it is too warm or shrink when exposed to lower temperatures. Depending on the type of beverage and other pharmaceutical products they store, glass bottles can be thicker or thinner. Large international companies that are considered brand names, usually have customized, possibly etched glass bottles.

The recycling of glass bottles is required by law, and the separation of the glass residues in households is essential for the process. Glass bottles do not affect the structure of the environment by their chemical composition, their only problem comes from the fact that they remain in the same form for millions of years, there will actually be no change in their structure. The necessity of recycling comes from the fact that a huge quantity of glass bottles are produced and deposited as garbage every year, which only leads to an overwhelmingly high pressure on the environment.

3. Metals

Some metals and metal alloys possess high structural strength per unit mass, making them useful materials for carrying large loads or resisting impact damage. Metal alloys can be engineered to have high resistance to shear, torque and deformation.

Types of Materials

Aluminium, Tin, Lead, Stainless steel.

Advantages

- Strong material
- Opaque
- Impermeable to liquids, gases, odours and bacteria
- Resistant to both low and high temperature.

Disadvantages

- Chemical reaction with drug products, i.e. not inert.
- Corrosion might occur from inside or outside. To overcome corrosion metal substances are coated, e.g. tin plate, made by coating low carbon steel sheet electronically with pure tin.

Most commonly used metal packaging material is aluminium because

- It can be used uncoated
- It is light weight
- It is ductible
- It is non-toxic
- Resistant to corrosion
- Sterilizable
- Can be shaped containers

Metal Cans

Metal cans have a number of advantages over other types of containers:

- They provide total protection of the contents.
- Metal is very resistant to chemical attack.
- They are tamperproof.
- They are convenient for presentation.

Constraints associated with use of metal cans include:

- They are heavier than other materials, except glass, and therefore have higher transport costs.
- The heat treatment associated with the use of metal cans is not suitable for small-scale production.

Uses: Metal containers are commonly used for the packaging of pharmaceutical products, food products, beverages, etc.

Thin Forms: Thin forms of paper, regenerated cellulose, metal foil and all types of plastics, plus filament reinforcement and a range of coatings or surface treatments to further enhance their performance can be combined in thousands of permutations to meet virtually any performance specification except direct load bearing and extreme levels of physical abuse.

4. Paper and Natural Fibres

In the case of paper and board, there is limited scope for improving pack geometry, and only a little more for improving materials processing and pack constructional detail. Improvement in material performance provides the principal opportunity to reduce costs. As paper is produced from natural fibres, its mechanical properties depend upon their individual strength, their length, orientation and the degree of inter-fibre bonding which can be achieved. Flow patterns in the lay-down of separate fibre layers are one aspect which can be improved by mechanical and electrostatic techniques. Current concerns with the chlorine content of paper mill effluents has focused much attention on the use of natural (i.e. unbleached) kraft pulp for packaging paper. This is inherently stronger than bleached grades, and allows some worthwhile down-gauging to be achieved. Paper and boards are used in various forms for packaging of pharmaceutical products. These are used as outer containers such as cartons and boxes. They provide mechanical protection to other containers (blister and strip packs of tablet and capsules, suppositories, syrup bottles, glass containers, etc.).

5. Rubber

The use of rubber is widespread, ranging from household to industrial products, entering the production stream at the intermediate stage or as final products. These are available in variety of composition so that a suitable material may be chosen depending on the compatibility of the product. Rubber is an elastic polymer that finds wide applications in the fabrications of closures for pharmaceutical packaging (vials, transfusion bottles antibiotic containers, etc.) and washers in number of products.

The most important advantage of rubber closure is their self sealability after penetration with a needle. They provide adequate protection to the packed product from microbial contamination. They are soft, elastic and easily fit on the container to give a perfect seal. They provide a hermetic seal to the container.

They can withstand high temperature and pressure of autoclaving.

Disadvantages: Good quality rubber closures are comparatively expensive. Certain rubber closures may show the problem with aging. Permeability of air and moisture varies on the material depending on the material of construction and these are not completely impermeable. Additives used during the manufacture of rubber closures may leach out into the product and cause deterioration. Rubber closures may adsorb or absorb active medicaments as well as excipients like preservatives so as to render them ineffective.

6. Corrugated Fibreboard

Corrugated fibreboard is a paper based construction material consisting of a fluted corrugated sheet and one or two liner board are made of paperboards. It is mainly used in manufacture of corrugated boxes and shipping containers. Paperboard and fibreboard are sometimes called cardboard.

Packaging Closures

- Plastic – wadless or lined, CR (child resistant), CT (continuous thread), snap fit.
- Metal – screw, ROPP (Roll on pilfer proof) Closures.
- Liner – cork, pulp board, EPE (Expand able poly ethylene); flowed in gasket – product contact materials/facings: PVDC, Saran, Saranex, Melinex, EPE, Vinyl, Foamed PVC.
- Induction heat seals.

Table 3.2: Resistance to these factors

Type of packaging	Puncture crush etc.	Sunlight	Air	Water	Heat	Odour	Insects	Rod-ents	Micro-organisms
Metal cans	*	*	*	*	#	*	*	*	*
Glass (bottle jar)	*	Coloured	*	*	*	*	*	*	*
Paper bag		*					#		
Cardboard	*	*			#		#		
Wood (box)	*	*			*		#	#	
Pottery (sealed lid)	*	*	*	*	*	*	*	*	*
Foil		*		#	#	*	#		
Plastic tub sealed	*	*		*	#	*	*	#	*
Cellulose uncoated			*	*		*	#		
Cellulose coated			*	*		*	*		*
Polyethylene									
Low-density			#	*		#	#		*
Stretch wrap				*					
Shrink wrap				*					
High density			*	*		*	#		*
Polypro-pylene			*	*		*	#		*
Polyester									
Plain			*	*		*	*		*
Metallized	*	*	*	*	*	*	#		*

* = good protection

\# = some protection

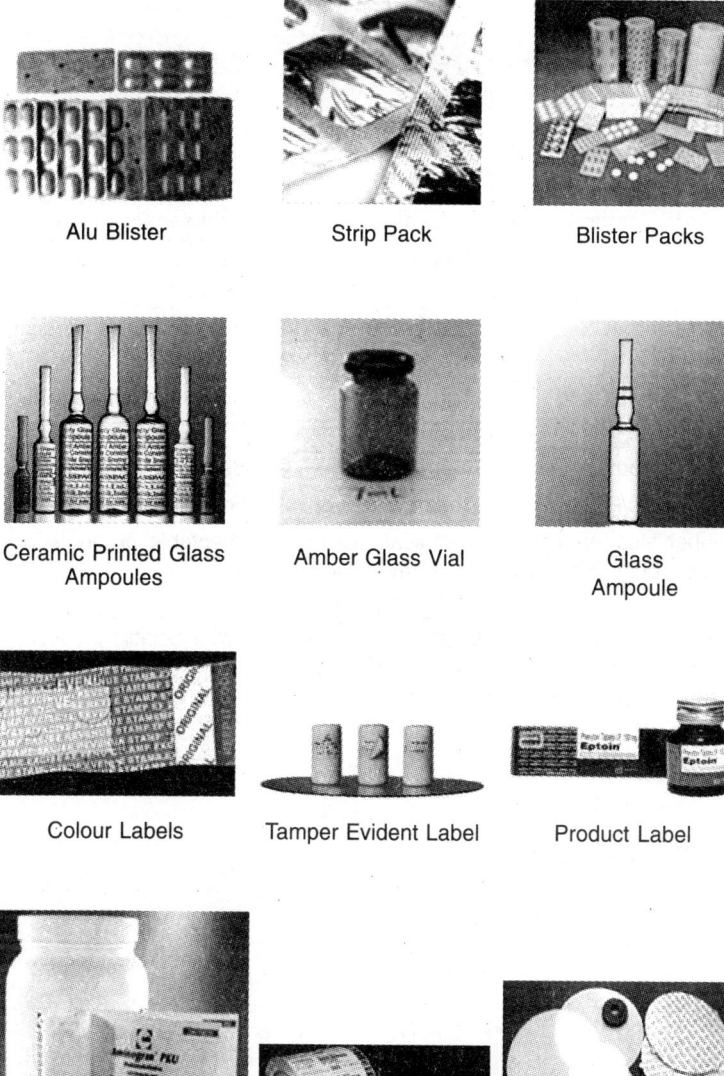

Alu Blister Strip Pack Blister Packs

Ceramic Printed Glass Ampoules Amber Glass Vial Glass Ampoule

Colour Labels Tamper Evident Label Product Label

Product Literature/ Leaf Let Bar Code Label Liners

Fig. 3.3: Type of packaging materials used by pharma industry

Table 3.3: Choosing containers and closures

Materials of Construction/Type	Critical Properties	Area of use
HDPE container	Good barrier to moisture, gas and light	All kind of product from solid orals and dry syrup
PET/PP (Amber)	Moderate barrier	Light sensitive products
Glass Bottles	High barrier	For highly sensitive products
Glass vials (USP I and II)	High barrier	For injectables product
Glass Bottles and vials (USP type III)	High barrier	Dry syrup, suspensions and powder for injection
Surface coated vials	High barrier	Sensitive products
PFS (glass/PE)	Moderate to high	For unit dose injectables
Rubber stopper, natural rubber, butyl, Halobutyl	Chemical resistant, low permeability, low water / solvent	Injectable products
Rubber stopper, natural rubber, butyl, Halobuty (legged and slotted)	Chemical resistant, low premeability, low water/solvent	Lyo injectable products

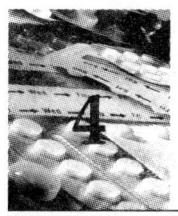

Polymers and Plastics

4.1 INTRODUCTION

Polymers are long chain giant organic molecules are assembled from many smaller molecules called monomers. Polymers consist of many repeating monomer units in long chains. A polymer is analogous to a necklace made from many small beads (monomers).

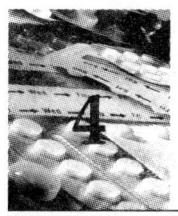

Fig. 4.1: Appearance of real linear polymer chain

25 nm

A polymer is a large molecule (macromolecule) composed of repeating structural units typically connected by covalent chemical bonds. While polymer in popular usage suggests plastic, the term actually refers to a large class of natural and synthetic materials with a wide variety of properties. Because of the extraordinary range of properties accessible in polymeric materials, they play an essential and ubiquitous role in everyday life-from plastics and elastomers . A simple example is polyethylene, whose repeating unit is based on ethylene (IUPAC name ethene) monomer. Most commonly, as in this example, the continuously linked backbone of a polymer used for the preparation of plastics consists mainly of carbon atoms. However, other structures do exist; for example, elements such as silicon form familiar materials such as silicones, examples being silly putty and waterproof plumbing sealant. The backbone of DNA is in fact based on a phosphodiester bond, and repeating units of polysaccharides (e.g. cellulose) are joined together by glycosidic bonds via oxygen atoms. Natural polymeric materials such as shellac, amber, and natural rubber have been in use for centuries. Biopolymers such as proteins and nucleic acids play crucial roles in biological processes. A variety of other natural polymers exist, such as cellulose, which is the main constituent of wood and paper. The list of synthetic polymers includes synthetic rubber, Bakelite, neoprene, nylon, PVC, polystyrene, polyethylene, polypropylene, polyacrylonitrile, PVB, silicone, and many more.

Homopolymers: Consist of chains with identical bonding linkages to each monomer unit. This usually implies that the polymer is made from all identical monomer molecules. These may be represented as: -[A-A-A-A-A-A]-

Polymers are Further Classified by the Reaction mode of Polymerization

Addition Polymers: The monomer molecules bond to each other without the loss of any other atoms. Alkene monomers are the biggest groups of polymers in this class.

Natural Polymers: Natural polymers are discussed in other web pages and include:

Proteins – silk, collagen, keratin.

Carbohydrates – cellulose, starch, glycogen.

DNA – RNA

Other Natural polymers: Rubber (hydrocarbon base) and silicones (alternating silicon and oxygen).

Polymer Synthesis

Polymerization is the process of combining many small molecules known as monomers into a covalently bonded chain. During the polymerization process, some chemical groups may be lost from each monomer. This is the case, for example, in the polymerization of PET polyester. The monomers are terephthalic acid ($HOOC-C_6H_4-COOH$) and ethylene glycol ($HO-CH_2-CH_2-OH$) but the repeating unit is $-OC-C_6H_4-COO-CH_2-CH_2-O-$, which corresponds to the combination of the two monomers with the loss of two water molecules. The distinct piece of each monomer that is incorporated into the polymer is known as a repeat unit or monomer residue.

Modification of Natural Polymers

Many commercially important polymers are synthesized by chemical modification of naturally occurring polymers. Prominent examples include the reaction of nitric acid and cellulose to form nitrocellulose and the formation of vulcanized rubber by heating natural rubber in the presence of sulfur.

Branch Point in a Polymer

An important microstructural feature determining polymer properties is the polymer architecture. The simplest polymer architecture is a linear chain: A single backbone with no branches. A related unbranching architecture is a ring polymer. A branched polymer molecule is composed of a main chain with one or more substituent side chains or branches. Special types of branched polymers include star polymers, comb polymers, brush polymers, dendronized polymers, ladders, and dendrimers. A good example of this effect is related to the range of physical attributes of polyethylene. High-density polyethylene (HDPE) has a very low degree of branching, is quite stiff, and is used in applications such as milk jugs. Low-density polyethylene (LDPE), on the other hand, has significant numbers of both long and short branches, is quite flexible, and is used in applications such as plastic films.

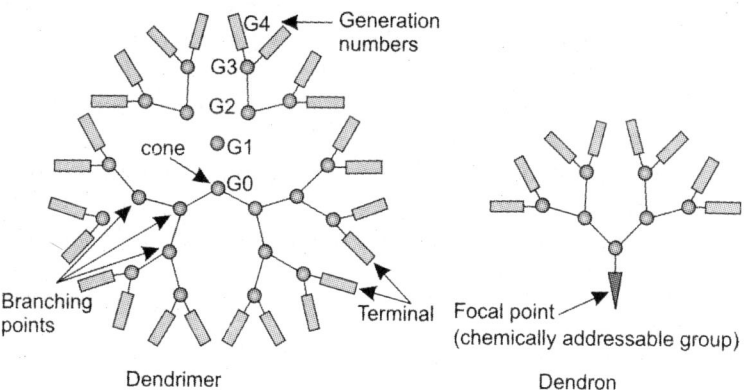

Fig. 4.2: Dendrimer and dendron

Dendrimer and Dendron

Dendrimers are a special case of polymer where every monomer unit is branched. This tends to reduce intermolecular chain entanglement and crystallization.

Chain Length

The physical properties of a polymer are strongly dependent on the size or length of the polymer chain. For example, as chain length is increased, melting and boiling temperatures increase quickly.

Monomer Arrangement in Copolymers

Monomers within a copolymer may be organized along the backbone in a variety of ways.

- Alternating copolymers possess regularly alternating monomer residues $[AB...]_n$.
- Periodic copolymers have monomer residue types arranged in a repeating sequence: $[A_nB_m...]_m$ being different from n.
- Statistical copolymers have monomer residues arranged according to a known statistical rule. A statistical copolymer in which the probability of finding a particular type of monomer residue at an particular point in the chain is independent of the types of surrounding monomer residue may be referred to as a truly random copolymer.
- Block copolymers have two or more homopolymer subunits linked by covalent bonds Polymers with two or three blocks of two distinct chemical species (e.g. A and B) are called diblock copolymers and triblock copolymers, respectively Polymers with three blocks, each of a different chemical species (e.g. A, B and C) are termed triblock terpolymers.
- Graft or grafted copolymers contain side chains that have a different composition or configuration than the main chain.

Tacticity

Tacticity describes the relative stereochemistry of chiral centers in neighboring structural units within a macromolecule. There are three types: isotactic (all substituents on the same side), atactic (random placement of substituents), and syndiotactic (alternating placement of substituents).

Polymer Morphology

Polymer morphology generally describes the arrangement of chains in space and microscopic ordering of many polymer chains.

Tensile Strength

The tensile strength of a material quantifies how much stress the material will endure before suffering permanent deformation. This is very important in applications that rely upon a polymer's physical strength or durability. For example, a rubber band with a higher tensile strength will hold a greater weight before snapping. In general, tensile strength increases with polymer chain length and crosslinking of polymer chains.

Young's Modulus of Elasticity

Young's Modulus quantifies the elasticity of the polymer. It is defined, for small strains, as the ratio of rate of change of stress to strain. Like tensile strength, this is highly relevant in polymer applications involving the physical properties of polymers, such as rubber bands. The modulus is strongly dependent on temperature.

Transport Properties

Transport properties such as diffusivity relate to how rapidly molecules move through the polymer matrix. These are very important in many applications of polymers for films and membranes.

Inclusion of Plasticizers

Inclusion of plasticizers tends to lower T_g and increase polymer flexibility. Plasticizers are generally small molecules that are chemically similar to the polymer and create gaps between polymer chains for greater mobility and reduced interchain interactions. A good example of the action of plasticizers is related to polyvinylchlorides or PVCs. A uPVC, or unplasticized polyvinyl chloride, is used for things such as pipes.

Standardized Polymer Nomenclature

There are multiple conventions for naming polymer substances. Many commonly used polymers, such as those found in consumer products, are referred to by a common or trivial name. The trivial name is assigned based on historical precedent or popular usage rather than a standardized naming convention. Both the American Chemical Society and IUPAC have proposed standardized naming conventions; the ACS and IUPAC conventions are similar but not identical. Examples of the differences between the various naming conventions are given in the below:

Common name	ACS name	IUPAC name
Poly (ethylene oxide) or PEO	Poly (oxyethylene)	Poly(oxyethene)
Poly (ethylene terephthalate) or PET	Poly(oxy-1,2-ethanediyloxycarbonyl-1,4-phenylenecarbonyl)	Poly (oxyethene-oxyterephthaloyl)
Nylon 6	Poly[amino (1-oxo-1,6 -hexanediyl)]	Poly[amino (1-oxohexan-1,6-diyl)]

In both standardized conventions, the polymer's names are intended to reflect the monomer(s) from which they are synthesized rather than the precise nature of the repeating subunit. For example, the polymer synthesized from the simple alkene ethene is called polyethylene, retaining the-ene suffix even though the double bond is removed during the polymerization process.

Polymer Degradation

A plastic item with thirty years of exposure to heat and cold, brake fluid, and sunlight. Notice the discolouration, swollen dimensions, and tiny splits running through the material. Polymer degradation is a change in the properties-tensile strength, colour, shape, molecular weight, etc. of a polymer or polymer-based product under the influence of one or more environmental factors, such as heat, light, chemicals and, in some cases, galvanic action. It is often due to the hydrolysis of the bonds connecting the polymer chain, which in turn leads to a decrease in the molecular mass of the polymer. These changes may be undesirable, such as changes during use, or desirable, as in biodegradation or deliberately lowering the molecular mass of a polymer. Such changes occur primarily because of the effect of these factors on the chemical composition of the polymer. Ozone cracking and UV degradation are specific failure modes for certain polymers. The susceptibility of a polymer to degradation depends on its structure. Epoxies and chains containing aromatic functionality are especially susceptible to UV degradation while polyesters are susceptible to degradation by hydrolysis. Carbon based polymers are more susceptible to thermal degradation than inorganically bound polymers such as Polydimethylsiloxane and are therefore not ideal for most high temperature applications. Polymer degradation may occur through galvanic action. In 1990, Michael Faudree discovered that imide-linked resins in CFRP (carbon fibre reinforced polymers) composites degrade when bare composite is coupled with an active metal in saline, i.e. salt water environments. Polymers affected include bismaleimides (BMI), condensation polyamides, triazines, and blends thereof. Degradation occurs in the form of dissolved resin and loose fibres. Hydroxyl ions are generated at the graphite cathode attacking the O-C-N bond in the polyamide structure. This phenomenon, that polymers can undergo galvanic corrosion like metals do have been referred to as the "Faudree Effect". Standard corrosion protection procedures were found to prevent polymer degradation under most conditions. The degradation of polymers to form smaller molecules may proceed by random scission or specific scission. The degradation of polyethylene occurs by random scission-a random breakage of the linkages (bonds) that hold the atoms of the polymer together. When heated above 450 DEGC it degrades to form a mixture of hydrocarbons. Other polymers-like polyalphamethylstyrene-undergo specific chain scission with breakage occurring only at the ends. They literally unzip or depolymerize to become the constituent monomer.

However, the degradation process can be useful from the viewpoints of understanding the structure of a polymer or recycling/reusing the polymer waste to prevent or reduce environmental pollution. Polylactic acid and polyglycolic acid, for example, are two polymers that are useful for their ability to degrade under aqueous conditions. A copolymer of these polymers is used for biomedical applications, such as hydrolysable stitches that degrade over time after they are applied to a wound. These materials can also be used for plastics that will degrade over time after they are used and will therefore not remain as litter. The sorting of polymer waste for recycling purposes may be facilitated by the use of the Resin identification codes developed by the Society of the Plastics Industry to identify the type of plastic.

Product Failure

In a finished product, such a change is to be prevented or delayed. Failure of safety-critical polymer components can cause serious accidents, such as fire in the case of cracked and degraded polymer fuel lines. Chlorine-induced cracking of acetal resin plumbing joints and polybutylene pipes has caused many serious floods in domestic properties, especially in the USA in the 1990s. Traces of chlorine in the water supply attacked vulnerable polymers in the plastic plumbing, a problem which occurs faster if any of the parts have been poorly extruded or injection molded. Attack of the acetal joint occurred because of faulty molding, leading to cracking along the threads of the fitting which is a serious stress concentration. Polymer oxidation has caused accidents involving medical devices. One of the oldest known failure modes is ozone cracking caused by chain scission when ozone gas attacks susceptible elastomers such as natural rubber and nitrile rubber. They possess double bonds in their repeat units which are cleaved during ozonolysis. Cracks in fuel lines can penetrate the bore of the tube and cause fuel leakage. If cracking occurs in the engine compartment, electric sparks can ignite the gasoline and can cause a serious fire. Fuel lines can also be attacked by another form of degradation: hydrolysis. Nylon 6, 6 is susceptible to acid hydrolysis, and in one accident, a fractured fuel line led to a spillage of diesel into the road. If diesel fuel leaks onto the road, accidents to following cars can be caused by the slippery nature of the deposit, which is like black ice.

4.2 PLASTICS

Any of various organic compounds produced by polymerization, capable of being molded, extruded, cast into various shapes and films, or drawn into filaments used as textile fibres or plastics are any of a group of synthetic or natural organic materials that may be shaped when soft and then hardened, including many types of resins, resinoids, polymers, cellulose derivatives, casein materials, and proteins: used in place of other materials, as glass, wood, and metals, in packaging, construction, decoration, etc. "Plastics are defined as the polymers (solid materials) which become mobile on heating and thus can be cast into moulds."

History

Plastics are polymers. The most simple definition of a polymer is something made of many units. Each link of the chain is the "mer" or basic unit that is made of carbon, hydrogen, oxygen, and/or silicon. To make the chain, many links or "mers" are hooked or polymerized together. Polymerization can be demonstrated by linking strips of construction paper together to make paper garlands or hooking together hundreds of paper clips to form chains. Polymers have been with us since the beginning of time. Natural polymers include such things as tar and shellac, tortoise shell and horns, as well as tree saps that produce amber and latex. These polymers were processed with heat and pressure into useful articles like hair ornaments and jewelry. Natural polymers began to be chemically modified during the 1800s to produce many materials. The most famous of these were vulcanized rubber, gun cotton, and celluloid. The first semisynthetic polymer produced was Bakelite in 1909 and was soon followed by the first synthetic fibre, rayon, which was developed in 1911.

The first man-made plastic – parkesine: The first man-made plastic was created by Alexander Parkes who publicly demonstrated it at the 1862 Great International Exhibition in London. The material called Parkesine was an organic material derived from cellulose that once heated could be molded, and retained its shape when cooled.

Celluloid: Celluloid is derived from cellulose and alcoholized camphor. John Wesley Hyatt invented celluloid as a substitute for the ivory in billiard balls in 1868.

Formaldehyde resins: Bakelite-after cellulose nitrate, formaldehyde was the next product to advance the technology of plastic. Around 1897, efforts to manufacture white chalkboards led to casein plastics (milk protein mixed with formaldehyde) Galalith and Erinoid are two early trade name examples.

In 1899, Arthur Smith received British Patent 16, 275, for "phenol-formaldehyde resins for use as an ebonite substitute in electrical insulation", the first patent for processing a formaldehyde resin. However, in 1907, Leo Hendrik Baekeland improved phenol-formaldehyde reaction techniques and invented the first fully synthetic resin to become commercially successful, trade named Bakelite.

- 1839 – Natural Rubber - method of processing invented by Charles Goodyear.
- 1843 – Vulcanite - Thomas Hancock.

Semi-synthetics

- 1839 – Polystyrene or PS discovered - Eduard Simon.
- 1862 – Parkesine - Alexander Parkes.
- 1863 – Cellulose Nitrate or Celluloid - John Wesley Hyatt.
- 1872 – Polyvinyl Chloride or PVC - first created by Eugen Baumann.
- 1894 – Viscose Rayon - Charles Frederick Cross, Edward John Bevan.

Thermosetting Plastics and Thermoplastics

- 1909 – First true plastic Phenol-formaldehyde trade named bakelite – Leo Hendrik Baekeland.
- 1926 – Vinyl or PVC – Walter Semon invented a plasticized PVC.

- 1927 – Cellulose acetate.
- 1933 – Polyvinylidene chloride or Saran also called PVDC– accidentally discovered by Ralph Wiley, a Dow Chemical lab worker.
- 1935 – Low-density polyethylene or LDPE – Reginald Gibson and Eric Fawcett.
- 1936 – Acrylic or Polymethyl Methacrylate.
- 1937 – Polyurethanes trade named Igamid for plastics materials and Perlon for fibres. Otto Bayer and co-workers discovered and patented the chemistry of polyurethanes.
- 1938 – Polystyrene made practical.
- 1938 – Polytetrafluoroethylene or PTFE trade named Teflon - Roy Plunkett.
- 1939 – Nylon and Neoprene considered a replacement for silk and a synthetic rubber respectively Wallace Hume Carothers.
- 1941 – Polyethylene terephthalate or Pet – Whinfield and Dickson.
- 1942 – Low Density Polyethylene.
- 1951 – High-density polyethylene or HDPE trade named Marlex – Paul Hogan and Robert Banks.
- 1951 – Polypropylene or PP - Paul Hogan and Robert Banks.
- 1964 – Polyamide
- 1970 – Thermoplastic Polyester this includes trademarked Dacron, Mylar, Melinex, Teijin and Tetoron.
- 1978 – Linear Low Density Polyethylene.
- 1985 – Liquid Crystal Polymers.

4.3 THE STRUCTURE OF POLYMERS

Many common classes of polymers are composed of hydrocarbons. These polymers are specifically made of small units bonded into long chains. Carbon makes up the backbone of the molecule and hydrogen atoms are bonded along the backbone. Below is a diagram of polyethylene, the simplest polymer structure.

There are polymers that contain only carbon and hydrogen. Polypropylene, polybutylene, polystyrene, and polymethylpentene are examples of these. Even though the basic makeup of many polymers is carbon and hydrogen, other elements can also be involved. Oxygen, chlorine, fluorine, nitrogen, silicon, phosphorous, and sulfur are other elements that are found in the molecular makeup of polymers. Polyvinyl chloride (PVC)

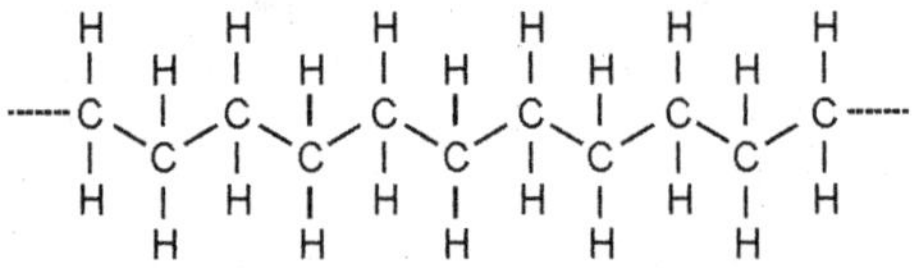

Fig. 4.3: Polymer structure (polyethylene)

contains chlorine. Nylon contains nitrogen and oxygen. Teflon contains fluorine. Polyester and polycarbonates contain oxygen. Vulcanized rubber and thiokol contain sulfur. There are also some polymers that, instead of having a carbon backbone, have a silicon or silicon-oxygen backbone. These are considered inorganic polymers.

4.4 RAW MATERIALS OF PLASTICS

Plastics are made from the following materials:

Plasticizers: They improve the softening, decrease brittleness and workability of plastics. They are organic substances.

Stabilizers: They prevent chemical degradation of plastics. By nature they are antioxidants.

Fillers: They increase the tensile strength of plastics. They are wood flour and glass wool.

Reinforcing agents: They increase its mechanical strength. Example is glass fibre.

Pigments: They are used to impart a particular colour to the plastic.

4.5 TYPES OF PLASTICS

Plastics are natural/synthetic materials. They are produced by chemically modifying natural substances or are synthesized from inorganic and organic raw materials. On the basis of their physical characteristics, plastics are usually divided into thermosets, elastomers and thermoplastics. These groups differ primarily with regard to molecular structure, which is what determines their differing thermal behavior. The following Table lists the characteristics of the various types of plastics.

Type of plastic	Molecular structure	Characteristics an applications
Thermosets		Thermosets are hard and have a very tight-meshed, branched molecular structure. Curing proceeds during shaping, after which it is no longer possible to shape the material by heating. Further shaping may then only be performed by machining. Thermosets are used, for example, to make light switches.
Elastomers		While elastomers also have a crosslinked structure, they have a looser mesh than thermosets, giving rise to a degree of elasticity. Once shaped, elastomers also cannot be reshaped by heating. Elastomers are used, for example, to produce automobile tires.
Thermoplastics		Thermoplastics have a linear or branched molecular structure which determines their strength and thermal behavior; they are flexible at ordinary temperatures. At approx. 120–180°C, thermoplastics become a pasty/liquid mass. The service temperature range for thermoplastics is considerably lower than that for thermosets. The thermoplastics polyethylene (PE), polyvinyl chloride (PVC) and polystyrene (PS) are used, for example, in packaging applications.

Thermosetting Polymer

A thermosetting plastic, also known as a thermoset, is polymer material that irreversibly cures. The cure may be done through heat (generally above 200°C (392°F)), through a chemical reaction (two-part epoxy, for example), or irradiation such as electron beam processing.

Thermoset materials are usually liquid or malleable prior to curing and designed to be molded into their final form, or used as adhesives. Others are solids like that of the molding compound used in semiconductors and integrated circuits (ICs).

According to IUPAC recommendation: A thermosetting polymer is a prepolymer in a soft solid or viscous state that changes irreversibly into an infusible, insoluble polymer network by curing. Curing can be induced by the action of heat or suitable radiation, or both. A cured thermosetting polymer is called a thermoset.

Types of Thermosetting Polymer

1. Bismaleimides (BMI): This is the most recent polymer this polymer is produced by the condensation reaction of a diamine with maleic anhydride.

2. Epoxy (Epoxide): Epoxy is used widely in numerous formulations and forms in the aircraft-aerospace industry. It is called "the work horse of modern day composites". Standard epoxies (90%) are based on bisphenol A diglycidyl ether formula.

3. Bakelite/Phenolic (PF): The limitations of celluloid led to the next major advance, known as "phenolic" or "phenol-formaldehyde" plastics. A chemist named Leo Hendrik Baekelund, a Belgian-born American living in New York state, was searching for an insulating shellac to coat wires in electric motors and generators. Baekelund found that mixtures of phenol (C_6H_5OH) and formaldehyde (HCOH) formed a sticky mass when mixed together and heated, and the mass became extremely hard if allowed to cool and dry. It means bakelite is a condensation polymer of phenol and formaldehyde. Bakelite is widely used for making moulded products.

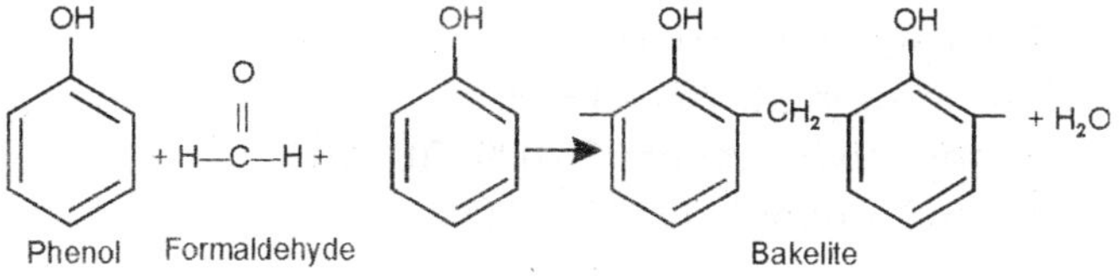

Fig. 4.4: Synthesis of bakelite

Bakelite was the first true plastic. It was a purely synthetic material, not based on any material or molecule found in nature. It was also the first "thermoset" plastic. Conventional "thermoplastics" can be molded and then melted again, but thermoset plastics form bonds between polymers when "cured", creating a tangled matrix that cannot be undone without destroying the plastic. Thermoplastics are tough and temperature resistant.

Bakelite was cheap, strong, and durable. It was molded into thousands of forms, such as electric switches, electric board, cameras, body, radios, telephones, buttons, clocks, and of course billiard balls. Phenolic plastics are still in widespread use. For example, electronic circuit boards are made of sheets of paper or cloth impregnated with phenolic resin.

General purpose molding compounds, engineering molding compounds and sheet molding compounds are the primary forms of phenolic. Phenolic is also used in some Honeycomb core (H/C) as the matrix binder. This Phenolic is used in many electrical applications such as breaker boxes, brake lining material and even, recently, combined with various reinforcements in the molding of an engine block-head assembly, called the polimotor. Phenolics may be processed by the various common techniques, including compression, transfer and injection molding.

Properties of Phenol-formaldehyde

- High-strength glass fiber reinforced
- Relative density 1.69–2.0
- Water absorption 24 h (%) 0.03–1.2
- Melting temperature (°C)
- Thermo set processing range (°F) C: 300–380 I: 330–390
- Molding pressure I–20

- Shrinkage 0.001–0.004
- Tensile strength 7000–18000
- Compressive strength 16,000–70,000
- Flexural strength 12,000–60,000

Applications and Usage

Although no longer extensively used as an industrial manufacturing material, Bakelite was used in a myriad of applications including saxophone mouthpieces, whistles, cameras, solid-body electric guitars, rotary-dial telephones, early machine guns, and appliance casings. The thermosetting plastic was at one point considered for the manufacture of coins, due to a shortage of traditional manufacturing material.

In 1943, Bakelite and other non-metal materials were tested for usage as a penny in the United States before the Mint settled on zinc coated steel. The foremost usage of Bakelite today is as a substitute for porcelain and other opaque ceramics in applications where fine detail is unimportant (other thermoset resins can capture detail more finely when molded) and durability over traditional ceramic compounds is desired. As such, a main continuing use for bakelite is in the area of board and tabletop games. Devices such as billiard balls, dominoes, Mahjongg tiles and other gaming tilesets, and movers/pieces for games like chess, checkers, and backgammon are constructed of Bakelite for the look, durability, fine polish, weight, and sound of the resulting pieces.

Dice are sometimes made of Bakelite for weight and sound, but the majorities are made of a thermoplastic such as ABS. It is also used to make the presentation boxes of luxury Breitling watches. Bakelite is also sometimes used as a substitute for metal in the construction of firearm magazines. Bakelite is also used in the mounting of metal samples in metallography. Phenolic resins have been commonly used in ablative heat shields.

4. Polyester: This is an extremely versatile, fairly inexpensive, polymer. Unsaturated polyester combines an unsaturated dibasic acid and a glycol dissolved in a monomer, generally styrene, including an inhibitor to stabilize the resin. Organic peroxides, such as methyl ethyl ketone peroxide (MEKP) and a promoter are combined with the resin to initiate a room temperature (RT) cure. In this liquid state, polyester may be processed by numerous methods, including Hand Layup (HLU), vacuum bag molding, spray-up and compression molded Sheet Molding Compound (SMC), etc. The resin can also be B-staged after application to chopped reinforcements and continuous reinforcement, pre-preg. Solid molding compounds in the form of pellets or granules are also used in processes such as compression and transfer molding.

5. Polyamide: This polymer is presently the most advanced of all TS matrices. It has characteristics of high temperature (H/T) physical and mechanical properties. It is available as uncured resin, prepreg, stock shapes, thin sheets, laminates, and machined parts. Along with the H/T properties, this polymer must be processed at very high temperatures and relative pressure to produce these characteristics. With prepreg materials, 600°F (316°C) to 650°F (343°C) temperatures and 200 psi (1,379 kPa) pressures are required. The entire cure profiles are inherently long as there are a number of intermediate temperatures dwells, duration of these are dependent on part size and thickness. The cut of PI is 450°F (232°C), highest of all TS, with short term exposure capabilities of 900°F (482°C). Normal operating temperatures range from cryogenic to 500°F (260°C).

Properties of Polyamide

- Good mechanical properties at H/T
- Good electrical properties
- High wear resistance
- Low creep at high temperatures
- Good compression with glass or graphite fibre reinforcement
- Good chemical resistance
- Inherently flame resistant
- Unaffected by most solvents and oils

Polyamide Film

Polyamide film possesses a unique combination of properties that make it ideal for a variety of applications in many different industries.

6. High-performance resin: The high-performance resin is used in electrical, wear resistant and as structural materials when combined with reinforcement for aircraft-aerospace applications, which are replacing heavier more expensive metals. High temperature processing causes some technical problems as well as higher costs compared to other polymers. Hysols PMR series is an example of this polymer.

7. Polyurethane (PUR): Polyurethanes are the single most versatile family of polymers there is. Polyurethanes can be elastomers, and they can be paints. They can be fibres, and they can be adhesives. They just pop up everywhere. A wonderfully bizarre polyurethane is spandex.

These thermosetting polymers are produced by combinations of polyisocyanate and polyol as well as other ingredients and reactive materials. Polyurethane plastics belong to the group that can be thermosetting or thermoplastic. Polyurethane is the only plastic which can be made in both rigid and flexible foams. Polyurethanes are called polyurethanes because in their backbones they have a urethane linkage.

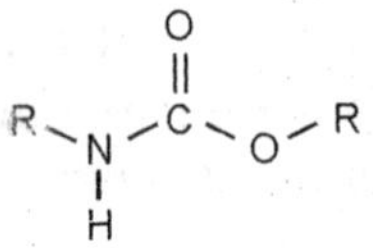

A urethane

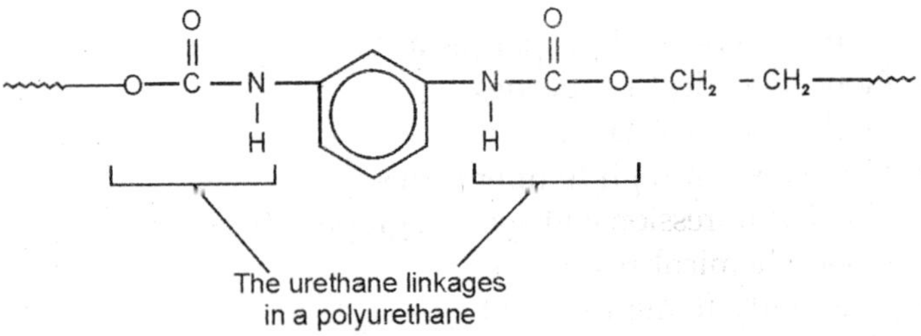

The urethane linkages
in a polyurethane

Fig. 4.5: Simple polyurethane

Polyurethanes can hydrogen bond very well, and thus can be very crystalline. For this reason they are often used to make block copolymers with soft rubbery polymers. These block copolymers have properties of thermoplastic elastomers.

Polyurethane Foam

Polyurethanes are the most well known polymers used to make foams. If you are sitting on a padded chair right now, the cushion is more than likely made of polyurethane foam. Polyurethanes are more than foam. Polyurethane foam structural core can be combined with glass-reinforced or graphite-reinforced composite laminates to produce a lightweight, strong, sandwich structure.

Spandex

One unusual polyurethane thermoplastic elastomer is spandex, which DuPont sells under the trade name Lycra. It has both urea and urethane linkages in its backbone. What gives spandex its special properties is the fact that it has hard and soft blocks in its repeat structure. The short polymeric chain of a polyglycol, usually about forty or so repeats units long, is soft and rubbery. The rest of the repeat unit, is the stretch with the urethane linkages, the urea linkages, and the aromatic groups, is extremely rigid. This section is stiff enough that the rigid sections from different chains clump together and align to form fibres. They are unusual fibres, as the fibrous domains formed by the stiff blocks are linked together by the rubbery soft sections. The result is a fibre that acts like an elastomer. This allows us to make fabric that stretches for exercise clothing and the like.

Properties: Due to the property of high elasticity, some polyurethane plastics are used in decorative and protective coatings. The high elasticity makes these polyurethane plastics resistant to a chemical attack. Also including heat resistance property.

Advantages

There are a wide variety of polyurethane adhesives and sealants available. They differ in terms of features such as bulk flexibility, resistance to oil or chemicals, heat resistance, gap filling and leveling, retaining, sealing, and thread locking.

Polyurethane adhesives and sealants with bulk flexibility form a layer that can bend or flex without cracking or delaminating.

Polyurethane adhesives and sealants that are resistant to oils and chemicals are not damaged by exposure to acids, alkalis, oils or fuel.

Heat resistant polyurethane adhesives and sealants are not damaged by prolonged exposure to raised temperatures.

Many are flame resistant, meaning that they resist ignition when exposed to high temperatures.

They reduce production costs and improve reliability by eliminating lock washers and other expensive locking devices.

These polyurethane adhesives and sealants also preserve on-torque and distribute the load over the entire engagement length of the fastener, effectively eliminating premature material fatigue and fastener failure.

General uses: The flexible polyurethane foam is used in mattresses, carpets, furniture, etc. The rigid polyurethane foam is used in chair shells, mirror frames and many more.

Application

They provide additional support in applications that deal with raised levels of sound, vibration or shock.

They are used in applications such as sealing fuel or oil tanks, and are used in chemical process vessels, piping, and fittings that are exposed to oil and corrosive mixtures.

In addition to providing bonding and protection, many polyurethane adhesives and sealants are used to level, fill gaps, and seal holes.

They vary based on the composition of the adhesive and its style (i.e. flowing liquid, viscous liquid, or compound paste). A common filling application is gap filling, which involves simply closing up gaps between two bonded substrates.

There are also leveling mastics, highly viscous polyurethane adhesives that are applied by trowel to give thick glue lines with gap-sealing properties. Typically, mastics are used to bond tiles to sub-flooring. They fill in gaps or irregularities in a surface before tile or other materials are applied.

Polyurethane adhesives and sealants with retaining properties are used to reliably retain cylindrical mating parts such as bearings, pulleys, couplings, rotors and gears.

These products eliminate the need for press or shrink fits and provide up to twice the shear strength of these methods of assembly on slip-fit parts.

Threadlocking or threadlocker polyurethane adhesives and sealants lock all kinds of threads that are subject to transverse and axial loads against vibrational loosening.

8. Silicone: Silicone is a unique, partly organic, polymer structure made of alternating silicon and oxygen atoms rather than the familiar carbon-to-carbon backbone characteristics of organic polymer. Silicone can be in the form of a liquid, gel, elastomer or solid. It has a broad temperature use range, elasticity, chemical resistance, good release properties, etc. In the area of composites, silicone is used as a sealant and coating material. It is often used as a reusable bag material for vacuum-bag curing of composite parts.

Miscellaneous

Urea-formaldehyde and melamine-formaldehyde, although not widely used in modern day composite applications, are characteristically used in molding compounds where some use of fillers and reinforcements occurs. Also, the urea resin is often used as the matrix binder in construction utility products such as particle board, wafer board, and plywood, which are true particulate and laminar composite structures.

Advantages and Disadvantages of Thermoset Polymers

Advantages

- Well established processing and application history.
- Overall, better economics than thermoplastic (TP) polymers.
- Better high temperature (H/T) properties.
- Good wetting and adhesion to reinforcement.

Disadvantages

- Resins and composite materials must be refrigerated.
- Long process cycles.
- Reduced impact – toughness.
- Poor recycling capabilities.
- More difficult repair ability.

Thermoplastic

A thermoplastic, also known as thermosoftening plastic, is a polymer that turns to a liquid when heated and freezes to a very glassy state when cooled sufficiently. Most thermoplastics are high-molecular-weight polymers whose chains associate through weak van der Waals forces (polyethylene); stronger dipole-dipole interactions and hydrogen bonding (nylon); or even stacking of aromatic rings (polystyrene). Thermoplastic polymers differ from thermosetting polymers (Bakelite) in that they can be remelted and remoulded. Many thermoplastic materials are addition polymers, e.g. vinyl chain-growth polymers such as polyethylene and polypropylene.

1. Cellulose

Uses : Wood, fibres (cotton, rayon, flax, hemp), component of shampoo thickeners

Monomer : Glucose

Morphology : Crystalline

Cellulose is one of many polymers found in nature. Wood, paper, and cotton all contain cellulose. Cellulose is an excellent fibre. Wood, cotton, and hemp rope are all made of fibrous cellulose. Cellulose is made of repeat units of the monomer glucose. This is the same glucose which your body metabolizes in order to live, but you

Fig. 4.6: Glucose

cannot digest it in the form of cellulose. Because cellulose is built out of a sugar monomer, it is called a polysaccharide.

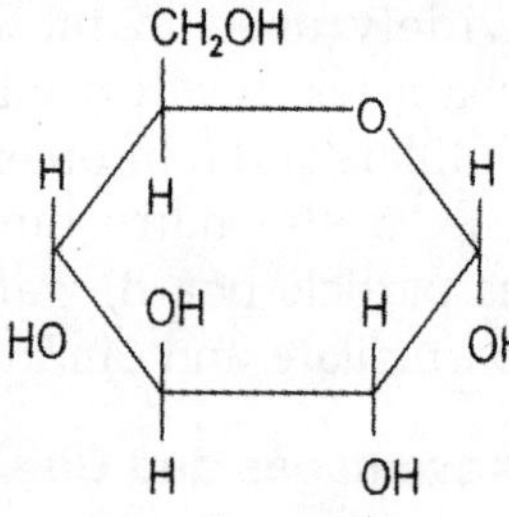

Cellulose is an organic compound with the formula $(C_6H_{10}O_5)n$, a polysaccharide consisting of a linear chain of several hundred to over ten thousand? ($1 \rightarrow 4$) linked D-glucose units. Cellulose has an important place in the story of polymers because it was used to make some of the first synthetic polymers, like cellulose nitrate, cellulose acetate, and rayon. Cellulose is the structural component of the primary cell wall of green plants, many forms of algae and the oomycetes. Some species of bacteria secrete it to form biofilms. Cellulose is the most common organic compound on Earth. About 33 percent of all plant matter is cellulose (the cellulose content of cotton is 90 percent and that of wood is 40–50 percent).

For industrial use, cellulose is mainly obtained from wood pulp and cotton. It is mainly used to produce paperboard and paper; to a smaller extent it is converted into a wide variety of derivative products such as cellophane and rayon. Converting cellulose from energy crops into biofuels such as cellulosic ethanol is under investigation as an alternative fuel source. Some animals, particularly ruminants and termites, can digest cellulose with the help of symbiotic micro-organisms that live in their guts. Humans can digest cellulose to some extent, however it is often referred to as 'dietary fibre' or 'roughage' (e.g. outer shell of Maize) and acts as a hydrophilic bulking agent for feces.

Commercial Products

Cellulose is the major constituent of paper, paperboard, and card stock and of textiles made from cotton, linen, and other plant fibres. Cellulose can be converted into cellophane, a thin transparent film, and into rayon, an important fibre that has been used for textiles since the beginning of the 20th century. Both cellophane and rayon are known as "regenerated cellulose fibres"; they are identical to cellulose in chemical structure and are usually made from dissolving pulp via viscose. A more recent and environmentally friendly method to produce rayon is the Lyocell process. Cellulose is the raw material in the manufacture of nitrocellulose (cellulose nitrate) which was historically used in smokeless gunpowder and as the base material for celluloid used for photographic and movie films until the mid 1930s. Cellulose is used to make water-soluble adhesives and binders such as methyl cellulose and carboxymethyl cellulose which are used in wallpaper paste. Microcrystalline cellulose (E460i) and powdered cellulose (E460ii) are used as inactive fillers in tablets and as thickeners and stabilizers in processed foods. Cellulose powder is for example used in Kraft Parmesean Cheese to prevent caking inside the tube. Cellulose is used in the laboratory as the stationary phase for thin layer chromatography. Cellulose fibres are also used in liquid filtration, sometimes in combination with diatomaceous earth or other filtration media, to create a filter bed of inert material. Cellulose is further used to make hydrophilic and highly absorbent sponges.

Cellulose based Plastics: Celluloid

Hyatt was something of an industrial genius who understood what could be done with such a shapeable, or "plastic", material and proceeded to design much of the basic industrial machinery needed to produce good-quality plastic materials in quantity. Since cellulose was the main constituent used in the synthesis of his new material, Hyatt named it "celluloid". It was introduced in 1863.

Celluloid is the name of a class of compounds created from nitrocellulose (or cellulose nitrate) and camphor, plus dyes and other agents. Generally regarded as the first thermoplastic. Celluloid is easily molded and shaped, and there are suggestions that it was initially made as an ivory replacement. Celluloid is highly flammable and also easily decomposes, and is no longer widely used. Its most common use today is the table tennis ball.

Formulation

A typical formulation of celluloid might contain roughly 70 to 80 parts nitrocellulose (cellulose nitrate) and 30 parts camphor. In addition, it may include 0 to 14 parts dye, 1 to 5 parts ethyl alcohol, and stabilizers and other agents to increase stability and reduce flammability. Other nitrocellulose-based plastics slightly predated celluloid. In particular, collodion, invented in 1848, dried to a celluloid-like film. It was used as a wound dressing and emulsion for photographic plates.

Applications

Items such as knife handles, fountain pen bodies, collars, cuffs, and toys were made from this material. It, however, burned easily and suffered from spontaneous decomposition.

It was therefore largely replaced by cellulose acetate plastics and later polyethylenes by the mid-twentieth century. The use of celluloid for early film however has been problematic for film preservation.

Products still made from celluloid include the table tennis ball, and some musical instrument accessories and parts, such as guitar picks and pick guards. In addition, cured celluloid is used in luxury pens produced by OMAS and other high-end pen manufacturers.

One of the first products was dental pieces. Sets of false teeth built around celluloid proved cheaper than existing rubber dentures. However, celluloid dentures tended to soften when hot, making tea drinking tricky, and the camphor taste tended to be difficult to suppress.

Celluloid's real breakthrough products were waterproof shirt collars, cuffs, and the false shirt fronts known as "dickies", whose unmanageable nature later became a stock joke in silent-movie comedies. They did not wilt and did not stain easily, and Hyatt sold them by trainloads. Corsets made with celluloid stays also proved popular, since perspiration didn't rust the stays, as it would if they had been made of metal.

Celluloid proved extremely versatile in its fields of application, providing a cheap and attractive replacement for ivory, tortoise-shell and bone. Traditional products that had used these materials were much easier to fabricate with plastics.

Some of the items made with cellulose in the 19th century were beautifully designed and implemented. For example, celluloid combs made to tie up the long tresses of hair fashionable at the time are now jewel-like museum pieces. Such pretty trinkets were no longer only for the rich.

Celluloid could also be used in entirely new applications. Hyatt figured out how to fabricate the material in a strip format for movie film. By the year 1900, movie film was a major market for celluloid.

Ping-pong balls, one of the few products still made with celluloid, sizzle and burn if set on fire, and Hyatt liked to tell stories about celluloid billiard balls exploding when struck very hard. These stories might have had a basis in fact, since the billiard balls were often celluloid covered with paints based on another, even more flammable, nitrocellulose product known as "collodion". If the balls had been imperfectly manufactured, the paints might have acted as primer to set the rest of the ball off with a bang.

Cellulose was also used to produce cloth. While the men who developed celluloid were interested in replacing ivory, those who developed the new fibres were interested in replacing another expensive material, silk.

Disadvantages

However, celluloid still tended to yellow and crack over time, and it had another, more dangerous defect: it burned easily and spectacularly, unsurprising given that mixtures of nitric acid and cellulose are also used to synthesize smokeless powder.

Rayon

Rayon is the oldest commercial man-made fibre. The US trade Commission defines rayon as "manmade textile fibres and filaments composed of regenerated cellulose". The process of making viscose was discovered by CF cross and EJ bevan in 1891. The process used to make viscose can either be a continuous or batch process. The batch process is flexible in producing a wide variety of rayons having broad versatility. Rayon's versatility is the result of the fibre being chemically and structurally engineered by making use of the properties of cellulose from which it is made. However, it is somewhat difficult to control uniformity between batches and it also requires high labor involvement. The continuous process is the main method for producing rayon. Three methods of production lead to distinctly different types of rayon fibres: viscose rayon, cuprammonium rayon and saponified cellulose acetate. Of the methods mentioned, the viscose method is relatively inexpensive and of particular significance in the production of non woven fabrics.

Structure of Rayon

In regenerated celluloses, the unit cell structure is an allotropic modification of cellulose (I), designated as cellulose (II), other allotropic modifications are also known as cellulose (III) and cellulose (IV). The structure of cellulose derivatives could be represented by a continuous range of states of local molecular order rather than definite polymorphic forms of cellulose which depend on the conditions by which the fibre is made. Rayon fibre properties will depend on:

- How cellulose molecules are arranged and held together.
- The average size and size distribution of the molecules.

Properties of Rayon

Variations during spinning of viscose or during drawing of filaments provide a wide variety of fibres with a wide variety of properties. These include:

- Fibers with thickness of 1.7 to 5.0 dtex, particularly those between 1.7 and 3.3 dtex, dominate large scale production.
- Tenacity ranges between 2.0 to 2.6 g/den when dry and 1.0 to 1.5 g/den when wet.
- Wet strength of the fibre is of importance during its manufacturing and also in subsequent usage. Modifications in the production process have led to the problem of low wet strength being overcome.
- Dry and wet tenacities extend over a range depending on the degree of polymerization and crystallinity. The higher the crystallinity and orientation of rayon, the lower is the drop in tenacity upon wetting.
- Percentage elongation-at-break seems to vary from 10 to 30% dry and 15 to 40% wet. Elongation-at-break is seen to decrease with an increase in the degree of crystallinity and orientation of rayon.
- Thermal properties: Viscose rayon loses strength above 149°C; chars and decomposes at 177 to 204°C. It does not melt or stick at elevated temperatures.
- *Chemical properties:* Hot dilute acids attack rayon, whereas bases do not seem to significantly attack rayon. Rayon is attacked by bleaches at very high concentrations and by mildew under severe hot and moist conditions. Prolonged exposure to sunlight causes loss of strength because of degradation of cellulose chains.
- Abrasion resistance is fair and rayon resists pill formation. Rayon has both poor crease recovery and crease retention.

Rayon Fibre Characteristics

- Highly absorbent
- Soft and comfortable
- Easy to dye
- Drapes well

The drawing process applied in spinning may be adjusted to produce rayon fibres of extra strength and reduced elongation. Such fibres are designated as high tenacity rayons, which have about twice the strength and two-third of the stretch of regular rayon. An intermediate grade, known as medium tenacity rayon, is also made. Its strength and stretch characteristics fall midway between those of high tenacity and regular rayon.

Some Major Rayon Fibre Uses

- *Apparel:* Accessories, blouses, dresses, jackets, lingerie, linings, millinery, slacks, sportshirts, sportswear, suits, ties, work clothes.
- *Home furnishings:* Bedspreads, blankets, curtains, draperies, sheets, slipcovers, tablecloths, upholstery.
- *Industrial uses:* Industrial products, medical surgical products, nonwoven products, tire cord.
- *Other uses:* Feminine hygiene products.

Advantages of Rayon

- High sheen
- Softer
- Relatively heat resistant
- Less elasticity then polyester

Disadvantages of Rayon

- Not colorfast
- Not as strong as polyester
- Less durable than polyester

2. Polyethylene

Uses   : Thermoplastics, fibres
Monomer   : Ethylene

Polymerization   : Free radical chain polymerization,
                       Ziegler-Natta polymerization, metall-
                       ocene catalysis polymerization
Morphology   : Highly crystalline (linear), highly
                       amorphous (branched)
Melting temperature : 137°C
Glass transition   : −130 to −80°C
temperature

Polyethylene (PE): Polyethylene is the most commonly used plastic in the world with annual consumption rates exceeding 50 billion pounds per year. The term polyethylene describes a huge family of resins obtained by polymerizing ethylene gas, $H_2C=CH_2$, and it is by far the largest volume commercial polymer. For such a versatile material, it has a very simple structure, the simplest of all commercial polymers. A molecule of polyethylene is nothing more than a long chain of carbon atoms, with two hydrogen atoms attached to each carbon atom.

This thermoplastic is available in a range of flexibilities and other properties depending on the production process, with high density materials being the most rigid. Polyethylene can be formed by a wide variety of thermoplastic processing methods and is particularly useful where moisture resistance and low cost are required. Low density polyethylene typically has a density value ranging from 0.91 to 0.925 g/cm³, linear low density polyethylene is in the range of 0.918 to 0.94 g/cm³, while high density polyethylene ranges from 0.935 to 0.96 g/cm³ and above.

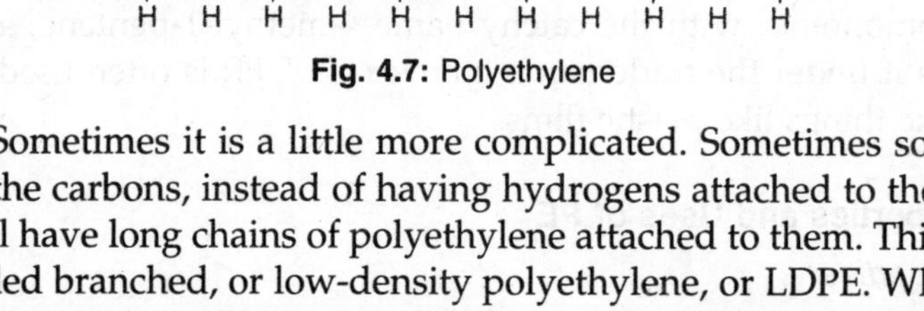

Fig. 4.7: Polyethylene

Sometimes it is a little more complicated. Sometimes some of the carbons, instead of having hydrogens attached to them, will have long chains of polyethylene attached to them. This is called branched, or low-density polyethylene, or LDPE. When there is no branching, it is called linear polyethylene, or HDPE. Linear polyethylene is much stronger than branched polyethylene, but branched polyethylene is cheaper and easier to make.

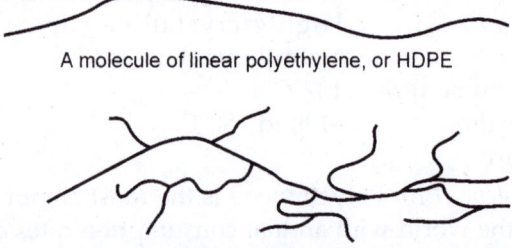

A molecule of linear polyethylene, or HDPE

A molecule of branched polyethylene, or LDPE

Fig. 4.8: Molecules of HDPE and LDPE

Linear polyethylene is normally produced with molecular weights in the range of 200,000 to 500,000, but it can be made even higher. Polyethylene with molecular weights of three to six million is referred to as ultra-high molecular weight polyethylene, or UHMWPE. UHMWPE can be used to make fibres which are so strong they replaced Kevlar for use in bullet proof vests. Large sheets of it can be used instead of ice for skating rinks.

Branched polyethylene is often made by free radical vinyl polymerization. Linear polyethylene is made by a more complicated procedure called Ziegler-Natta polymerization. UHMWPE is made using metallocene catalysis polymerization.

But Ziegler-Natta polymerization can be used to make LDPE, too. By copolymerizing ethylene monomer with a alkyl-branched comonomer such as one gets a copolymer which has short hydrocarbon branches. Copolymers like this are called linear low-density polyethylene, or LLDPE. BP produces LLDPE using a comonomer with the catchy name 4-methyl-1-pentene, and sells it under the trade name Innovex. LLDPE is often used to make things like plastic films.

Properties and Uses of PE

Properties

Polyethylene is cheap, flexible, durable and chemically resistant. It is light, versatile synthetic resin made from the polymerization of ethylene. While PE has low resistance to chemical attack, it was found later that a PE container could be made much more robust by exposing it to fluorine gas, which modified the surface layer of the container into the much tougher "polyfluoroethylene". Polyethylene is resistant to concentrated acids, alkalies and many organic solvents.

General Uses

Polyethylene is a member of the important family of polyolefin resins. It is the most widely used plastic in the world, being made into products ranging from clear food wrap and shopping bags to detergent bottles and automobile fuel tanks. It can also be slit or spun into synthetic fibres or modified to take on the elastic properties of a rubber.

Polyethylene is probably the polymer we see most in daily life. Polyethylene is the most popular plastic in the world. This is the polymer that makes grocery bags, shampoo bottles, children's toys, and even bullet proof vests. LLDPE is often used to make things like plastic films. UHMWPE can be used to make fibres which are so strong they replaced Kevlar for use in bullet proof vests. Large sheets of it can be used instead of ice for skating rinks.

PE Generics

- HDPE
- LDPE
- LLDPE
- EVA
- PE, unspecified
- MDPE
- HDPE, HMW
- XLPE
- LMDPE, etc.

Advantages of PE

- Processability, good
- Food contact acceptable
- Antioxidant
- ESCR, high (stress crack resist)

- Copolymer
- Density, low–impact resistance, good
- Density, high–toughness, good.

Disadvantages of PE

- High thermal expansion
- Poor weathering resistance
- Subject to stress cracking
- Difficult to bond
- Flammable
- Poor temperature capability
- Low strength/stiffness.

Typical PE Applications

- Film
- Packaging
- Bags
- Piping
- Containers
- Industrial applications
- Packaging, food
- Laminates
- Master batch.

Major Polyethylene Compounds

Low-density polyethylene: LDPE is similar to HDPE but its less molecular structure renders it less chemically resistant. It is more translucent and is used mainly for squeeze applications. The price is usually higher than HDPE for the same type of container.

LDPE is prepared from gaseous ethylene under very high pressures and high temperatures in the presence of oxide initiators. These processes yield a polymer structure with both long and short branches. Because the branches prevent the polyethylene molecules from packing closely together in hard, stiff, crystalline arrangements, LDPE is a very flexible material. Its melting point is approximately 110°C (230°F).

Uses: Principal uses are in packaging film, trash and plastic bags, agricultural mulch, wire and cable insulation, squeeze bottles, toys, and house wares.

Very low density polyethylene (VLDPE): Densities between 0.890 and 0.915. Applications include disposable gloves, shrink packages, vacuum cleaner hoses, tuning, bottles, shrink wrap, diaper film liners and other health care products.

Linear low density polyethylene (LLDPE): The structure has a linear backbone, but it has short, uniform branches that, like the longer branches of LDPE, prevent the polymer chains from packing closely together. Overall, LLDPE has similar properties to LDPE and competes for the same markets. Densities between 0.916 and 0.930.

The main advantages of LLDPE are that the polymerization conditions are less energy-intensive and that the polymer's properties may be altered by varying the type and amount of its chemical ingredients. Properties include good flex life, low warpage, and improved stress-crack resistance.

Uses: Applications include films for ice, trash, garment, and produce bags.

High density polyethylene (HDPE): A linear polymer, High Density Polyethylene (HDPE) is prepared from ethylene by a catalytic process. The absence of branching results in a more closely packed structure with a higher density and somewhat higher chemical resistance than LDPE. High Density Polyethylene is also somewhat harder and more opaque and it can withstand rather higher temperatures (120°C for short periods, 110°C continuously). High density polyethylene lends itself particularly well to blow molding.

HDPE is extremely economical and usually approved by the FDA for food products. It has a good moisture barrier and is impact resistant. HDPE is translucent in its natural state, but may have colorant added. It is compatible with a wide range of products including acids but not solvents. When flame treated it is an excellent choice for silk-screening. It cannot stand up to hot fill of over about 160°C.

Products include blow-molded bottles for milk and household cleaners; blow-extruded grocery bags, construction film, and agricultural mulch; and injection-molded pails, caps, appliance housings, and toys.

Polyethylene 300 (HDPE – High Density Polyethylene) is a rigid material which is available in large sheets for general use in plant engineering, tank construction and the wastewater industry, where all round chemical resistance and weather ability are required. This is a good food grade general purpose polyethylene, making it a great choice for use in commercial kitchens.

General uses: HDPE is used more often to make containers, plumbing, and automotive fittings.

Features and Benefits of HDPE

- Excellent abrasion resistance.
- Very low co-efficient of friction.
- Very high surface release properties.
- High chemical resistance.
- Excellent impact resistance.
- Very good damping properties.
- Good wear resistant material.
- Cheaper than nylon.
- Weldable (suitable for fabrication).
- Light weight (easy to handle without special equipment).
- Physiologically inert (approved for food applications).
- Electrical insulation.
- Weatherproof
- Chemical resistance - resists corrosive chemicals (e.g. Sulphuric acid, caustic soda).
- Withstands temperatures of −50 to +80°C

Applications of HDPE

- Componentry in direct contact with foodstuffs.
- Cutting and chopping boards.
- Commercial cutting boards in abattoirs, meat works and fish markets.
- Spacers between steel plates.
- Washers
- Butchers preparation tables.
- Poultry processing plants

High molecular weight polyethylene (HMWPE): Polyethylene 500 (HMWPE - High Molecular Weight Polyethylene) has excellent mechanical properties, rigidity and creep resistance and these qualities make this polyethylene ideal for use in the food industry as cutting and chopping boards, underlays in food preparation and machined parts.

Features and Benefits of HMWPE

- Mechanical parts
- Light weight
- Physiologically inert (approved for food and beverage applications)
- Electrical insulation
- Weatherproof
- Chemical resistance (resists corrosive chemicals)
- Excellent mechanical properties
- Rigidity
- Creep resistance
- Withstands temperatures of −100 to +80°C.

Applications for HMWPE

- Machined parts
- Guides and fixtures
- Gears and rollers
- Cutting and chopping boards
- Vacuum table
- Food and beverage industry.

Ultra High Molecular Weight Polyethylene (UHMWPE)

Linear polyethylene can be produced in ultra high molecular weight versions, with molecular weights of 3,000,000 to 6,000,000 atomic units, as opposed to 500,000 atomic units for HDPE. These polymers can be spun into fibres and then drawn, or stretched, into a highly crystalline state, resulting in high stiffness and a tensile strength many times that of steel. Yarns made from these fibres are woven into bulletproof vests.

Polyethylene 7000 (UHMWPE – Ultra High Molecular Weight Polyethylene) is formulated for optimum sliding characteristics and resistance to wear and abrasion. This polyethylene is virtually unbreakable and reduces friction, wear, clogging and noise when compared with metal. This plastic product never needs lubrication. Problems with cohesive, wet or sticky materials can be overcome with the use of UHMWPE in industrial situations ranging from fine foods to the mining industry. Polyethylene 7000 is rated better than carbon steel for sliding abrasion applications and is another of our plastic products which comes under the umbrella of engineering plastics.

Properties and Benefits of UHMWPE

- Impact strength
- Very high dielectric strength
- Chemical resistant (will not corrode)
- Abrasion resistant
- Low coefficient of friction
- No lubrication required
- Electrical insulation
- Weatherproof
- Light weight
- Approved for the food and beverage industries.

Applications for UHMWPE

- Mechanical transmission support products
- Mechanical bearing parts
- Food machine equipment
- Flow promotion
- Packaging
- Assembly
- Chemical production
- Conveying
- Elevating
- Chain wear guide strip/profiles
- Slides on boat trailers (black)
- Bulk storage
- Materials handling
- Liners for tanks and bins/hoppers/chutes

- Withstands temperatures of − 260 to + 90°C
- Trucking industry (truck trays)

Ethylene copolymers: Ethylene can be copolymerized with a number of other compounds.

Ethylene-ethyl acrylate (EEA): Properties range from rubbery to tough ethylene-like properties. Applications include hot melt adhesives, shrink wrap, produce bags, bag-in-box products, and wire coating.

Ethylene-methyl acrylate (EMA): Produced by addition of methyl acrylate monomer (40% by weight)with ethylene gas. Tough, thermally stable olefin with good elastomeric characteristics. Applications include food packaging, disposable medical gloves, heat-sealable layers, and coating for composite packaging.

Ethylene-vinyl acetate copolymer (EVA): Ethylene-vinyl acetate copolymer (EVA), for instance, is produced by the copolymerization of ethylene and vinyl acetate under pressure, using free-radical catalysts. Many different grades are manufactured, with the vinyl acetate content varying from 5 to 50% by weight.

Properties and use

EVA copolymers are more permeable to gases and moisture than polyethylene, but they are less crystalline and more transparent, and they exhibit better oil and grease resistance. Ethylene vinyl acetate has low-temperature flexibility and is used in tough films and as a component of multiplayer constructions for low-temperature heat sealing. Principal uses are in packaging film, adhesives, toys, tubing, gaskets, wire coatings, drum liners, and carpet backing. The ethylene-acrylic acid and ethylene-methacrylic acid ionomers are transparent, semicrystalline, and impervious to moisture. They are employed in automotive parts, packaging film, footwear, surface coatings, and carpet backing. One prominent ethylene-methacrylic acid copolymer is Surlyn, which is made into hard, tough, abrasion-resistant golf-ball covers. Other important ethylene copolymers are the ethylene-propylene copolymers.

Cross-linked Polyethylene

Cross-linked polyethylene, commonly abbreviated PEX or XLPE, is a form of polyethylene with cross-links. It is formed into tubing, and is used predominantly in hydronic radiant heating systems, domestic water piping and insulation for high tension (high voltage) electrical cables. It is also used for natural gas and offshore oil applications, chemical transportation, and transportation of sewage and slurries. Recently, it has become a viable alternative to polyvinyl chloride (PVC), chlorinated polyvinyl chloride (CPVC) or copper pipe for use as residential water pipes.

Uses

PEX has become a contender for use in residential water
· plumbing because of its flexibility. It can be bent into a wide-radius turn if space permits, or by using elbow; PVC, CPVC and copper all require elbow joints.

· PEX Tubing is widely used to replace copper in plumbing applications. Typically, red PEX tubing is used for hot water while blue PEX tubing is used for cold water.

· The advantageous properties of PEX also make it a candidate for progressive replacement of metal and thermoplastic pipes, especially in long-life applications.

3. Poly (ethylene terephthalate)

Uses	: Thermoplastics, fibres
Monomer	: Ethylene glycol and dimethyl terephthalate
Polymerization	: Transesterification
Morphology	: Highly crystalline
Melting temperature	: 265°C
Glass transition temperature	: 74°C

Polyesters are the polymers, in the form of fibres, that were used back in the seventies to make all that wonderful disco clothing, the kind you see being modeled on the right.

But since then, the nations of the world have striven to develop more tasteful uses for polyesters, like those nifty shatterproof plastic bottles that hold your favourite refreshing beverages, polyesters can be both plastics and fibres. Another place you find polyester is in balloons. Not the cheap ones that you use for water balloons, those are made of natural rubber.

Polyesters have hydrocarbon backbones which contain ester linkages, hence the name.

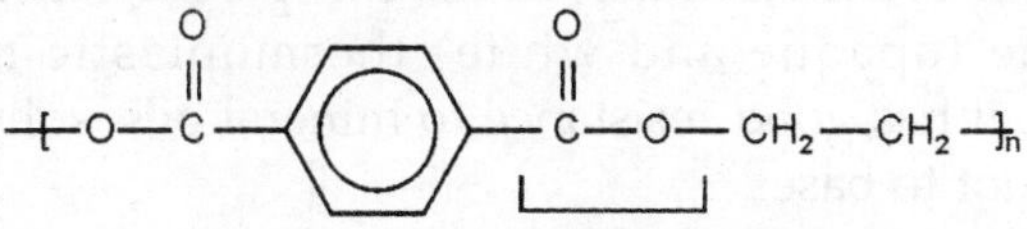

Fig. 4.9: Structure of poly (ethylene terephthalate)

The structure in the picture is called poly (ethylene terephthalate), or PET for short, because it is made up of ethylene groups and terephthalate groups.

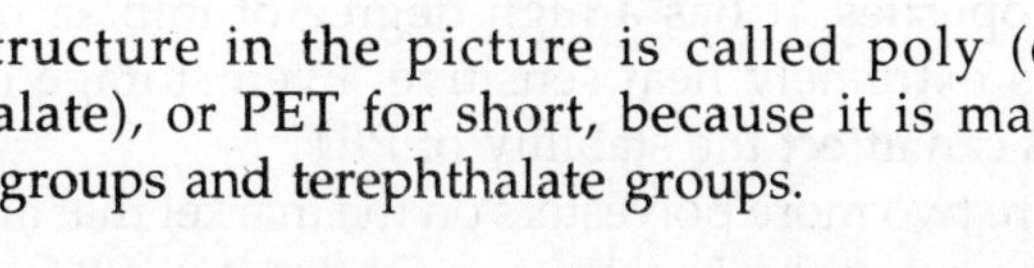

Fig. 4.10: Structure of polyethylene terephthalate

PET has too low a glass transition temperature, that is the temperature at which the PET becomes soft. Now reusing a soft drink bottle requires that the bottle be sterilized before it is used again. This means washing it at really high temperatures, temperatures too high for PET. Filling a jar with jelly is also carried out at high temperatures. There is a new kind of polyester that is just the thing needed for jelly jars and returnable bottles. It is poly (ethylene naphthalate), or PEN. PEN has a higher glass transition temperature than PET. That's the temperature at which a polymer gets soft. The glass transition temperature of PEN is high enough so that it can withstand the heat of both sterilizing bottle washing and hot strawberry jelly.

Properties and Uses

The semi-crystalline PET has good strength, ductility, stiffness and hardness. The amorphous PET has better ductility but less stiffness and hardness.

PET (polyethylene terephthalate) PET has good barrier properties against oxygen and carbon dioxide. Therefore, it is utilized in bottles for mineral water. Other applications include food trays for oven use, roasting bags, audio/video tapes as well as mechanical components.

PET exists both as an amorphous (transparent) and as a semi-crystalline (opaque and white) thermoplastic material. Generally, it has good resistance to mineral oils, solvents and acids but not to bases.

PET transparent films. Crystal clear bottles for soft drinks have excellent clarity and very good alcohol and essential oil barrier properties. It has a high degree of impact resistance but PET is extremely heat sensitive. Even storage of empty containers can affect the stability of PET.

There are two more polyesters on the market that are related to PET. There is poly (butylene terephthalate) (PBT) and poly (trimethylene terephthalate). They are usually used for the same type of things as PET, but in some cases these perform better. These are also used in food packaging and ORS packaging.

Polyethylene Products

Polyethylene is available in several grades. All the grades have similar properties and perform along similar lines, but as the grades of these plastic products increase, so does the quality, performance and of course the price, as is the case with most plastic products and their grades. When the molecular weight increases in the polyethylene family, their characteristics also increase and enhanced performance is achieved. All the polyethylenes are lightweight and have good chemical resistance and do not absorb water. Polyethylenes are used where componentry is required to be in direct contact with food stuffs and also is made into parts subject to high impact stresses. Some of the different grades of polyethylene are listed below with a few of their specific applications and benefits.

Disadvantages

Very susceptible to heat degradation. Excessive shear heat should be avoided – therefore low screw speed and back pressure required. For optimum clarity, mould temperature should be kept between 10–50°C (50–120°F).

4. Polypropylene

Uses	: Thermoplastics, fibres, thermoplastic elastomers.
Monomer	: Propylene
Polymerization	: Ziegler-Natta polymerization, metallocene catalysis polymerization.
Morphology	: Highly crystalline (isotactic), highly amorphous (atactic).
Melting temperature	: 174°C (100% isotactic).
Glass transition temperature	: –17°C

Prior to 1954 most attempts to produce plastics from polyolefins had little commercial success. PP invented in 1955 by Italian Scientist FJ Natta by addition reaction of propylene gas with a stereospecific catalyst titanium trichloride. Polypropylene is one of those rather versatile polymers out there. It serves double duty, both as a plastic and as a fibre.

As a plastic it is used to make things like dishwasher-safe food containers. It can do this because it does not melt below 160°C, or 320°F. Polyethylene, a more common plastic, will anneal at around 100°C, which means that polyethylene dishes will warp in the dishwasher.

As a fibre, polypropylene is used to make indoor-outdoor carpeting, the kind that you always find around swimming pools and miniature golf courses. It works well for outdoor carpet because it is easy to make colored polypropylene, and because polypropylene does not absorb water, like nylon does. Structurally, it is a vinyl polymer, and is similar to polyethylene, only that on every other carbon atom in the backbone chain

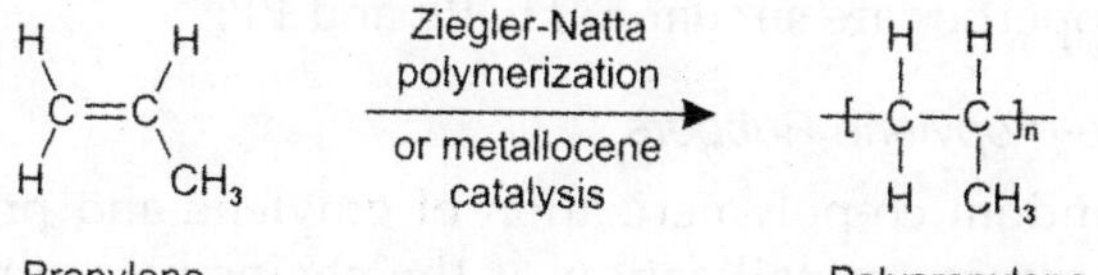

Fig. 4.11: Synthesis of polypropylene

has a methyl group attached to it. Polypropylene can be made from the monomer propylene by Ziegler-Natta polymerization and by metallocene catalysis polymerization.

Most polypropylene we use is isotactic. This means that all the methyl groups are on the same side of the chain, like this:

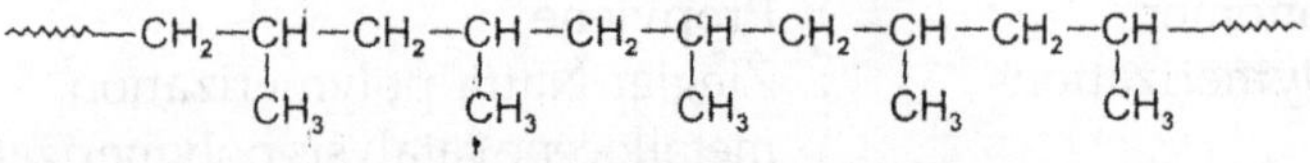

$$\text{~~~—CH}_2\text{—CH—CH}_2\text{—CH—CH}_2\text{—CH—CH}_2\text{—CH—CH}_2\text{—CH—~~~}$$
$$\quad\quad\quad\text{CH}_3\quad\quad\text{CH}_3\quad\quad\text{CH}_3\quad\quad\text{CH}_3\quad\quad\text{CH}_3$$

Fig. 4.12: Isotactic polypropylene

But sometimes atactic polypropylene is also used. Atactic means that the methyl groups are placed randomly on both sides of the chain like this:

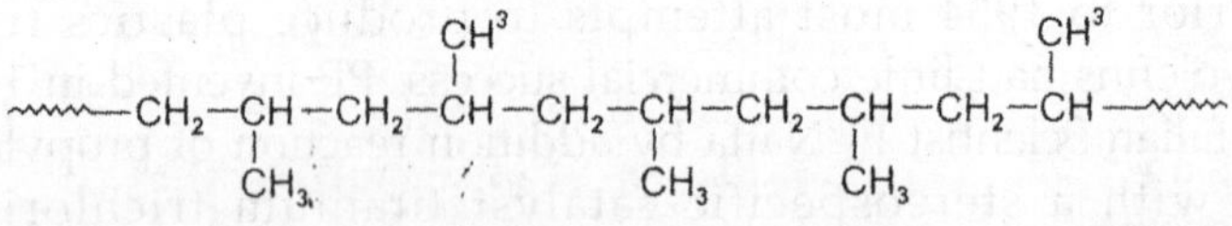

$$\quad\quad\quad\quad\quad\quad\text{CH}^3\quad\quad\quad\quad\quad\quad\quad\quad\text{CH}^3$$
$$\text{~~~—CH}_2\text{—CH—CH}_2\text{—CH—CH}_2\text{—CH—CH}_2\text{—CH—CH}_2\text{—CH—~~~}$$
$$\quad\quad\quad\text{CH}_3\quad\quad\quad\quad\quad\text{CH}_3\quad\quad\text{CH}_3$$

Fig. 4.13: Atactic polypropylene

Most kinds of rubber have to be crosslinked to give them strength, but not polypropylene elastomers. Elastomeric polypropylene, as this copolymer is called, is a kind of thermoplastic elastomer.

Copolymers of Polypropylene

Ethylene-propylene Copolymers

Small amount of PP can lower crystallinity of linear HDPE.

Polyallomers (block copolymers)

- Blocks of PE and PP polymers allows crystallization to take place.
- Properties are similar to HDPE and PP.

Ethylene-propylene Rubbers

- Random co-polymerization of ethylene and propylene prevents crystallization of the chains by suppressing regularity of molecules.

- Resulting polymers are amorphous having low Tg (between –110°C and –20°C depending on % of PE and PP).
- Polymers are rubbery at room temperature.
- Conventional vulcanization allows for use as commercial rubber, thermoplastic rubbers, TPR.

Disadvantages

- High thermal expansion
- UV degradation
- Poor weathering resistance
- Subject to attack by chlorinated solvents and aromatics
- Difficulty to bond or paint
- Oxidizes readily
- Flammable

One of the main drawbacks to polypropylene is the product has a resistance to the addition of paint or ink once the cooling process has completed. This can make the raw material more difficult to work with, especially in applications where the polypropylene is being used to create household products, such as shelf organizers. Manufacturers have to be very careful to add the right amount of color at just the right time in the cooling process, or the material will be much more susceptible to cracking.

When it comes to the use of polypropylene in carpeting and upholstery, textile manufacturers have to be constantly aware of the temperature of the machinery while the fibre is going through the process. If the fibre becomes too hot, there is a tendency to break and jam on the rollers of many types of textile machinery. Carding, spinning, twisting, and warping machinery must be watched closely to ensure the refined fibre does not jam and begin to collect around a roller. When this happens, the material has a tendency to melt and harden into a substance that is extremely difficult to chip away.

The finished product must also be given extra care as well. Polypropylene does have a tendency to shrink after being woven into a pattern or design. Allowing for the average rate of shrinkage of the polymer makes it possible for manufacturers to accurately judge the amount of polypropylene yarn or woven sheets of material to purchase. When this is done, it is much easier to calculate the correct amount of trimming that can be done and still produce a product with the proper dimensions.

Abd pointed out such flaws as its notch sensitivity in impact properties, which is a tendency to crack or split easily in areas with small radii. PP's clarity is poorer than amorphous resins such as polystyrene, polycarbonate or PET. Its chemical resistance also makes bonding difficult as well as decorating with paint, labels and ink. A low-melt viscosity yields a narrow processing window for thermoforming and blow molding and it tends to warp and shrink more than most other materials due to high crystallinity.

Properties of Polypropylene

Polypropylene has an excellent balance of mechanical properties, melt flow, colour stability and moisture barrier properties.

PP's proportion mixes thermal, chemical and electrical properties with moderate strength. Because it has such a hard, high-gloss surface, it is ideally suited to environments where there is concern for bacteria build-up or build-up that can interfere with flow. It is these properties that make it appealing for industries such as food, medical and beauty aids.

The single property where PP outperforms almost all other materials is chemical resistance. The saturated olefinic chains yield resistance to most oils and solvents, as well as water-based chemicals, soaps, and moderate acids and bases. Few other materials with the strength properties of PP, and certainly none in the same price range, can match the chemical resistance of PP.

The material's chemical resistance also defends against aqueous, salts or alkaline solutions.

Advantages of Polypropylene
- Low cost
- Excellent flexural strength
- Good impact strength
- Processable by all thermoplastic equipment
- Low coefficient of friction

- Excellent electrical insulation
- Good fatigue resistance
- Excellent moisture resistance
- Service temperature to 126°C
- Very good chemical resistance

PP features good insulating properties, but dielectric strength shows some degree of change at elevated temperatures. Excellent track, arc resistance and dielectric strength allow PP to be used extensively in electrical applications. It can also be modified to be conductive or antistatic.

As a homopolymer, PP can be used in temperatures ranging from 30°F to 210°F, depending on specific chemistry; copolymers in the range from –20°F to 180°F.
PP's higher melting point (174°C) as one of its advantages as compared to other thermoplastics such as ABS, polyethylene and polystyrene. Other benefits include: a lower cost per volume and lower specific gravity, and good fatigue resistance. PP is useful at a wide variety of molecular weights, to allow proper viscosity for blow molding and sheet extrusion, right up to high-speed injection molding.

PP's benefits, in injection molding, it produces high-quality parts at high speed and it is the only low-cost resin capable of producing living hinges. PP's low temperature impact strength is poor as is its resistance to UV.

Applications of Polypropylene

Polypropylene is commonly spun into fibres, injection molded, cast into thin films, extruded into sheet and profiles and blow molded. Polypropylene has a high tensile strength when the molecules are oriented, and relatively low melt strength; these are the primary requirements for fibre markets.

The combination of excellent chemical resistance, a good balance of physical properties and low cost makes PP an attractive material for automotive applications. With a melting point of 174°C, PP can be reinforced for use in underhood applications, where temperature resistance is crucial. These include air duct work and covers for batteries and other components.

PP's clarity, microwave and freezer properties, impact properties, and FDA-approved status for its widespread use in the food, medical and beauty aid industries. She cites such applications as trays, cups, lids, clamshell packaging, sterilization trays, single-dose medication and other product packaging.

What makes polypropylene unique is its potential to replace higher-priced, clear PVC and PETG applications.

One of the most overlooked applications for PP is thin film, which is often oriented or biaxially oriented. These films are used in items such as candy wrappers and cigarette package wrappers. The extreme chemical resistance of PP leads to another unique application – landfill liners and impoundment caps. Here, very thick extruded sheets are used to prevent landfill chemicals from leaching into the environment.

Other applications for molded PP include housewares, rigid packaging containers, toys, disposable medical syringes, video cassette cases, appliance housing/outdoor furniture and luggage. Non-woven applications include insulation wrap, disposable diapers, automotive interiors and medical textiles.

5. Poly (vinyl chloride)

Uses	: Thermoplastics
Monomer	: Vinyl chloride
Polymerization	: Free radical chain polymerization
Morphology	: Highly amorphous, ~11% crystallinity
Glass transition temperature	: ~84°C

PVC is a semi rigid material that has extremely good resistance to oils but is vulnerable to solvents. PVC is unstable at temperatures over 160 degrees and will distort. It has good drop impact resistance. PVC has side chains incorporating chlorine molecules, which form strong bonds.

Structurally, PVC is a vinyl polymer. It is similar to polyethylene, but on every other carbon in the backbone chain, one of the hydrogen atoms is replaced with a chlorine atom. It's produced by the free radical polymerization of vinyl chloride.

In other words PVC stands for "POLY VINYL CHLORIDE". It is a polymer of vinyl chloride (CH_2=CHCl). It is prepared by heating vinyl chloride at 60°C in the presence of hydrogen peroxide. Monomer is vinyl chloride.

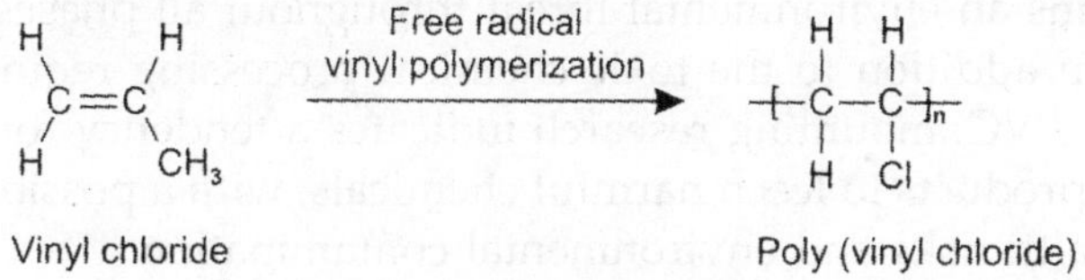

Fig. 4.14: Synthesis of PVC

Uses

Poly (vinyl chloride) is the plastic known at the hardware store as PVC. This is the PVC from which pipes are made, and PVC pipe is everywhere. The plumbing in your house is probably PVC pipe, unless it is an older house. PVC pipe is what rural high schools with small budgets use to make goal posts for their football fields. But there's more to PVC than just pipe. The "vinyl" siding used on houses is made of poly (vinyl chloride). Inside the house, PVC is used to make linoleum for the floor. In the seventies, PVC was often used to make vinyl car tops.

PVC is useful because it resists two things that hate each other: fire and water. Because of its water resistance it is used to make raincoats and shower curtains, and of course, water pipes. It has flame resistance, too, because it contains chlorine. When anybody try to burn PVC, chlorine atoms are released, and chlorine atoms inhibit combustion.

Polyvinyl chloride, better known as PVC or vinyl, is an inexpensive plastic so versatile it has become completely pervasive in modern society. The list of products made from polyvinyl chloride is exhaustive, ranging from phonograph records to drainage and potable piping, water bottles, cling film, credit cards and toys. More uses include window frames, rain gutters, wall paneling, doors, wallpapers, flooring, garden furniture, binders and even pens. Even imitation leather is a product of polyvinyl chloride. In fact, it's hard to turn anywhere without seeing some form of this plastic.

Disadvantages

In 1913, polyvinyl chloride became the first synthetic product ever patented. However, its diversity is now in question, as it comes from a highly toxic production industry and potentially remains an environmental threat throughout all phases of its life. In addition to the toxic chemical processing required to make PVC, mounting research indicates a tendency for some PVC products to leech harmful chemicals, with a possible link to health risks and environmental contamination.

Additionally, polyvinyl chloride is not biodegradable, a fact that manufacturers promote as a plus, while environmentalists count it among many of polyvinyl chloride's drawbacks. They point to the ever-growing massive amounts of discarded PVC products and shrinking landfills, and the potential for long-term leeching that could lead to ground water contamination. Polyvinyl chloride should not be burned, as it can release harmful gas, and recycling is difficult because of the diverse additives used in various products.

Though polyvinyl chloride products have been used without apparent problems to human health for many years, the concern is that growing toxic waste created by the process, possible leaching, and PVC's non-biodegradable status will eventually and inevitably lead to problems that could be catastrophic. The conservative trend is headed towards environmentally friendly, biodegradable alternatives. Among others, these include wood, paper, copper, steel, and clay. Chlorine-free plastics, such as polyethylene (PE), polypropylene (PP) and polyisobutylene, may also be preferred over PVC, although most of these are not biodegradable.

Advantages

PVC is the most widely used polymer for cables production in Europe. It is mainly dominant in the low voltage and some specialist applications. Telecommunication is also an important application for PVC. PVC cables have a number of benefits, such as:

- Good electrical and insulation properties over a wide temperature range.

- Inherent fire safety
- Excellent durability and long-life expectancy.
- Easy processing characteristics to achieve desired specification for end-products.
- Cost-effectiveness
- Recyclability - no cross-linking therefore the ability to be reprocessed back into cable applications, see further down.
- Compares favourably to alternative materials using LCA methodologies primarily due to lower usage of non-renewable resources, i.e. 43% derived from oil/gas and 57% derived from salt.
- Highly resistant to degradation by ultraviolet light.
- Cheap

Benefits of PVC

The use of PVC compounds in medical device manufacture during the last 50 years has demonstrated its great ability to satisfy the demanding requirements of the healthcare industry. Historically, PVC was introduced into flexible tubing and containers as a replacement for natural rubber and glass. It began to dominate the market when the need for single use pre-sterilised components became recognised.

PVC is the most widely used thermoplastic material in medical devices due to its:

Safety: Before medical devices can be used all the components must be fully understood from a toxicological point of view. Consequently all the materials used to make such components have to be thoroughly tested and assessed in the EU before being accepted. Experience based on all available knowledge from international environmental and healthcare authorities shows that PVC is safe. It is the best material existing today which optimises all performance and safety requirements at lowest cost.

Chemical stability: Material used in medical applications must be capable of accepting or conveying a variety of liquids without themselves undergoing any significant changes in composition or properties.

Biocompatibility: Whenever plastics are used in direct contact with the patient's tissue or blood, a high degree of compatibility is essential between the tissue/blood and the material. The significance of this property increases with time over which plastic is in contact with the tissue or blood. PVC is characterised by high biocompatibility, and this can be increased further by appropriate surface modification.

Clarity and transparency: Because of its physical properties, products made from PVC can be formulated with excellent transparency to allow for continual monitoring of fluid flow. If colour-coded application is needed, virtually any colour can be created.

Flexibility, durability and dependability: Not only does PVC offer the flexibility necessary for applications such as blood bags and IV containers, but can also be relied upon for its strength and durability, even under changing temperatures and conditions.

Sterilizability: The absence of sources of infection is a fundamental requirement in medical product applications. PVC products can be easily sterilized using such methods as steam, radiation or ethylene oxide.

Compatibility: PVC is compatible with virtually all pharmaceutical products in healthcare facilities today. It also has excellent water and chemical resistance, helping to keep solutions sterile.

Resistance to chemical stress cracking: PVC's resilience helps assure that medical products function consistently, for extended use, in demanding applications. Ease of processing PVC can easily be extruded to make IV tubing, thermoformed to make 'blister' packaging or blow moulding to make hollow rigid containers. This versatility is a major reason why PVC is the material of choice for medical product and packaging designers.

Low cost: The use of PVC plays a big role in containing rising healthcare costs. With PVC accounting for almost one-third of medical plastics currently in use, a switch to an alternative could cost the healthcare community hundreds of million of euro. No less important for the wide variety of applications of

PVC are its printability, its transparency or translucency as required by the application, its low tendency to form microvoids (significant for gloves) and its gloss. These qualities help to maintain the safety of patients and medical staff, while also limiting the cost of healthcare. Indeed, PVC is the best material to meets the performance, safety and cost criteria for a wide variety of medical applications today, especially those intended for single use. As a result, almost one third of all plastic-based disposable medical devices used in hospitals are made from PVC. In addition to its specific healthcare benefits, PVC's very versatile properties mean that it is used in a broad range of other applications. For example, within a hospital it may be used in water and drainage pipes and in fire resistant cabling in electrical and telecommunications equipment.

It also offers specific advantages in other healthcare applications such as:

- Flooring in operating theaters - PVC helps eliminate cross-infection due to seamless joints.
- PVC coated mattress covers - hygienic and easy to clean.
- Easily fabricated oxygen tents, relying on the welding characteristics of PVC combined with good transparency.
- Furniture covered by a PVC film is easy to clean and helps reducing the risks of infection.

PVC in Packaging

Several simple properties have made PVC invaluable as one of the key plastics used in modern day packaging to protect and preserve products. It is flexible, light, cost-effective, transparent, tough and safe. PVC requires less fuel to manufacture and transport when compared with other packaging materials such as metal or glass, and protects against contamination by helping to prevent the spread of germs during manufacture, distribution and display, particularly in the form of cling film. This prevents unnecessary wastage as it ensures food lasts longer. Approximately 500,000 tons of PVC is used in packaging across Europe each year. Its major packaging applications are rigid film (about 60%), flexible film such as cling film (11%) and closures (3%).

PVC provides a very versatile and cost-efficient material for the production of:

- Blisters and presentation trays
- Toiletries
- Toothpaste tubes
- Salad packs
- Bottle sleeving
- Mobile phone accessories
- Cash containers

Other Vinyl Polymers

Polyvinylidene chloride (PVDC, Saran TM): PVDC is an excellent barrier to moisture and gases. It is commonly used as a household wrap and as an added layer for many other resins.

Ethylene-vinyl alcohol (EVOH): Introduced in the mid-70s, EVOH is one of the best barriers to gases in the plastics industry. But EVOH loses these properties when exposed to moisture. Often used as an interior coating for juice containers and food packaging, EVOH is fully recyclable in its multi-layered form.

6. Polystyrene

Uses	: Thermoplastics
Monomer	: Styrene
Polymerization	: Free radical chain polymerization (atactic), Ziegler-Natta polymerization (syndiotactic)
Morphology	: Highly amorphous (atactic), highly crystalline (syndiotactic)
Melting temperature	: 270°C (syndiotactic)
Glass transition temperature	: 100°C

Polystyrene is an inexpensive and hard plastic, and probably only polyethylene is more common in your everyday life. PS has a wide range of properties including versatility, rigidity, clarity, and brittleness. It is a poor barrier to oxygen and water vapor. But the most unique property of PS is thermoforming, the ability to form and foam. Two familiar products made of foamed PS are coffee cups and fast food clam shell containers. Used in a variety of applications because of its low cost and easy ability to be processed, PS is often used in automobiles, insulation, disposables, packaging, toys, construction, electronics, and housewares. PS is also used for sour cream and cottage cheese containers, and horticultural products such as trays, packs, and flats.

Polystyrene is a vinyl polymer. Structurally, it is a long hydrocarbon chain, with a phenyl group attached to every other carbon atom. Polystyrene is produced by free radical vinyl polymerization, from the monomer styrene.

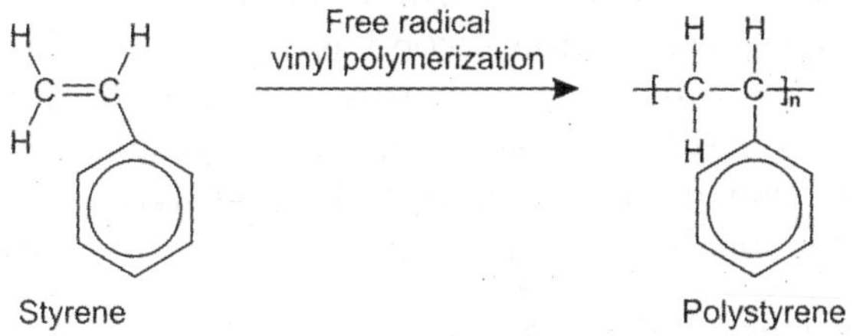

Styrene   Polystyrene

Fig. 4.15: Synthesis of polystyrene

Polystyrene is also a component of a type of hard rubber called poly(styrene-butadiene-styrene), or SBS rubber. SBS rubber is a thermoplastic elastomer.

The Polystyrene of the Future

There's a new kind of polystyrene out there, called syndiotactic polystyrene. It is different because the phenyl groups on the polymer chain are attached to alternating sides of the polymer backbone chain. "Normal" or atactic polystyrene has no order with regard to the side of the chain on which the phenyl groups are attached. Syndiotactic polystyrene is made by metallocene catalysis polymerization. Stronger, not as brittle, and capable of taking harder impacts without breaking than regular polystyrene. This material is called high-impact polystyrene, or HIPS for short.

Properties

PS has a wide range of properties including versatility, rigidity, clarity, and brittleness. It is a poor barrier to oxygen and water vapour. But the most unique property of PS is thermoforming, the ability to form and foam.

Advantages of Polystyrene

Using polystyrene insulation offers both heat loss reduction and water prevention. Polystyrene is an excellent insulator. Since a great deal of the cost of running a home is bound up with the costs of heating and cooling, polystyrene is a good choice for energy efficiency – and this also applies to building a conservatory. The material is moisture resistant, so it's unlikely that any water or water vapour will penetrate it. There are two places polystyrene might be use when building a conservatory. The first is within the dwarf wall at the base of the conservatory; the second is within the floor. Using polystyrene will keep moisture out and heat in. Once polystyrene has been treated, the advantages of lightness and superior insulation may well make polystyrene the perfect choice for insulating conservatory.

Disadvantages of Polystyrene

Its a poor barrier to oxygen and water vapour. Some forms of polystyrene can be expensive compared with other methods of insulation. They may also degrade when exposed to sunlight or ultra high temperatures, though this should be of little concern within a conservatory structure. However, the main disadvantage of using polystyrene for insulation is that it is flammable. In order to use it safely it must be treated with some sort of flame retardant, which sends the cost up again.
- Energy efficient
- Cost effective
- Flammable

Applications

Polystyrene is a "polymer of styrene". Polymers are large molecules consisting of adjoined identical molecules, and styrene is a colorless, oily liquid. When polystyrene is made, its structure is that of a rigid transparent thermoplastic, resembling stiff white foam. It is one of the most common types of plastic, and it can be found in the home, in the office, at industrial sites, and just about any other place you would find plastics. Businesses rely on polystyrene for a number of uses, including manufacturing, packaging, and construction.

Plastic forks, DVD cases, the outside housing of computers, radios, model cars, toys, rulers, and hair combs and the housings of things like hairdryers, and kitchen appliances are all made from hard polystyrene. It is found frequently in the food industry and used as a disposable transportation system to keep hot and cold foods at desired temperatures. Disposable and reusable items can be made from polystyrene as it is cheap but durable.

PS has a wide range of properties including versatility, rigidity, clarity, and brittleness.

It's a poor barrier to oxygen and water vapor. But the most unique property of PS is thermoforming, the ability to form and foam.

Two familiar products made of foamed PS are coffee cups and fast food clam shell containers. Used in a variety of applications because of its low cost and easy ability to be processed.

PS is often used in automobiles, insulation, disposables, packaging, toys, construction, electronics, and house wares. PS is also used for sour cream and cottage cheese containers, and horticultural products such as trays, packs, and flats.

The packaging industry is also a fan of polystyrene. Foam peanuts and other polystyrene packaging materials keep delicate items safely ensconced in boxes, and expanded polystyrene (EPS) is a popular item for both individuals and businesses. Electronics, glassware, and chemicals are all kept safe with EPS. Foam peanuts can be poured loosely into boxes to house any shape of item, or EPS can be easily formed by manufactures to fit products exactly and provide the safest possible packaging.

Polystyrene is also found in the building business. Polystyrene block is used as an energy efficient means for constructing both homes and businesses. Polystyrene block form construction is touted as providing homes with even temperatures and fewer drafts. This type of construction also reduces noise, heating and cooling bills, and general maintenance. Durability and strength is also offered by this type of block form construction. The polystyrene is used in conjunction with reinforced concrete and is therefore a winner in the battle against weather calamities.

Whatever the industry, polystyrene is likely to show up in at least some capacity. It is durability, range of hardness and flexibility, as well as it is low cost make it a popular material for a number of projects. As an insulator, protector, and product with the ability to conform to any shape, it is hard to beat as a universal manufacturing material, and it will likely be found in a full range of industries for years to come.

7. Poly (methyl methacrylate)

Uses : Thermoplastics
Monomer : Methyl methacrylate
Polymerization : Free radical vinyl polymeri-
zation
Morphology : Amorphous
Glass transition temperature : 120°C

Poly (methyl methacrylate), which lazy scientists call PMMA, it is clear and colourless polymer used extensively for optical applications. It is available commercially in both pellet and sheet form. Outstanding properties include weatherability and scratch resistance. The most serious deficiencies are low impact strength and poor chemical resistance.

It is a clear plastic, used as a shatterproof replacement for glass. The barrier at the ice rink, which keeps hockey pucks from flying in the faces of fans, is made of PMMA. The chemical company Rohm and Haas makes windows out of it and calls it Plexiglas. Ineos Acrylics also makes it and calls it Lucite. Lucite is used to make the surfaces of hot tubs, sinks, and the ever popular one piece bathtub and shower units, among other things.

When it comes to making windows, PMMA has another advantage over glass. PMMA is more transparent than glass. When glass windows are made too thick, they become difficult to see through. But PMMA windows can be made as much as 13 inches (33 cm) thick, and they are still perfectly transparent. This makes PMMA a wonderful material for making large aquariums, whose windows must be thick in order to contain the high pressure millions of gallons of water.

PMMA is more than just plastic and paint. Often lubricating oils and hydraulic fluids tend to get really viscous and even gummy when they get really cold. This is a real pain when you are trying to operate heavy equipment in really cold weather. But when a little bit PMMA is dissolved in these oils and fluids, they do not get viscous in the cold, and machines can be operated down to –100°C (–150°F), that is, presuming the rest of the machine can take that kind of cold.

PMMA is a vinyl polymer, made by free radical vinyl

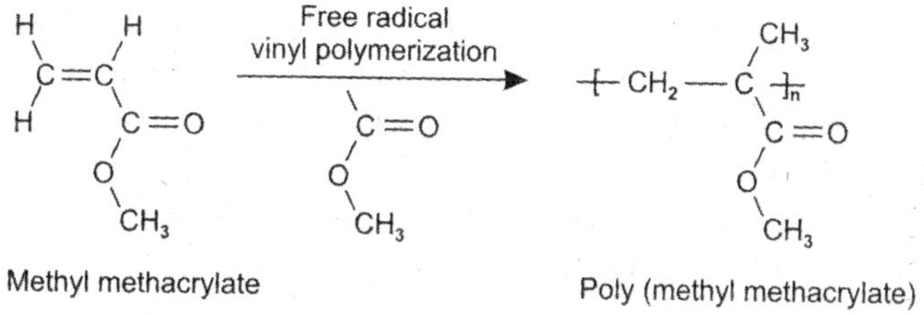

Methyl methacrylate   Poly (methyl methacrylate)

Fig. 4.16: Synthesis of poly (methyl methacrylate)

polymerization from the monomer methyl methacrylate.

PMMA is a member of a family of polymers which chemists call acrylates, but the rest of the world calls acrylics.

Properties

- Hard
- Rigid
- Transparent (very clear to see through)
- Softening point at 120°C
- Tougher than polystyrene but less tough than abs (acrylobutylstyrene) polymer.
- Absorbs very little visible light but there is a 4% reflection at each polymer-air interface for normal incident light.
- PMMA is a polar material and has a rather high dielectric constant and power factor.
- A good electrical insulator at low frequencies but less satisfactory at higher frequencies.
- Good water resistance.
- PMMA prepared by free radical polymerization is amorphous and is therefore soluble in solvents with

similar solubility parameters such as benzene, toluene, chloroform, methylene chloride, esters, ethyl acetate, and amyl acetate.

- PMMA has good resistance to alkalis (sodium hydroxide, etc.), aqueous inorganic salts (the pacific ocean) and dilute acids.
- PMMA has a better resistance to hydrolysis than PMA probably by virtue of the shielding of the methyl group.
- PMMA's outstanding good outdoor weather resistance is remarkably superior to other thermoplastics.
- When heated about 200°C, decomposition becomes appreciable and at 350 – 450°C, a nearly quantitative yield of monomer is readily obtained. Thus, the recovery of monomer from scrap is feasible.
- Because it is a thermoplastic, it can be molten and molded (at 100 to 150°C) into anything we want.

Advantages

Outstanding weathering and resistance to UV radiation. Transparent. High gloss and hardness. Good rigidity. Dimensionally stable. Good abrasion resistance – surface scratches can be polished out. PMMA has another advantage over glass. PMMA is more transparent than glass. Another polymer used as an unbreakable glass substitute is polycarbonate. But PMMA is cheaper.

Disadvantages

Not a tough material in comparison with engineering plastics, notch sensitive and generally brittle. Although not attacked by alcohol alone, alcohol with carbon tetrachloride and ether will cause swelling. Dissolved by most aromatic and chlorinated hydrocarbons. Water absorption is low but can have a considerable effect on dimensions and a lesser one on mechanical properties.

Applications

It is used in the formation of Sinks, baths, knobs and batons. Displays and signs. Aircraft glazing, technical models, tap tops and accessories. Automotive rear light housings, automotive components such as badges, steering wheel insignia and fascia panels.

Plastic Optical Fibre abbreviated POF, typically uses PMMA as the core material, and fluorinated polymers for the clad material. In large-diameter fibres, 96% of the cross-section is the core that allows the transmission of light.

It is being focused on for the following fields in particular:
- Digital home appliance interfaces
- Home networks
- Car networks
- Illuminations

Non-textile Applications

– Sheets
– Glass replacement

8. Polycarbonate of Bisphenol

Uses   : Compact discs, lightweight eye glasses, shatterproof glass
Monomer   : Bisphenol A
Polymerization   : Interfacial polymerization
Morphology   : Amorphous
Glass transition temperature : 150°C

Polycarbonate, or specifically polycarbonate of bisphenol A, is a clear plastic used to make shatterproof windows, lightweight eyeglass lenses, and such. General Electric makes this stuff and sells it as Lexan.

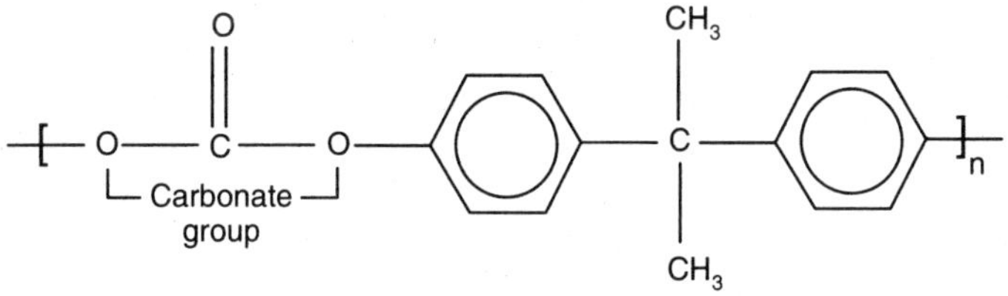

Fig. 4.17: Polycarbonate

Polycarbonate is a versatile, tough plastic used for a variety of applications, from bulletproof windows to compact disks (CDs).

Polycarbonates are a particular group of thermoplastic polymers. They are easily worked, moulded, and thermoformed; as such, these plastics are very widely used in the modern chemical industry. Their interesting features (temperature resistance, impact resistance and optical properties) position them between commodity plastics and engineering plastics.

Polycarbonates received their name because they are polymers having functional groups linked together by carbonate groups (-O-(C=O)-O-) in a long molecular chain. Also carbon monoxide was used as a C1-synthon on an industrial scale to produce diphenyl carbonate, being later trans-esterified with a diphenolic derivative affording poly (aromatic carbonate)s. Polycarbonate has a glass transition temperature of about 150°C (302°F), so it softens gradually above this point and flows above about 300°C (572°F).

Synthesis

Polycarbonate can be synthesized from bisphenol A and phosgene (carbonyl dichloride, $COCl_2$). The first step in the synthesis of polycarbonate from bisphenol A is treatment of bisphenol A with sodium hydroxide.

Properties

- Lightweight
- High-performance
- Possesses a unique balance of toughness
- Dimensional stability, optical clarity
- High heat resistance and
- Excellent electrical resistance

Because of these attributes, polycarbonate is used in a wide variety of common products including digital media (e.g. CDs, DVDs), electronic equipment, automobiles, construction glazing, sports safety equipment and medical devices. The durability, shatter-resistance and heat-resistance of polycarbonate also make it an ideal choice for tableware as well as reusable bottles and food storage containers that can be conveniently used in the refrigerator and microwave (APME).

Advantages

Polycarbonate is a versatile, tough plastic used for a variety of applications, from bulletproof windows to compact disks (CDs). The main advantage of polycarbonate over other types of plastic is unbeatable strength combined with light weight. While acrylic is 17% stronger than glass, polycarbonate is nearly unbreakable. Bulletproof windows and enclosures as seen inside banks or at drive-throughs are often made of polycarbonate. Add to this the advantage that polycarbonate is just one-third the weight of acrylic, or one-sixth as heavy as glass, and the only drawback is that it is more expensive than either acrylic or glass.

Applications

Polycarbonate is becoming more common in housewares as well as laboratories and in industry, especially in applications where any of its main features-high impact resistance, temperature resistance, optical properties are required.

Main transformation techniques for polycarbonate resins:

- Extrusion into tubes, rods and other profiles.
- Extrusion with cylinders into sheets (0.5–15 mm (0.020–0.59 in) and films (below 1 mm (0.039 in), which can be used directly or manufactured into other shapes using thermoforming or secondary fabrication techniques, such as bending, drilling, routing, laser cutting, etc.
- injection molding into ready articles.

Typical Injected Applications

- Compact discs, DVDs, Blu-ray Discs
- Drinking bottles
- Drinking glasses
- Lab equipment, research animal enclosures
- Lighting lenses, sunglass/eyeglass lenses, safety glasses, automotive headlamp lenses
- MP3/Digital audio player cases
- Ocarinas
- Toys (particularly hard wearing toys such as spinning tops/RC Cars, etc).

Typical Sheet/Film Application

- *Advertisement:* Signs, displays, poster protection.
- *Building:* Domelights, flat or curved glazing, and sound walls.
- *Computers:* Laptops and computer cases.
- *Industry:* Machined or formed, cases, machine glazing, riot shields, visors, instrument panels.
- *Hobby:* Machined into fins, gyro mounts, and flybar locks for use with radio-controlled helicopters.

For use in applications exposed to weathering or UV-radiation, a special surface treatment is needed. This either can be a coating (e.g. for improved abrasion resistance), or a coextrusion for enhanced weathering resistance.

Some polycarbonate grades are used in medical applications and comply with both ISO 10993-1 and USP Class VI standards (occasionally referred to as PC-ISO). Class VI is the most stringent of the six USP ratings. These grades can be sterilized using steam at 120°C, gamma radiation or the ethylene oxide (EtO) method. However, scientific research indicates possible problems with biocompatibility.

In the automotive industry, injection moulded polycarbonate can produce very smooth surfaces that make it well suited for direct (without the need for a basecoat) metalised parts such as decorative bezels and optical reflectors. Its uniform mould shrinkage results in parts with greater accuracy than those made of polypropylene. However, due to its susceptibility to environmental stress cracking, its use is limited to low stress applications.

Being based on bisphenol A (a substance obtained from phenol, which in turn is based on benzene) pricing is largely dependent on phenol and benzene pricing.

Bisphenol A

Bisphenol A (BPA) is a key building block of polycarbonate plastic. In recent years a number of researchers from government agencies, academia and industry worldwide have studied the potential for low levels of BPA to migrate from polycarbonate products into foods and beverages. These studies consistently show that the potential migration of BPA into food is extremely low, generally less than 5 parts per billion, under conditions typical for uses of polycarbonate products.

BPA, is an organic compound with two phenol functional groups. It is a difunctional building block of several important plastics and plastic additives.

Suspected of being hazardous to humans since the 1930s, concerns about the use of bisphenol A in consumer products were regularly reported in the news media in 2008 after several governments issued reports questioning its safety, and some retailers have removed products containing it from their shelves. A 2010 report from the FDA raised further concerns regarding exposure of fetuses, infants, and young children.

Synthesis

Bisphenol A was first reported by AP Dianin in 1891. It is prepared by the condensation of acetone (hence the suffix A in the name) with two equivalents of phenol. The reaction is catalyzed by an acid, such as hydrochloric acid (HCl) or a sulfonated polystyrene resin. Typically, a large excess of phenol is used to ensure full condensation:

$$(CH_3)_2CO + 2\ C_6H_5OH \rightarrow (CH_3)_2C(C_6H_4OH)_2 + H_2O$$

A large number of ketones undergo analogous condensation reactions. The method is efficient and the only by-product is water.

Use

Bisphenol A is used primarily to make plastics, and products containing bisphenol A-based plastics have been in commerce for more than 50 years.

It is a key monomer in production of epoxy resin sand in the most common form of polycarbonate plastic.

Polycarbonate plastic, which is clear and nearly shatter-proof, is used to make a variety of common products including baby and water bottles, sports equipment, medical and dental devices, dental fillings and sealants, eyeglass lenses, CDs and DVDs, and household electronics.

BPA is also used in the synthesis of polysulfones and polyether ketones, as an antioxidant in some plasticizers, and as a polymerization inhibitor in PVC.

Epoxy resins containing bisphenol A are used as coatings on the inside of almost all food and beverage cans, however, due to BPA health concerns, in Japan epoxy coating was mostly replaced by PET film.

Bisphenol A is also a precursor to the flame retardant, tetrabromobisphenol A, and was formerly used as a fungicide. Bisphenol A is a preferred color developer in thermal paper and in carbonless copy paper. BPA-based products are also used in foundry castings and for lining water pipes.

9. Polyacrylonitrile

Uses   : Fibres, precursor for carbon fibre
Monomer   : Acrylonitrile
Polymerization   : Free radical chain polymerization
Morphology   : Highly crystalline
Melting temperature   : 319°C
Glass transition temperature   : 87°C

Polyacrylonitrile (PAN) is a resinous, fibrous, or rubbery organic polymer. Almost all polyacrylonitrile resins are copolymers made from mixtures of monomers; with acrylonitrile as the main component. PAN fibres are the chemical precursor of high-quality carbon fibre. Poly (acrylonitrile) is most commonly used in fibre form. Since it softens only slightly below its thermal degradation temperature, it must be processed by wet or dry spinning rather than melt spinning.

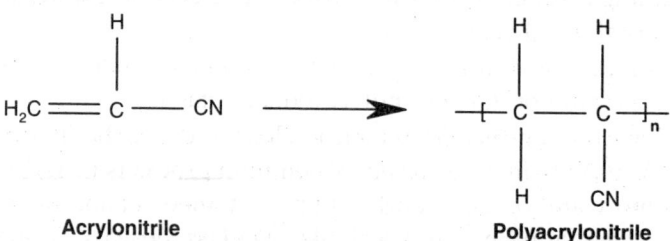

Acrylonitrile   **Polyacrylonitrile**

Fig. 4.18: Polymerization of acrylonitrile

It is a component repeat unit in several important copolymers, such as styrene-acrylonitrile or SAN and ABS plastic. Hard, relatively insoluble, and high-melting materials produced by the polymerization of acrylonitrile, as shown in the reaction below.

Also, sometimes we make copolymers of acrylonitrile and vinyl chloride. These copolymers are flame-retardant, and the fibres made from them are called modacrylic fibres.

But the slew of copolymers of acrylonitrile does not stop there. Poly (styrene-co-acrylonitrile) (SAN) and poly (acrylonitrile-co-butadiene-co-styrene) (ABS), are used as plastics.

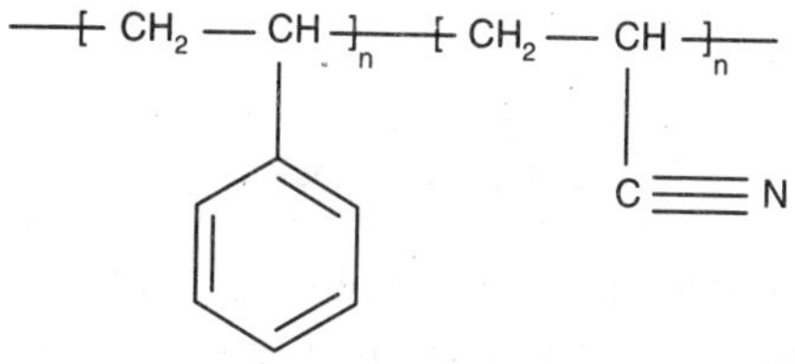

$$\left[CH_2 - CH \right]_n \left[CH_2 - CH \right]_n$$

Fig. 4.19: SAN

SAN is a simple random copolymer of styrene and acrylonitrile. But ABS is more complicated. It's made by polymerizing styrene and acrylonitrile in the presence of polybutadiene. Polybutadiene has carbon-carbon double bonds in it, which can polymerize, too. So we end up with a polybutadiene chain with SAN chains grafted onto it, see below.

ABS is very strong and lightweight. It is strong enough to be used to make automobile body parts. Using plastics like ABS makes automobiles lighter, so they use less fuel, and therefore they pollute less.

ABS is a stronger plastic than polystyrene because of the nitrile groups of its acrylonitrile units. The nitrile groups are very polar, so they are attracted to each other. This allows opposite charges on the nitrile groups to stabilize each other like you see in the picture on the left. This strong attraction holds ABS chains together tightly, making the material stronger. Also the rubbery polybutadiene makes ABS tougher than polystyrene.

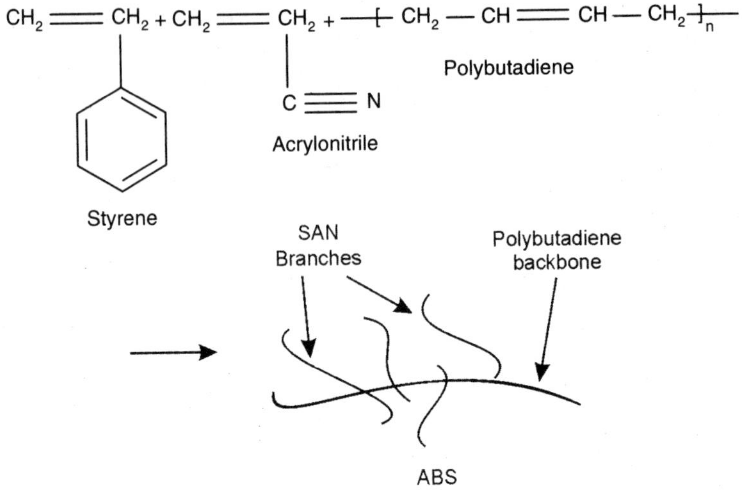

$$CH_2 = CH_2 + CH_2 = CH_2 + -\!\!\left[CH_2 - CH = CH - CH_2 \right]_n -$$

Polybutadiene

$C \equiv N$

Acrylonitrile

Styrene

SAN Branches

Polybutadiene backbone

ABS

Fig. 4.20: Synthesis of ABS

Polyacrylonitrile is a vinyl polymer, and a derivative of the acrylate family of polymers. It is made from the monomer acrylonitrile by free radical vinyl polymerization.

Applications

Homopolymers of polyacrylonitrile have been used as fibres in hot gas filtration systems, and even fibre reinforced concrete. Copolymers containing polyacrylonitrile are often used as fibres to make knitted clothing, like socks and sweaters, as well as outdoor products like tents and similar items.

It is chemically modified to make the carbon fibres found in plenty of both high-tech and common daily applications such as civil and military aircraft primary and secondary structures, missiles, solid propellant rocket motors, pressure vessels, fishing rods, tennis rackets, badminton rackets and high-tech bicycles.

Polyacrylonitrile is used for very few products an average consumer would be familiar with, except to make another polymer, carbon fibre.

10. Acrylonitrile Butadiene Styrene (ABS)

Acrylonitrile Butadiene Styrene (ABS) is the polymerization of Acrylonitrile, Butadiene and Styrene monomers. Chemically, this thermoplastic family of plastics is called "terpolymers", in that they involve the combination of three different monomers to form a single material that draws from the properties of all three (ABS is an amorphous thermoplastic blend. The recipe is 15–35% acrylonitrile, 5–30% butadiene and 40–60% styrene. Depending on the blend different properties can be achieved). Acrylnitrile contributes with thermal and chemical resistance, and the rubber like butadiene gives ductility and impact strength. Styrene gives the glossy surface and makes the material easily machinable and less expensive.

Generally, ABS has good impact strength also at low temperatures. It has satisfactory stiffness and dimensional stability, glossy surface and is easy to machine. If UV-stabilizators are added, ABS is suitable for outdoor applications. ABS has good dimensional stability and electrical insulating properties.

Features

Full list of features including; flame retardant, heat resistance, high, impact resistance, good, impact resistance.

Properties

Common properties including; density, tensile strength, flexural modulus.

ABS Resistance

- Excellent resistance (no attack) to glycerine, inorganic salts, alkalis, many acids, most alcohols and hydrocarbons.
- Limited resistance (moderate attack and suitable for short term use only) to weak acids.
- Poor resistance (not recommended for use with) strong acids and solvents, ketones, aldehydes, esters, and some chlorinated hydrocarbons.

ABS Fabrication

- It can be thermo-formed, pressure formed, blow molded, sheared, sawed, drilled, or even "cold stamped".
- Joints can be ultrasonic welded, thermo-welded, and chemically bonded.
- Impact resistant

- Commonly used for telephone bodies, safety helmets, piping, furniture, car components, TV casings, radios, control panels, and similar.
- Valve bodies, material handling equipment.

Applications

Full list of applications including; Automotive Applications, Electrical/Electronic Applications.

11. Polypropylene (PP)

Prior to 1954 most attempts to produce plastics from polyolefins had little commercial success. PP invented in 1955 by Italian Scientist FJ Natta by addition reaction of propylene gas with a stereospecific catalyst titanium trichloride. Isotactic polypropylene was stereospecific (molecules are arranged in a definite order in space). Polypropylene is similar in manufacturing method and in properties to PE.

Polymerization of PP

- Polypropylene produced with low pressure process (Ziegler).
- Polypropylene produced with linear chains.
- Polypropylene is similar in manufacturing method and in properties to PE.

Differences between PP and PE

- *Density:* PP = 0.90; PE = 0.941 to 0.965
- *Melt Temperature:* PP = 176 0C; PE = 110°C
- *Service Temperature:* PP has higher service temperature
- *Hardness:* PP is harder, more rigid, and higher brittle point.
- *Stress Cracking:* PP is more resistant to environmental stress cracking.

Advantages and Disadvantages of Polypropylene

1. Advantages
   - Low cost
   - Excellent flexural strength
   - Good impact strength
   - Processable by all thermoplastic equipment
   - Low coefficient of friction

- Excellent electrical insulation
- Good fatigue resistance
- Excellent moisture resistance
- Service temperature to 126°C
- Very good chemical resistance.

2. Disadvantages
   - High thermal expansion
   - UV degradation
   - Poor weathering resistance
   - Subject to attack by chlorinated solvents and aromatics
   - Difficulty to bond or paint
   - Oxidizes readily
   - Flammable.

Copolymers of Polypropylene

- Ethylene-propylene copolymers
  - Small amount of PP can lower crystallinity of linear HDPE.
- Polyallomers (block copolymers)
  - Blocks of PE and PP polymers allows crystallization to take place.
  - Properties are similar to HDPE and PP.
- Ethylene-propylene rubbers
  - Random co-polymerization of ethylene and propylene prevents crystallization of the chains by suppressing regularity of molecules.
  - Resulting polymers are amorphous having low Tg (between –110°C and –20°C depending on % of PE and PP).
  - Polymers are rubbery at room temperature.
  - Conventional vulcanization allows for use as commercial rubber, thermoplastic rubbers, TPR.

Polyolefin Polybutylene

- History
  - PB invented in 1974 by Witco Chemical.
  - Ethyl side groups in a linear backbone.

- Description
  - Linear isotactic material.
  - Upon cooling the crystallinity is 30%.
  - Post-forming techniques can increase crystallinity to 55%.
  - Formed by conventional thermoplastic techniques.
- Applications (primarily pipe and film areas)
  - High performance films.
  - Tank liners and pipes.
  - Hot-melt adhesive.
  - Coextruded as moisture barrier and heat-sealable packages.

Polyolefin Polymethylpentene (PMP)

- Description
  - Crystallizes to 40–60%.
  - Highly transparent with 90% transmission.
  - Formed by injection molding and blow molding.
- Properties
  - Low density of 0.83 g/cc; High transparency.
  - Mechanical properties comparable to polyolefins with higher temperature properties and higher creep properties.
  - Low permeability to gasses and better chemical resistance.
  - Attacked by oxidizing agents and light hydrogen carbon solvents.
  - Attacked by UV and is quite flammable.
- Applications
  - Lighting elements (Diffusers, lenses reflectors), liquid level.
  - Food packaging containers, trays and bags.

12. Aluminium Oxynitride

ALONIDE™ Aluminium Oxynitride is a transparent ceramic powder with surface areas from 0.9–7.5 m^2/g range. It is also available in Ultra high purity and high purity and coated and dispersed forms.

High surface area aluminium oxynitride nano layers can also be achieved using thin film by sputtering targets and evaporation technology using pellets, rod and foil. Nano-powders are analyzed for chemical composition by ICP, particle size distribution (PSD) by laser diffraction, and for Specific Surface Area (SSA) by BET multi-point correlation techniques. Research into applications for Aluminium Oxynitride includes use in aerospace to take advantage of its transparent properties due to and firmness, thermal conductivity, controllable thermal expansion and low density and for use in other coatings, plastics, and wire. Aluminium Oxynitride is generally immediately available in most volumes. Additional technical, research and safety (MSDS) information is available.

Aluminium is a Block P, Group 13, Period 3 element. The electronic configuration is [Ne] $3s^2$ $3p^1$. In its elemental form aluminium's CAS number is 7429–90–5. The aluminium atom has a radius of 143.2.pm and it's van der Waals radius is 200.pm. Aluminium is a silvery-white metal that possesses many desirable characteristics. It is light, nonmagnetic and nonsparking. It stands second among metals in the scale of malleability, and sixth in ductility. It is extensively used in many industrial applications where a strong, light, easily constructed material is needed. Although it is electrical conductivity is only about 60% that of copper, it is used in electrical transmission lines because of its light weight. Pure aluminium is soft and lacks strength, but alloyed with small amounts of copper, magnesium, silicon, manganese, or other elements impart a variety of useful properties. These alloys are of vital importance in the construction of modern aircraft and rockets. Aluminium, evaporated in a vacuum, forms a highly reflective coating for both visible light and radiant heat. They are used to coat telescope mirrors. Aluminium is available as metal and compounds with purities from 99 to 99.9999% (ACS grade to ultra-high purity); metals in the form of foil, sputtering target, and rod and compounds as submicron and nanopowder.

Application

A transparent scratchproof watch case closure element, wherein it is realized by sintering a pressed part or an injected part having a general shape similar to that of said closure element, said part being formed essentially of a powder or of a mixture of powders of ceramic material wherein said closure element is transparent in the visible spectrum, and wherein said closure element is made of aluminium oxynitride having the composition $Al_{23}-1/x$ $O_{27}+x$ N_5-x, X being between 0.429 and 2.

A new type of transparent armor made of aluminium could one day replace glass in military vehicles. The product is called aluminium oxynitride. It is being tested by the Army and the University of Dayton Research Institute in Ohio. The material is a ceramic compound with a high compressive strength and durability, according to an Army statement issued this week. It performs better than the multilayered glass products currently in use, and its about half the weight. It is virtually scratch-resistant Engineers here are testing a new kind of transparent armor – stronger and lighter than traditional materials that could stop armor-piercing weapons from penetrating vehicle window.

13. Nylon (polyamide)

Nylon is a generic designation for a family of synthetic polymers known generically as polyamides. Nylons are one of the most common polymers used as a fibre. Nylon is found in clothing all the time, but also in other places, in the form of a thermoplastic. Nylon's first real success came with it is use in women's stockings, in about 1940. They were a big hit, but

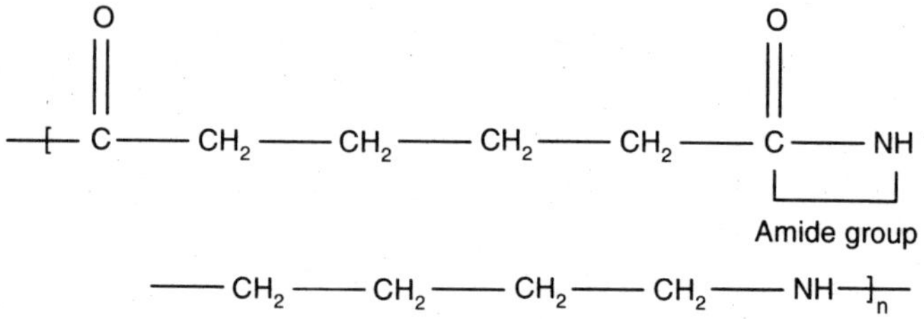

Fig. 4.21: Nylon

they became hard to get, because the next year the United States entered World War II, and nylon was needed to make war materials, like parachutes and ropes. But before stockings or parachutes, the very first nylon product was a toothbrush with nylon bristles.

Nylons are also called polyamides, because of the characteristic amide groups in the backbone chain. Proteins, such as the silk nylon was made to replace, are also polyamides. These amide groups are very polar, and can hydrogen bond with each other. Because of this, and because the nylon backbone is so regular and symmetrical, nylons are often crystalline, and make very good fibres. First produced on February 28, 1935 by Wallace Carothers at DuPont. Nylon is one of the most commonly used polymers.

Nylon Fibre

The Federal Trade Commission's definition for Nylon Fibre: A manufactured fibre in which the fibre forming substance is a long-chain synthetic polyamide in which less than 85% of the amide-linkages are attached directly (-CO-NH-) to two aliphatic groups.

- A synthetic thermoplastic fibre (Nylon melts/glazes easily at relatively low temperatures).
- Round, smooth and shiny filament fibres.
- Cross sections can be either (i) trilobal – to imitate silk or (ii) multilobal – to increase staple like appearance and hand.
- Its most widely used structures are multifilament, monofilament, staple or tow and is available as partially drawn or as finished filaments.
- Regular nylon has a round cross section and is perfectly uniform. The filaments are generally completely transparent unless they have been delustered or solution dyed. Thus, they are microscopically recognized as glass rods.
- Molecular chains of nylon are long and straight variations but have no side chains or linkages. Cold drawing can align the chains so they are oriented with the lengthwise direction and are highly crystalline.

- Nylon is related chemically to the protein fibres silk and wool. They both have similar dye sites but nylon has many fewer dye sites than wool.

Characteristics

- Variation of luster: nylon has the ability to be very lustrous, semilustrous or dull.
- Durability: its high tenacity fibres are used for seatbelts, tire cords, ballistic cloth and other uses.
- High elongation.
- Excellent abrasion resistance.
- Highly resilient (nylon fabrics are heat-set).
- Paved the way for easy-care garments.
- High resistance to insects, fungi, animals, as well as molds, mildew, rot and many chemicals.
- Used in carpets and nylon stockings.
- Melts instead of burning.
- Used in many military applications.
- Good specific strength.
- Transparent under infrared light (–12dB).

Use in Composites

Nylon can be used as the matrix material in composite materials, with reinforcing fibres like glass or carbon fibre, and has a higher density than pure nylon. Such thermoplastic composites (25% glass fibre) are frequently used in car components next to the engine, such as intake manifolds, where the good heat resistance of such materials makes them feasible competitors to metals. Some of the terpolymers based upon nylon are used every day in packaging. Nylon has been used for meat wrappings and sausage sheaths.

Nylon 6, 6

Uses	: Fibers, thermoplastics
Monomers	: Adipic acid and hexamethylene diamine
Polymerization	: Acid catalyzed condensation polymerization
Morphology	: Highly crystalline

Melting temperature   : 280°C
Glass transition temperature : 50°C

Nylon 6-6, also referred to as nylon 6, 6, is a type of nylon. Nylon comes in many types, the two most common for textile and plastics industries are: nylon 6 and nylon 6, 6.

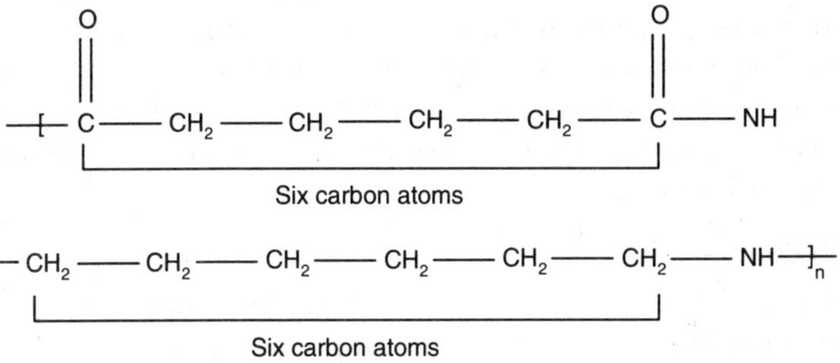

Fig. 4.22: Nylon 6, 6

Composition

Nylon 6, 6 is made of hexamethylene diamine and adipic acid, which give nylon 6, 6 a total of 12 carbon atoms and it's name.

Physical Properties

1. Nylon 6, 6 has a melting point of 280°C, high for a synthetic fibre, though not a match for polyesters or aramids such as Kevlar. This fact makes it the most resistant to heat and friction and enables it to withstand heatsetting for twist retention.

2. It is long molecular chain results in more sites for hydrogen bonds, creating chemical "springs" and making it very resilient.

3. It has a dense structure with small, evenly spaced pores. This means that nylon 6, 6 is difficult to dye, but once dyed it has superior colour fastness and is less susceptible to fading from sunlight and ozone and to yellowing from nitrous oxide.

Applications

- Carpet fibre
- Apparel

- Airbags
- Tires
- Ropes
- Conveyor Belts
- Hoses

Nylon 6, 6's longer molecular chain and denser structure qualifies it as a premium nylon fibre, specified most often by professional architects and designers for use in commercial settings like offices, airports, and other places that get a lot of wear and tear. It is also an excellent choice for residential carpet applications.

Nylon 6

Uses   : Fibres, thermoplastics
Monomers   : Caprolactam
Polymerization   : Ring opening polymerization
Morphology   : Highly crystalline
Melting temperature   : 215°C
Glass transition temperature : 40°C

Caprolactam molecule used to synthesize Nylon 6 by ring opening polymerization. Nylon 6 or polycaprolactam is a polymer developed by Paul Schlack at IG Farben to reproduce the properties of nylon 6, 6 without violating the patent on its production. Unlike most other nylons, nylon 6 is not a condensation polymer, but instead is formed by ring-opening polymerization. This makes it a special case in the comparison between condensation and addition polymers. Its competition with nylon 6, 6 and the example it set have also shaped the economics of the synthetic fibre industry. It was given the trademark **Perlon** in the year 1952. It is a semicrystalline polyamide.

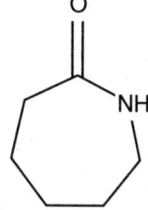

Fig. 4.23: Caprolactam

Properties

Nylon 6 fibres are tough, possessing high tensile strength, as well as elasticity and lustre. They are wrinkle-proof and highly resistant to abrasion and chemicals such as acids and alkalis. The fibres can absorb up to 2.4% of water, although this lowers tensile strength.

Applications

Nylon 6 is used as thread in bristles for toothbrushes, surgical sutures, and strings for acoustic and classical musical instruments, including guitars, violins, violas, and cellos. It is also used in the manufacture of a large variety of threads, ropes, filaments, nets, and tire cords, as well as hosiery and knitted garments. It can also be used in gun frames, which are made with a composite of Nylon 6 and other polymers. It has the potential to be used as a technical nutrient.

14. Aramids

Aramids are a family of nylons, including Nomex® and Kevlar®. Kevlar® is used to make things like bullet proof vests and puncture resistant bicycle tires. Blends of Nomex® and Kevlar® are used to make fireproof clothing. Nomex® is what keeps the monster truck and tractor drivers from burning to death should their fire-breathing rigs breathe a little too much fire. Thanks to Nomex®, an important part of American culture can be practiced safely. (Polymers play another part in the monster truck show in the form of elastomers from which those giant tires are made.) Nomex®–Kevlar® blends also protect fire fighters.

Kevlar® is a polyamide, in which all the amide groups are separated by para-phenylene groups, that is, the amide groups attach to the phenyl rings opposite to each other, at carbons 1 and 4.

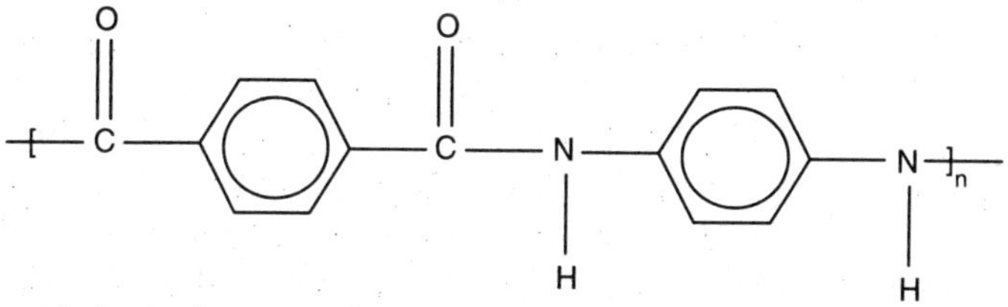

In kevlar the aromatic groups are all linked into the backbone chain through the 1 and 4 positions. This is called *para*-linkage.

Fig. 4.24: Aramides (Kevlar®)

Nomex®, on the other hand, has meta-phenylene groups, that is, the amide groups are attached to the phenyl ring at the 1 and 3 positions.

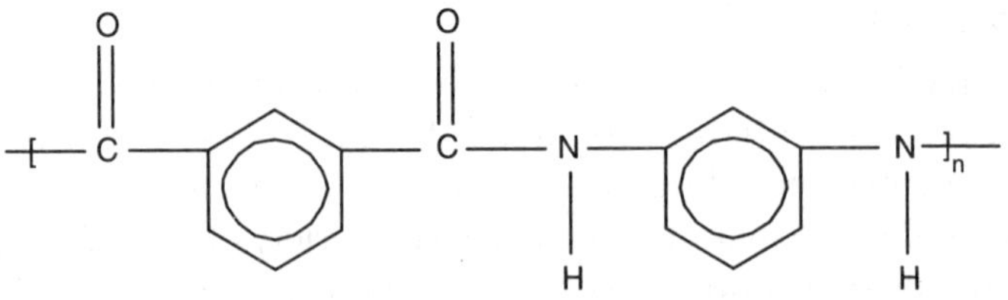

In nomex the aromatic groups are all linked into the backbone chain through the 1 and 3 positions. This is called *meta*-linkage.

Fig. 4.25: Armode (Nomex®)

Kevlar® is a very crystalline polymer. It took a long time to figure out how to make anything useful out of Kevlar® because it would not dissolve in anything. So processing it as a solution was out.

Aramids are used in the form of fibres. They form into even better fibres than non-aromatic polyamides, like nylon 6, 6.

4.6 RESIN IDENTIFICATION CODE

The SPI resin identification coding system is a set of symbols placed on plastics to identify the polymer type. It was developed by the Society of the Plastics Industry (SPI) in 1988, and is used internationally. The primary purpose of the codes is to allow efficient separation of different polymer types for recycling. The symbols used in the code consist of arrows that cycle clockwise to form a rounded triangle and enclosing a number, often with an acronym representing the plastic below the triangle. When the number is omitted, the symbol is known as the universal Recycling Symbol, indicating generic recyclable materials. In this case, other text and labels are used to indicate the material(s) used. Previously recycled resins are coded with an "R" prefix (for example, a PETE bottle made of recycled resin could be marked as RPETE using same numbering).

Contrary to misconceptions, the number does not indicate how hard the item is to recycle, nor how often the plastic was recycled. It is an arbitrary number and has no other meaning aside from identifying the specific plastic. The Unicode character encoding standard includes the resin identification codes, between code points U+2673 and U+2679 inclusive. The generic material recycling symbol is encoded as code point U+267A.

4.7 AVAILABILITY OF RECYCLING FACILITIES

Use of the recycling symbol in the coding of plastics has led to on going consumer confusion about which plastics are readily recyclable. In most communities throughout the United States, PETE and HDPE are the only plastics collected in municipal recycling programs. Some regions, though, are expanding the range of plastics collected as markets become available. A quarter of the solid waste from homes is plastic materials-some of which may be recycled as shown in the Table 4.1.

Table 4.1: Plastics that are recycled

Recycle Code	Abbreviation and Chemical Name of Plastic	Types of Uses and Examples
1.	PET-polyethylene terephthalate	Clear, 2 liter beverage bottles
2.	HDPE-High density polyethylene	Milk jugs, detergent bottles, some water bottles.
3.	PVC - Polyvinyl chloride	Saran wrap, plastic drain pipe, shower curtains, some water bottles
4.	LDPE - Low density polyethylene	Plastic bags, garment bags, coffee can lids.
5.	PP - Polypropylene	Aerosol can tops, rigid bottle caps, candy wrappers, bottoms of bottles.
6.	PS - Polystyrene	Hard clear plastic cups, foam cups, eating utensils, deli food containers, some packing popcorn.
7.	Other	Biodegradable, Some packing popcorn.

4.8 PLASTICS AND PACKAGING

Plastic is so versatile, it can be used for a variety of packaging purposes. If the product needs to be well protected, the plastic can be rigid and tough. If, on the other hand, the packaging needs to be convenient to carry, the plastic can be flexible or, a combination of the two can be achieved. Furthermore, the packaging can be designed into any shape or size desired and it can be clear or any colour imaginable.

Plastic packaging helps keep people, the earth, and animals healthy in a number of ways. For example, plastic packaging is used by medical facilities to dispose of needles and other items that may be contaminated. Similarly, fragile medical devices are often shipped in plastic containers because they can be precisely designed to prevent them from being damaged during shipping. Intravenous bags are also made with special see-through plastic to help the medical staff monitor the flow and intake of important nutrients and medicines.

Plastic is also used to store a variety of goods commonly found in the home. By creating shatterproof bottles with plastic, family members are protected from harm if the product should accidentally fall. Leak proof and child-resistant packaging can also be created with plastic.

Advantages and Disadvantages of Plastics

As we all know, plastics are all around us. We use plastics for a wide variety of products, from water bottles to body replacement parts. While these products are beneficial in many ways, they are also harmful.

Advantages of Plastics

1. Recyclable – Plastics can be melted and used to make other products.
2. Can be incinerated – Plastics can be melted down and may be able to generate electricity.
3. Durable – Plastics can take the wear and tear of everyday life without falling apart.
4. Resistant to the environment – Plastics are able to endure a variety of weather conditions without disintegrating.
5. Plastics are lighter than steel and other materials that they replace. They also lower vehicle weight significantly thus reducing fuel consumption.

6. Plastics have superior formability. This enables a function to in effect be produced in a single manufacturing process (e.g. injection moulding) rather than combining separate components in a more complex process. This reduces the total production cost for vehicle manufacturers.

7. Plastic components are an important way for manufacturers to differentiate products in a market where price and quality are increasingly uniform.

8. Injection moulding tools cost less than the tools used to manufacture components in metal, thus reducing unit cost.

9. Plastics work well in the vehicle's deformation zones, which are designed to give way and absorb impact in a collision.

10. Plastics are easily combined with other materials.

11. Plastics have better sound absorption than steel and sheet metal.

Disadvantages of Plastics

1. *Flammable:* This is definitely an advantage in that they can be melted down, however smoldering plastics can release toxic fumes into the environment.

2. *Cost of recycling:* While recycling is a plus, recycling is a very costly endeavor.

3. *Volume:* In the United States 20% of our landfill is made up of plastics. As more products are being made of plastics, where will this lead us in the future?

4. *Durability:* This is an advantage as well as a disadvantage. Plastics are extremely durable, which means that they last a long time. Those plastics in the landfill will be there for years.

Plastics make our lives easier, however is their cost on the environment worth it? We can only hope that soon someone will invent a way to safely and cheaply melt and reuse plastics.

Table 4.2: Plastic packaging resins

Resin Codes	Descriptions	Properties	Product Applications	Products Made with Recycled Content
♳ 1 PET	Polyethylene Terephthalate (PET, PETE). PET is clear, tough, and has good gas and moisture barrier properties. This resin is commonly used in beverage bottles and many injection-molded consumer product containers. Cleaned, recycled PET flakes and pellets are in great demand for spinning fibre for carpet yarns, producing fibrefill fibre for carpet yarns, and geo-textiles. Nickname: Polyester.	Clear and optically smooth surfaces for oriented films and bottles. Excellent barrier to oxygen, water, and carbon dioxide. High impact capability and shatter resistance. Excellent resistance to most solvents. Capability for hot-filling.	Plastic bottles for soft drinks, water, juice, sports drinks, beer, mouthwash, catsup and salad dressing. Food jars for peanut butter, jelly, jam and pickles. Ovenable film and micro-wavable food trays. In addition to packaging, PET's major uses are textiles, mono-filament, carpet, strapping, films, and engineering moldings.	Fiber for carpet, fleece jackets, comforter fill, and tote bags. Containers for food, beverages (bottles), and non-food items. Film and sheet. Strapping
♴ 2 HDPE	High Density Polyethylene (HDPE). HDPE is used to make many types of bottles. Unpigmented bottles are translucent, have good barrier properties and stiffness, and are well suited to packaging products with a short shelf life such as milk. Because HDPE has good chemical resistance, it is used for packaging many household and industrial chemicals such as	Excellent resistance to most solvents. Higher tensile strength compared to other forms of polyethylene. Relatively stiff material with useful temperature capabilities.	Bottles for milk, water, juice, cosmetics, shampoo, dish and laundry detergents, and household cleaners. Bags for groceries and retail purchases. Cereal box liners. Reusable shipping containers. In addition to packaging, HDPE's major uses are in	Bottles for non-food items, such as shampoo, conditioner, liquid laundry detergent, household cleaners, motor oil and antifreeze. Plastic lumber for outdoor decking, fencing and picnic tables. Pipe, floor tiles, buckets,

Contd...

Contd...

Resin Codes	Descriptions	Properties	Product Applications	Products Made with Recycled Content
	detergents and bleach. Pigmented HDPE bottles have better stress crack resistance than unpigmented HDPE.		injection molding applications, extruded pipe and conduit, plastic wood composites, and wire and cable covering.	crates, flower pots, garden edging, film and sheet, and recycling bins.
PVC	**Polyvinyl Chloride (PVC, Vinyl)** In addition to its stable physical properties, PVC has good chemical resistance, weatherability, flow characteristics and stable electrical properties. The diverse slate of vinyl products can be broadly divided into rigid and flexible materials.	High impact strength, brilliant clarity, excellent processing performance. Resistance to grease, oil and chemicals.	Rigid packaging applications include blister packs and clamshells. Flexible packaging uses include bags for bedding and medical, shrink wrap, deli and meet wrap and tamper resistance. In addition to packaging, PVC's major uses are rigid applications such as pipe, siding, window frames, fencing, decking and railing. Flexible applications include medical products such as blood bags and medical tubing, wire and cable insulation, carpet backing, and flooring.	Pipe, decking, fencing, paneling, gutters, carpet backing, floor tiles and mats, resilient flooring, mud flaps, cassette trays, electrical boxes, cables, traffic cones, garden hose, and mobile home skirting. Packaging, film and sheet, and loose-leaf binders.

Contd...

Contd...

Resin Codes	Descriptions	Properties	Product Applications	Products Made with Recycled Content
△ 4 LDPE	**Low Density Polyethylene (LDPE)** LDPE is used predominately in film applications due to its toughness, flexibility and relative transparency, making it popular for use in applications where heat sealing is necessary. LDPE also is used to manufacture some flexible lids and bottles as well as in wire and cable applications. Includes Linear Low Density Polyethylene (LLDPE).	Excellent resistance to acids, bases and vegetable oils. T o u g h - n e s s , flexibility and relative transparency (good combination of properties for packaging applications requiring heat sealing.	Bags for dry cleaning, newspapers, bread, frozen foods, fresh produce, and household garbage. Shrink wrap and stretch film. Coatings for paper milk cartons and hot and cold beverage cups. Container lids. Toys. Squeezable bottles (e.g., honey and mustard). In addition to packaging, LDPE's major uses are in injection molding applications, adhesives and sealants, and wire and cable coverings.	Shipping envelopes, garbage can liners, floor tile, paneling, furniture, film and sheet, compost bins, trash cans, landscape timber, and outdoor lumber.
△ 5 PP	**Polypropylene (PP)** PP has good chemical resistance, is strong, and has a high melting point making it good for hot-fill liquids. This resin is found in flexible and rigid packaging, fibres, and large molded parts for automotive and consumer products.	Excellent optical clarity in biaxially oriented films and stretch blow molded containers. Low moisture vapor transmission. Inertness toward acids, alkalis and	Containers for yogurt, margarine, takeout meals, and deli foods. Medicine bottles. Bottle caps and closures. Bottles for catsup and syrup. In addition to packaging, PP's major uses are in fibres, appliances and consumer products, including durable applications such as automotive and carpeting.	Products Made with Recycled Content* Automobile applications, such as battery cases, battery signal lights, battery cables, brooms and brushes, ice scrapers, oil funnels, and bicycle racks.

Contd...

Contd...

Resin Codes	Descriptions	Properties	Product Applications	Products Made with Recycled Content
⬖ 6 PS	**Polystyrene (PS)** PS is a versatile plastic that can be rigid or foamed. General purpose polystyrene is clear, hard and brittle. It has a relatively low melting point. Typical applications include protective packaging, food-service packaging, bottles, and food containers. PS is often combined with rubber to make high impact polystyrene (HIPS) which is used for packaging and durable applications requiring toughness, but not clarity.	most solvents. Excellent moisture barrier for short shelf life products. Excellent optical clarity in general purpose form Significant stiffness in both foamed and rigid forms. Low density and high stiffness in foamed applications. Low thermal conductivity and excellent insulation properties in foamed form.	Food service items, such as cups, plates, bowls, cutlery, hinged takeout containers (clamshells), meat and poultry trays, and rigid food containers (e.g., yogurt). These items may be made with foamed or non-foamed PS. Protective foam packaging for furniture, electronics and other delicate items. Packing peanuts, known as "loose fill." Compact disc cases and aspirin bottles. In addition to packaging, PS's major uses are in agricultural trays, electronic housings, cable spools, building insulation, video cassette cartridges, coat hangers, and medical products and toys.	Garden rakes, storage bins, shipping pallets, sheeting, trays. Thermal insulation, thermometers, light switch plates, vents, desk trays, rulers, and license plate frames. Cameras or video cassette casings. Foamed foodservice applications, such as egg shell cartons. Plastic mouldings (i.e., wood replacement products). Expandable polystyrene (EPS) foam protective packaging.
⬖ 7 OTHER	**Other:** Use of this code indicates that a package is made with a resin other than the six listed above, or is made of more than one resin and used in a multi-layer combination.	Dependent on resin or combination of resins.	Three- and five-gallon reusable water bottles, some citrus juice and catsup bottles. Oven-baking bags, barrier layers, and custom packaging.	Bottles and plastic lumber applications.

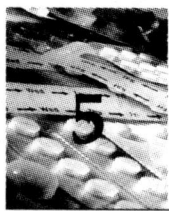

Glass

5.1 INTRODUCTION

Glass is the composition of inorganic compound which are formed by melting different compound like sand, soda-ash, lime stone, cullet (broken glass). Glass is known around 3000BC in the east European countries. It is used as glass-ware by Egyptian around 1500BC and they are made by sand-core method. Through the years and with more knowledge of its technology, glass has become the most widely used drug packaging material. The origin of the first synthetic glass is unknown; however, Egyptians were known to mold figurines from sand and silicon dioxide.

The American Heritage dictionary defines glass as a large class of materials with highly variable mechanical and optical properties, which solidify from the molten state without crystallization, that are typically based on silicon dioxide, boric oxide, aluminium oxide, or phosphorous pentoxide, that are generally transparent or translucent, and that are regarded physically as supercooled liquids rather than fine liquids.

American Society for Testing and Materials (ASTM) defines glass as an inorganic product of fusion that has cooled to a rigid condition without crystallizing. ASTM further states that glass is typically hard and brittle and has a conchoidal fracture. Glass may be colourless or coloured. It is transparent but may be made opaque or translucent. Glass is non-crystalline, is amorphous in structure, and may be formed from both organic and inorganic materials.

Glass is manufactured at very high temperatures and it has the properties of a viscous liquid. With the properties of a viscous liquid, hot glass can be formed into many commonly used forms with precision and accuracy. As a result of its non-crystalline nature, it affords a unique transparent property that is maintained because it does not crystallize upon cooling.

Glass is used in pharmaceutical and cosmetic industry for many years. They are used as a effective container last 40 years, plastic takes place of glass container and glass face competition with plastic. Glass is mainly used in pharmaceuticals and toiletry industries (9.2% and 5% respectively).

There are a variety of uses of glass, one use being a pharmaceutical packaging material. Glass is favored over other types of packaging material because its transparent property enables it to provide good visualization of contained material. Another good quality of glass is its excellent resistance to attack by most liquids, and, therefore, it resists interaction with contained products. It is also totally impermeable to gases, and it can be sterilized with any appropriate process. Glass, when properly coloured, also provides protection to a product from light.

Selection of Glass as Packaging Materials for the Pharmaceutical Products

Glass is mostly used in pharmaceuticals because they fulfill all the requirements needed for it like:
- They must protect the preparation from environment.
- They must be non-reacting with the product.
- They must not impart to the product tastes or odours.
- They must be FDA approved.
- They must be economical.
- They are providing good product presentation.
- They are made all the required size container.
- No change on aging.

Properties of Glass

These are the main characteristics of glass:
- Solid and hard material.
- Disordered and amorphous structure.
- Fragile and easily breakable into sharp pieces.

- Transparent to visible light.
- Inert and biologically inactive material.
- Glass is 100% recyclable and one of the safest packaging materials due to its composition and properties.

Glass is used for architecture application, illumination, electrical transmission, instruments for scientific research, optical instruments, domestic tools and even textiles. Glass does not deteriorate, corrode, stain or fade and therefore is one of the safest packaging materials.

5.2 PRODUCTION OF GLASS

Glass is a hard material normally fragile and transparent common in our daily life. It is composed mainly of sand (silicates, SiO_2) and an alkali.

These materials at high temperature (i.e. molten viscous state) fuse together; then they are cooled rapidly forming a rigid structure, however not having enough time to form a crystalline regular structure.

Depending on the final use and application the composition of the glass and cooling rate will vary to achieve the adequate properties for the specific application.

These are the basic components used in the manufacturing of glass:
1. **Sand (SiO_2 silica):** In its pure form it exists as a polymer, $(SiO_2)n$.
2. **Soda ash (sodium carbonate Na_2CO_3):** Normally SiO_2 softens up to 2000°C, where it starts to degrade (at 1713°C most of the molecules can already move freely). Adding soda will lower the melting point to 1000°C making it more manageable.
3. Limestone (calcium carbonate or $CaCO_3$) or dolomite ($MgCO_3$).

Also known as lime, calcium carbonate is found naturally as limestone, marble, or chalk. The soda makes the glass water-soluble, soft and not very durable. Therefore lime is added increasing the hardness and chemical durability and providing insolubility of the materials. Other materials and oxides can be added to increase properties (tinting, durability, etc.), produce different effects, colours, etc.

5.3 TYPES OF GLASS

The USP and NF described the various types of glass depending on the material used. They are classified into the following types:

1. Type I   Borosilicate glass
2. Type II Treated soda-lime glass
3. Type III Regular soda-lime glass
4. Type IV NP-general purpose soda-lime

1. Type I Borosilicate Glass

It is a highly resistant glass composed with silicon dioxides with calcium and sodium oxide. This type of glass is produced by replacing the sodium oxide flux by boric oxide and some of lime by alumina in the basic components of glass. The borosilicate glass has a high melting point and can withstand high temperature.

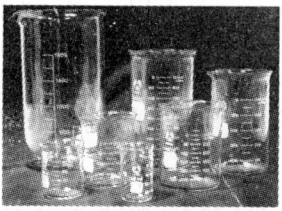

Fig. 5.1: Borosilicate glass

Typical composition of borosilicate glass is:

Silicon dioxide (SiO_2)	66–72%
Alumina (Al_2O_3)	04–10%
Sodium oxide (Na_2O) or	07–10%
Potassium oxide (K_2O)	07–10%
Boric oxide (B_2O_3)	09–11%
Calcium oxide (CaO)	01–05%
Barium oxide (BaO)	00–03%

And small quantities of magnesium oxide, ferric oxide and titanium oxide. They are manufactured at higher temperature 1700–1750°C.

Manufacturing Process

Borosilicate glass is created by adding boron to the traditional glassmaker's frit of silicate sand, soda and ground lime. Since borosilicate glass melts at a higher temperature than ordinary silicate glass, some new techniques were required for industrial production. Borrowing from the welding trade, burners combining oxygen with natural gas were required.

Uses

The refractory properties and physical strength of borosilicate glass make it ideal for use in high-durability laboratory equipment such as beakers and test tubes. In addition, borosilicate glass warps minimally when exposed to heat, allowing a borosilicate container to provide accurate measurements of volume over time.

During the mid-twentieth century, borosilicate glass tubing was used to pipe coolants (often distilled water) through high power vacuum tube-based electronic equipment, such as commercial broadcast transmitters.

Glass cookware is another common usage. Borosilicate glass measuring cups, featuring screen printed markings providing graduated measurements, are widely used in American kitchens.

Aquarium heaters are sometimes made of borosilicate glass. Due to its high heat resistance, it can tolerate the significant temperature difference between the water and the nichrome heating element.

Many high-quality flashlights use borosilicate glass for the lens. This allows for a higher percentage of light transmittance through the lens compared to plastics and lower-quality glass.

Specialty marijuana and tobacco pipes are made from borosilicate glass. The high heat resistance makes the pipes more durable. Most premanufactured glass guitar slides are also made of borosilicate glass.

New lampworking techniques led to artistic applications such as contemporary glass marbles. The modern studio glass movement has responded to colour. "The availability of colours began to increase when companies such as Glass Alchemy introduced the Crayon Colours, which brought a whole new vivacity to the glass industry."Borosilicate is commonly used in the glassblowing form of lampworking and the artists create a range of products ranging from jewelry, kitchenware, to sculpture as well as for artistic glass tobacco pipes.

Borosilicate glass is sometimes used for high-quality beverage glassware. Borosilicate glass lends kitchen- and glassware increased durability along with microwave and dishwasher compatibility.

Most astronomical reflecting telescope glass mirror components are made of borosilicate glass because of its low coefficient of expansion with heat. This makes very precise optical surfaces possible that change very little with temperature, and matched glass mirror components that "track" across temperature changes and retain the optical system's characteristics.

The optical glass most often used for making instrument lenses is Schott BK-7 (or the equivalent from other makers), a very finely made borosilicate crown glass. It is also designated as 517642 glass after its 1.517 refractive index and 64.2 Abbe number. Other less costly borosilicate glasses, such as Schott B270 or the equivalent, are used to make "crown glass" eyeglass lenses. Ordinary lower-cost borosilicate glass, like that used to make kitchenware and even reflecting telescope mirrors, cannot be used for high-quality lenses because of the striations and inclusions common to lower grades of this type of glass.

Borosilicate is also a material of choice for evacuated tube solar thermal technology, because of its high strength and heat resistance. Borosilicate glasses also find application in the semiconductor industry in the development of microelectro-mechanical systems (MEMS), as part of stacks of etched silica wafers bonded to the etched borosilicate glass. The thermal insulation tiles on the Space Shuttle are coated with a borosilicate glass. Lighting manufacturers use borosilicate glass in their refractors.

These glasses are used for immobilisation and disposal of radioactive wastes. In most countries high-level radioactive waste has been incorporated into alkali borosilicate or phosphate vitreous waste forms for many years and vitrification is an established technology. Vitrification is a particularly attractive immobilization route because of the high chemical durability of the vitrified glass product. This characteristic has been used by industry for centuries. The chemical resistance of glass can allow it to remain in a corrosive environment for many thousands and even millions of years.

Pharmaceutical Uses

Borosilicate glasses are used for manufacturing of laboratory glasswares, owenwares and containers for alkalisensitive products. Also used for the infusion fluid blood and plasma.

Additionally, borosilicate tubing is used as the feedstock for the production of parenteral drug packaging, such as vials and pre-filled syringes, and is also used for the production of ampoules and dental cartridges. The chemical resistance of borosilicate glass minimizes the migration of sodium ions from the glass matrix thus making it well suited for injectable drug applications. This type of glass is typically referred to as USP/EP JP Type I.

Advantages

This types of glasses are suitable for the packaging of parenteral preparations and alkali sensitive materials.

Disadvantages

Main disadvantage of these glasses are their higher cost. These are difficult to melt and mould (high melting point).

2. Type II Treated Soda-lime Glass

These types of glass are made by commercial soda-lime glass that has been de-alkalized, or treated to remove surface alkali. This process is known as sulphur treatment and virtually prevents "weathering" of empty bottles. This glass is considerably cheaper than borosilicate glass.

Manufacturing Process

This type of glass is prepared from soda lime glass by treating its surface with moist sulphur dioxide at a temperature above 500°C. The acidic gases neutralises the surface alkali to produce a layer of sodium sulphate which can be easily removed by washing. The process is known as sulphuring and the glass prepared by the processes is known as sulphured glass.

Dealkalization is a process of surface modification applicable to glasses containing alkali ions, wherein a thin surface layer is created that has a lower concentration of alkali ions than is present in the underlying, bulk glass. This change in surface composition commonly alters the observed properties of the surface, most notably enhancing corrosion resistance.

Many commercial glass products such as containers are made of soda-lime glass, and therefore have a substantial percentage of sodium ions in their internal structure. Since sodium is an alkali element, its selective removal from the surface results in a dealkalized surface. A classic example of dealkalization is the treatment of glass containers, where a special process is used to create a dealkalized inside surface that is more resistant to interactions with liquid products put inside the container. However, the term dealkalization may also be generally applied to any process where a glass surface forms a thin surface layer that is depleted of alkali ions relative to the bulk. A common example is the initial stages of glass corrosion or weathering, where alkali ions are leached from the surface region by interactions with water, forming a dealkalized surface layer.

A dealkalized surface may have either no alkali remaining or may just have less than the bulk. In silicate glasses, dealkalized surfaces are also often considered "silica-rich" since the selective removal of alkali ions can be thought to leave behind a surface composed primarily of silica (SiO_2). To be precise, dealkalization does not generally involve the outright removal of alkali from the glass, but rather its replacement with protons (H^+) or hydronium ions (H_3O^+) in the structure through the process of ion-exchange.

Pharmaceutical Uses

This type of glass is used for alkali sensitive products and parenteral products.

Advantages

These type of glasses are cheaper than borosilicate glasses. These are also suitable for the parenteral preparations. The surface of the glass is fairly resistant to attack by water for period of time.

3. Type III Regular Soda-lime Glass

It is the most common type of glass prepared from silica, soda-ash and lime stone.

Typical composition of soda-lime glass is:

Silicon dioxide	66–75%
Sodium oxide	12–19%
Calcium oxide	06–10%
Potassium oxide	less than 01%
Magnesium oxide	less than 01%
Aluminium oxide	less than 01%

It is cheaper compare to borosilicate glass and having low melting point. It contains higher concentration of alkali oxides and can impart alkalinity to aqueous preparations.

Regular soda-lime glass, also called soda-lime-silica glass, is the most prevalent type of glass, used for windowpanes, and glass containers (bottles and jars) for beverages, food, and some commodity items. Glass bakeware is often made of tempered soda-lime glass.

Manufacturing Process

Soda-lime glass is prepared by melting the raw materials, such as sodium carbonate (soda), lime, dolomite, silicon dioxide (silica), aluminium oxide (alumina), and small quantities of fining agents (e.g., sodium sulfate, sodium chloride) in a glass furnace at temperatures locally up to 1675°C. The temperature is only limited by the quality of the furnace superstructure material and by the glass composition. Green and brown bottles are obtained from raw materials containing iron oxide. Relatively inexpensive minerals such as trona, sand, and feldspar are used instead of pure chemicals. The mix of raw materials is termed batch.

Properties and Uses

Soda-lime glass is divided technically into glass used for windows, called float glass or flat glass, and glass for containers, called container glass. Both types differ in the application, production method (float process for windows, blowing and pressing for containers) and chemical composition Float glass has a higher magnesium oxide and sodium oxide content as compared to container glass, and a lower silica, calcium oxide, and aluminium oxide content. From this follows a slightly higher quality of container glass concerning the chemical durability against water, which is required especially for storage of beverages and food.

Pharmaceutical Uses

These glasses are used for the preparation of containers of required shape.

These glasses are used for the preparation of containers of all solid dosage form and oil injections.

Advantages

1. These are quite cheap
2. Low melting point
3. Easily molded into required shape

Disadvantages

Sodalime glass is not suitable for packaging of injectibles and liquid medicaments because;

1. It librates alkali in aqueous preparations.
2. It is not resistant to sudden change in temperature.
3. Flakes separate out easily.
4. Its surface loses some of it is brilliance.

4. Type IV NP- General Purpose Soda-lime

This type of glass made by soda-lime glass. In this glass supplied non-parenteral products.

Pharmaceutical Uses

These glasses are used for the packaging of non-parenteral products, intended for oral or topical use.

5.4 OTHER TYPES OF GLASS

Other than above glass some other types of glass are used they are:

1. Neutral glass
2. Coloured glass

Neutral Glass

This glass is regarded as an intermediate between the borosilicate and soda-lime glass. It is softer than borosilicate glass and can be molded into various shapes.

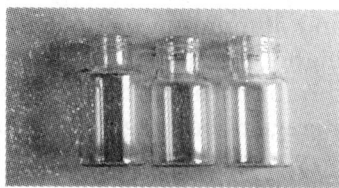

Fig. 5.2: Neutral glass

Typical composition of neutral glass is:

Silicon dioxide	72–75%
Boric oxide	07–10%
Aluminium oxide	04–06%
Sodium oxide	06–08%
Potassium oxide	0.5–02%
Barium oxide	02–04%

It is highly resistant to autoclaving and weathering. It is cheaper to borosilicate glass.

Uses: For the manufacturing of parenteral preparations.

Coloured Glass

Coloured glass is generally used for drugs which are sensitive to light. Such glass provide protection from light in the range of 290–455 nm.

They are formed by:

Amber: Addition of carbon and sulphur or iron and manganese dioxide.

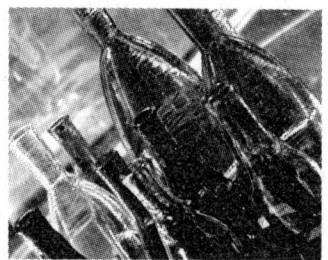

Fig. 5.3: Coloured glass

Yellow: Compounds of cadmium and sulphur.

Blue: Various shades of blue, cobalt oxide or occasionally copper (cupric) oxide.

Green: Achieved by addition iron oxide, manganese dioxide and chromium dioxide.

Opal: Fluorides or phosphates.

5.5 FACTORS OTHER THAN USP TYPE

- The filling processing steps that the container has to withstand are important. If lower thermal expansion of the container is required in the process, several options are available. A typical tubing formed container with thinner and more uniform walls will withstand thermal shock better than a molded glass container in the same expansion range. The physical design of the container also plays a part in the amount of thermal and mechanical shock resistance it exhibits. It is frequently necessary to make a compromise between high resistance to mechanical shock and high resistance to thermal shock.

- Light sensitivity: If the products to be packaged are light sensitive, amber glass must be used.

- If a product is sensitive to the presence of a particular ion, the composition of the glass container should be considered. For example, if a container was precleaned for environmental sampling and used to test for metal ions, it would not be feasible to measure low levels of metals such as sodium or calcium as the ions are in the container matrix and would eventually bloom back to the surface.

- The interaction of glass and aqueous solutions is extremely complex. Extractable and corrosion resistance as well as chemical resistance need to be addressed.

5.6 MANUFACTURING OF GLASS CONTAINERS

Glass containers can be fabricated by certain basic processes.

1. Blown glassware based on either press and blow or blow and blow principals.

2. Tubular glassware – a tube of glass is first produced and subsequently cut and shaped by a separate process.

3. Pressed glassware – Rarely use for packaging container.

- **Blown glass**

Flow Chart 5.1: Process (blow) for bottles

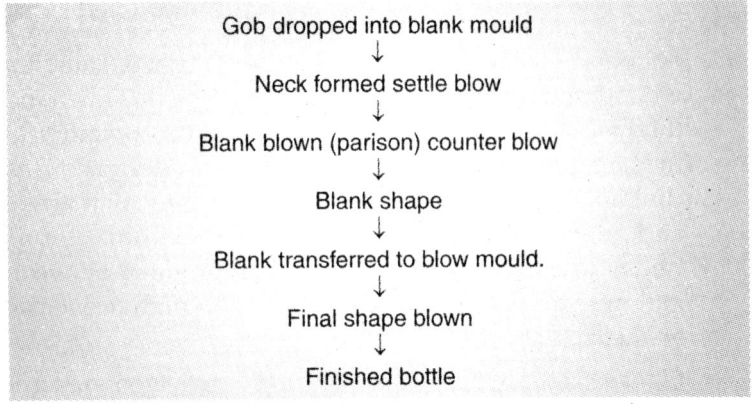

Gob dropped into blank mould
↓
Neck formed settle blow
↓
Blank blown (parison) counter blow
↓
Blank shape
↓
Blank transferred to blow mould.
↓
Final shape blown
↓
Finished bottle

- **The press and blow process (jars)**

Flow Chart 5.2: Process of press and blow process (jars)

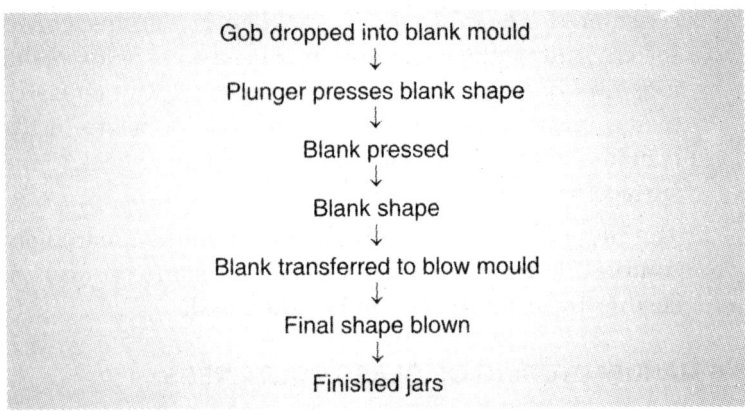

Gob dropped into blank mould
↓
Plunger presses blank shape
↓
Blank pressed
↓
Blank shape
↓
Blank transferred to blow mould
↓
Final shape blown
↓
Finished jars

5.7 FEATURES OF GLASS CONTAINERS

- *Design and decoration:* This may involves two basic concept—Aesthetic appeal and functional efficiency.
- *Production line handling:* This include cleaning, filling, capping, labeling, etc.
- *Strength:* This depends on design, weight, and distribution.

- *Consumer convenience:* They are easily rest on hand, used anywhere (bathroom kitchen).
- *Reuse:* They are reclosable and use after use of other.
- *Capacity:* They having capacity to moulded to the desired size and shape.
- *Cost:* They having lower cost.
- *Recyclability:* Glass is recyclable.
- *Decorative:* Brilliant effects may be achieved by ceramic printing.

5.8 TEST FOR GLASS CONTAINERS

- *Thermal shock test:* Glass sample is placed in an upright position in a tray which is immersed into hot water for a given time, then transferred into a cold water bath. Samples are examined before and after the tests for outside surface cracks or breakage.
  - Temperature range for hot 80–60°C for cold 30–40°C
- *Internal bursting pressure test:*
  - Instrument use - American glass research increment pressure tester.
  - Procedure - Bottle filled with water and then placed inside the test chamber. A sealing head is applied and the pressure is automatically raised by series of increments. Each increment is held for a set time. Bottle checked and pressure is continued increased until bottle is finally bursts.
- *Vertical load test:* The bottle is placed between a fixed platform and a hydraulic vertical load is applied and pressure registered on pressure gauge.

5.9 ADVANTAGES AND DISADVANTAGES OF GLASS CONTAINERS

Advantages

Glass container used in pharmaceuticals over the other packaging materials because they having following advantages.

- They are chemically inert so they are used in wide range or pharmaceuticals.

- They are strong and rigid and they are handled at high speed production line operation.
- They provide good product protection and presentation to the contents from contamination and form other environmental factors, i.e. heat, air, dust and moisture.
- Coloured glass provides protection against light.
- They are moulded into desired size and shape.
- They are cheap.
- There are different types of glass available so choice are available on their compatibility with the drug (dosages form) to be packed.
- They are easily sterilized so they are used for the parenteral preparations.
- They are provided easy product identification because it is transparent.
- They are easy to clean.
- No effect of time duration (No change on aging).
- They are non-corrosive.
- They are FDA approved.
- Impart no odour and taste to the product.

Disadvantages

- It is fragile and breaks easily so need special precautions when handling and transporting.
- It is heavier than other containers, their transportation expanses are higher.
- It may cracks when sudden change of temperature.
- Some container impart alkalinity so need special precautions when selecting to the particular formation
- Less pressure and safety and impact resistance.

5.10 USES OF GLASS CONTAINERS

General Uses

Creating new uses for glass, and enhancing existing materials, is essential to the glass industry's future. Needed improvements include:

- Design of "smart windows" that react to natural lighting conditions and temperatures (specialty glass sector).

- Development of lighter-weight, impact-resistant containers and flat glass (container and flat glass sectors).
- Development of fibre glass that compacts and rebounds easily (fibre glass sector).
- Development of new optical fibre designs and components capable of transmitting greater amounts of information (specialty glass sector).

Pharmaceutical Uses

Type I Glass Containers are used for the packaging of:
- Chemical
- Glassware's
- Human-blood and blood components
- Alkali sensitive preparations.

Type II Glass containers are used for the packaging of:
- Alkali sensitive preparations
- Human blood and blood products
- Parenterals use.

Type III Glass containers are used for the packaging of:
- Medicine bottle for solid medicaments
- For non-aqueous preparations
- Parenteral preparation.

Type IV Glass containers are used for the packaging of:
- Use for oral
- Use for topical.

Neutral glass:
- Use for the packaging of liquid preparations
- Use for the packaging of solid preparations.

Coloured glass:
- Use for the packaging of light sensitive products
- Not used for the packaging of parenterals.

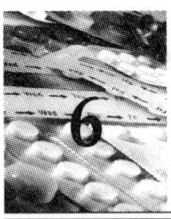

6 Metal Packaging

6.1 INTRODUCTION

A metal is a chemical element that is a good conductor of both electricity and heat and forms cations and ionic bonds with non-metals.

Ancient boxes and cups, made from silver and gold, were much too valuable for common use. Metal did not become a common packaging material until other metals, stronger alloys, thinner gauges and coatings were eventually developed. One of the new metal's that allowed metal to be used in packaging was tin. Tin is a corrosion-resistant metal, and ounce-for-ounce, its value is comparable to silver. However, tin can is "plated" in very thin layers over cheaper metals, and this process made it economical for containers. Since food was now safe within metal packaging, other products were made available in metal boxes. The invention of cans also required the invention of the can opener! Initially, a hammer and chisel was the only method of opening cans. Collapsible, soft metal tubes, today known as "flexible packaging".

Advantages of Metal Packaging

Metal packaging was invented more than a century ago. Since then it has undergone constant changes and improvements in order to adapted to the needs of modern consumers.

It's main advantages are as follows:

1. Full impermeability to the passage of gases and air as compared to other packaging materials, meaning a long shelf-life.

2. Tamper evidence and total protection against intentional damage to the finished product (poisoning or contamination, biological terrorism).
3. Full compatibility with the strictest demands for direct contact with food, medicine, sprays, paints, etc.
4. Low losses in all stages of filling, sealing, packing, distribution, and sale.
5. High speed production rates (for both manufacture and user).
6. Good heat transfer.
7. High-quality and varied graphic capabilities.
8. Possibility of interesting shapes.
9. Fully recyclable, environmental friendly packaging.

Disadvantages

Metal is heavier than plastic or glass.

Applications

Some metals and metal alloys possess high structural strength per unit mass, making them useful materials for carrying large loads or resisting impact damage. Metal alloys can be engineered to have high resistance to shear, torque and deformation.

The two most commonly used structural metals, iron and aluminium, are also the most abundant metals in the Earth's crust.

Metal packaging offers a comprehensive range of advantages in the near and long term. These have been grouped under the following sections:

1. Cans prevent waste.
2. Cans keep consumers safe and healthy.
3. Cans are cost effective and economical through the supply chain.
4. Cans are produced from viable sources of raw materials
5. Cans are the packaging recycling champions.
6. Cans use resources with care consistently achieving– "more with less".

6.2 ALUMINIUM

Aluminium (Al) is the most abundant metal on this planet which is silvery-whitish in appearance. There are several aluminium properties that makes aluminium, one of the most heavily used element. It has the symbol Al and its atomic number is 13. It is not soluble in water under normal circumstances. It makes up about 8% by weight of the Earth's solid surface.

Physical Properties

Atomic weigh and atomic number: The atomic weight of aluminium is 26.98 and its atomic number is 13.

Melting and Boiling Point: Aluminium melts when it is heated up to the temperature of 660.2°C and it will start boiling if the temperature is raised up to 2,467°C.

Strength and weight: Aluminium, in its purest form is a soft metal and very light in weight.

Heat and electrical conductivity: Aluminium is counted among the very good conductors of heat and electricity.

Chemical properties: Chemical aluminium properties mainly concern with chemical characteristics of aluminium such as it's reactivity, behavior towards acids, effect of temperature and pressure on reactivity, etc. Certain facts about chemical aluminium properties can be listed as follows:

Aluminium can form various salts which are soluble by reacting with certain mineral acids. Hydrogen gas is generated in this process.

The compounds which contain oxygen, get reduced when reacted with aluminium in the presence of high temperature.

Aluminium in the molten state reacts vigorously when brought in contact with water.

Aluminium forms a thin layer of oxide on its surface which protects it from being affected by open air, water, certain chemicals and solutions.

There are numerous other aluminium properties which are of particular use in a number of chemical and industrial applications. Aluminium is mainly obtained from its oxide ores and can be very economically recycled. These unique aluminium properties make aluminium one of the most important metal for industrial advancement.

Natural Occurrence

In the Earth's crust, aluminium is the most abundant (8.3% by weight) metallic element and the third most abundant of all elements (after oxygen and silicon).

Production and Refinement

Although aluminium is the most abundant metallic element in the Earth's crust, it is never found in free, metallic form, and it was once considered a precious metal more valuable than gold. Aluminium is a strongly reactive metal that forms a high-energy chemical bond with oxygen.

Recycling

Aluminium is 100% recyclable without any loss of its natural qualities. Recovery of the metal via recycling has become an important facet of the aluminium industry. The presence of aluminium can be detected in qualitative analysis using aluminon.

Advantages

They provide attractiveness of tin at lower cost. Aluminium is a light metal hence shipment cost of the product is low.

Disadvantages

Any substance that reacts with the oxide coating can cause corrosion.

Applications

Aluminium packaging via its unique combination of properties contributes to the efficient fabrication, storage, distribution, retailing and usage of many products. It can contain, protect, decorate or even dispense products as diverse as soft drinks and soaps, pet foods and snack foods, tobacco and toiletries, chocolates and chilled foods, tablets and take-away meals -even tennis balls and welding rods. Aluminium packaging has become part of everyday life. Depending upon the application, aluminium can be used to replace other materials like copper, steel, zinc, tin plate, stainless steel, titanium, wood, paper, concrete and composites.

Packaging of Aluminium

Corrosion resistance and protection against UV light combined with moisture and odour containment plus the fact that aluminium is non-toxic and will not leach or taint the products has resulted in the widespread use of aluminium foils and sheet in food packaging and protection. The most common use of aluminium for packaging has been in aluminium beverage cans. Aluminium cans now account for around 15% of the global consumption of aluminium.

Other Applications of Aluminium

Ladders, High pressure gas cylinders, Sporting goods, Machined components, Road barriers and signs, Furniture, Lithographic printing plates.

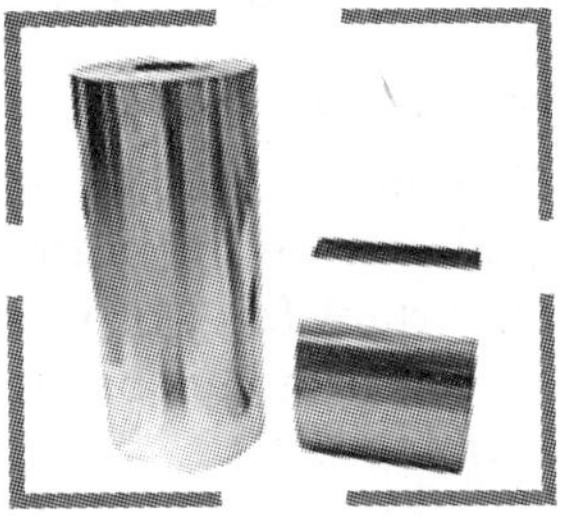

6.3 ALUMINIUM FOIL

Fig. 6.1: Aluminium foil

Aluminium as a metal is widely used in making aluminium foil, which in turn is, used an efficient packaging material. Aluminium foil is prepared out of aluminium in the form of thin sheets, which is about 0.02 mm in thickness. The foil is extremely pliable as a result of which it can be bent or wrapped around objects with great ease. Usually, an extremely thin layer, usually around 0.0065 mm is laminated to other materials like plastics and paper to make packaging material (Aluminium is produced in commercial foils as thin as 0.0065 mm (or 6.5 μm). Material thicker than 0.2 mm is called sheet or strip).

Aluminium Foil as a Packaging Material

Aluminium foil was used as a packaging material shortly after its initial production way back in 1913. Aluminium foil is one of the major flexible packaging material and is used all over the world in the protection and packaging of foods, cosmetics and chemical products. About 85% of all aluminium foil produced is used in some form of packaging. The major packaging applications of aluminium foil are:

- Household foil, 35%
- Laminated foil, 30% and
- Formed containers, 28.5%.

Aluminium foil does not harbour or promote the growth of bacteria, is sterile following the thermal treatment during its production process. It is also an ideal protection against product tampering – whether as an extended bottle neck foil or as a secure closure diaphragm.

Aluminium foil is impervious to light, gases, oils and fats, volatile compounds and water vapour. These properties combined with high formability, heat and cold resistance, non toxicity, strength and reflectivity to heat and light mean aluminium foil is used in many applications. These applications include:

- Pharmaceutical packaging
- Food protection and packaging
- Insulation
- Electrical shielding
- Laminates

Manufacture

Aluminium foil is produced by rolling sheet in gots cast from molten aluminium, then re-rolling on sheet and foil rolling mills to the desired thickness, or by continuously casting and cold rolling. To maintain a constant thickness in aluminium foil production, beta radiation is passed through the foil to a sensor the other side. If the intensity becomes too high, then the rollers adjust, increasing the thickness. If the intensities become too low and the foil has become too thick, the rollers apply more pressure, causing the foil to be made thinner. The continuous casting method is much less energy intensive and has become the preferred process. For thicknesses below 0.025 mm (0.001 in), two layers are usually put together for the final pass and afterwards separated which produces foil with one bright side and one matte side. The two sides in contact with each other are matte and the exterior sides become bright, this is done to reduce tearing, increase production rates, control thickness, and get around the need for a smaller diameter roller. Some lubrication is needed during the rolling stages; otherwise the foil surface can become marked with a herringbone pattern. These lubricants are sprayed on the foil surface before passing through the mill rolls. Kerosene based lubricants are commonly used, although oils approved for food contact must be used for foil intended for food packaging.

Aluminium becomes work hardened during the cold rolling process and is annealed for most purposes. The rolls of foil are heated until the degree of softness is reached, which may be up to 340°C for 12 hours. During this heating, the lubricating oils are burned off leaving a dry surface. Lubricant oils may not be completely burnt off for hard temper rolls, which can make subsequent coating or printing more difficult.

Properties

Aluminium foil has a highly reflective side and a more matte side. This is due to a common manufacturing process. As the foil is easy to tear, it is sent through machines in pairs. The side where the foil comes in contact with the other sheet is more matte than the other side.

Aluminium foils thicker than 0.025 mm (0.001 in) are impermeable to oxygen and water. Foils thinner than this become slightly permeable due to minute pinholes caused by the production process.

Benefits of Aluminium Foil as a Packaging Material

- Excellent impermeability to water vapour and gases.
- Extends shelf life.
- Uses less storage space.
- Generates less waste than many other packaging materials.
- Used as the barrier component in flexible cans.
- Acts as a barrier to oxygen, light, and odour.
- Nontoxic and hygienic.
- Greaseproof and non-absorptive to liquids.

- Ultraviolet radiations increase the forming of rancidity in certain foods and pharmaceutical products. Since foil is a good barrier to this radiation, resisting loss in flavour and appearance, and showing development of rancidity and staleness, it is widely used in storing food and pharmaceutical items.
- The aluminium packaging foil can be coated for protection, decoration, or heat sealing.

Applications of Aluminium Foil in Packaging

- Aluminium foil is used for pharmaceutical blister packages.
- It is used in the aseptic drink box.
- Suited for packaging medicinal oils.
- Suitable for packing ointments, grease-base cosmetics.
- As an effective barrier to light, aluminium foil is used extensively to package photographic materials and other light-sensitive products.
- It is used to make long life packs for dairy products, drinks, and many other sensitive foods.
- Aluminium foil trays and containers are used to bake cakes and pies.
- It is also used to pack takeaway meals, ready snacks and long life pet foods.
- Aluminium foil is used for wrapping food in order to preserve it in refrigerator.
- Candy-bar and chewing gum wraps make use of many of the desirable properties of aluminium foil.

Transparent Aluminium

Transparent aluminium is a state of aluminium achieved by bombarding a thin (50 nm) Al foil with soft X-ray laser radiation (wavelength 13.5 nm). The short laser pulse knocks out a core L-shell electron from every aluminium atom without breaking the crystalline structure of the metal making it transparent to soft X-rays of the same wavelength. This phenomenon is called saturable absorption. The thus produced transient state of aluminium is as dense as ordinary matter but can only exist for an extremely short period of time, as the energy required to maintain the high temperature which would be necessary to hold it in this state would be enormous. To create transparent aluminium, more power than is used by an entire city had to be focused into a dot with a diameter of less than one-twentieth of a thickness of a human hair, and then could only maintain the transparent state for 40 femtoseconds.

6.4 COLLAPSIBLE TUBES

Collapsible, soft metal tubes, today known as "flexible packaging", were first used for artists paints in 1841. Toothpaste was invented in the 1890s and started to appear in collapsible metal tubes. But food products really did not make use of this packaging form until the 1960s. Later, aluminium was changed to plastic for such food items as sandwich pastes, cake icings and pudding toppings. The metal tube's pre-eminent position is due to its unique qualities and characteristics: it is non-porous, light in weight, sanitary, durable, versatile, non-refillable, decorative, easy to handle, has a long shelf life and is adaptable to modern mass production methods and to automatic packaging. It is thus eminently suited for dispensing, in easily controlled portions, medicinal and pharmaceuticals, cosmetics, shaving creams, dentifrices, spread-type food products, and household and industrial items such as lubricants, adhesives and similar products. More than 40 standard sizes of tubes are available in sizes ranging in diameter from 3/8 to 2 inches, in length from 2 to 10 inches and in capacity from 3/4 dram to 16 ounces in aluminium, lead, tin, tin-coated lead and tin-lead alloy. Product compatibility largely determines the type of metal to be employed.

Collapsible Tube Packaging

Tubes find wide usage for packing adhesives/glues, toothpastes and other cosmetics, art colours/fabric paints, pharmaceuticals and oil paints.

Features of Standard Collapsible Tubes

- Plain or Printed in one or maximum 4 colours.
- Internally lacquered.

- Latex-lined to prevent leakage in the case of water based products.
- With open nozzle, closed nozzle or elongated nozzle.
- With or without caps of the desired type, style and colour.

Quality Features

- Superior protection, keeping the contents fresh and unadulterated through long periods of intermittent use.
- Tubes are of inconsequential weight, leak-proof, sturdy and indestructible.
- Economically advantageous.
- Compatible with a wide variety of substances.
- Can take on a protective coating.
- Corrosion resistant.
- Non-toxic and can be recycled.

Aluminium Collapsible Tubes

The collapsible aluminium tube embodies over 60% of the collapsible tubes used in a wide spectrum of industries. Aluminium is resilient to a variety of products and wherever essential, it can be given a protective/decorative coating. At the same time, the use of aluminium tube is highly economical. In fact, collapsible aluminium tube is considered as a critical packaging material for the protection of sensitive pharmaceuticals, medicines, foods and aggressive chemicals. Available in all diameters and lengths ranging from 10 to 57 mm, with options for different types of nozzles, lacquers and external finishes. These tubes are fabricated using highest purity aluminium, which can be easily recycled after use.

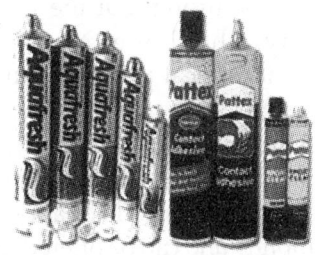

Fig. 6.2: Aluminium collapsible tubes

Applications

Aluminium tubes that finds wide application in several industries across the world. Tubes for packing pharmaceutical products, cosmetics, toothpastes, adhesives, paints and other products. Aluminium Collapsible Tube for Pharmaceutical Industry a wide range of collapsible tubes that is made from high quality aluminium. Durable in quality, these tubes are hygienically made to be used in pharmaceutical industry. We have designed our products in sizes to meet different packaging specifications, including critical tolerances for wall, annealing, coatings and seals.

Aluminium collapsible tube for artist paints: Aluminium collapsible used in the packaging of artist paints.

Aluminium collapsible tubes for ointments, cosmetics and adhesives: Aluminium collapsible tubes are widely used in packaging of ointments, cosmetics and adhesives across the globe. Superior in quality, these products are known for their durability and can be offered in different sizes.

Aluminium collapsible tubes long nozzel: These replaced tin tubes throughout the world and reduced the cost to 20%. Today, the Long Nozzle is used for adhesives and pharmaceutical products, such as eye ointments and surgical adhesives.

Aluminium collapsible tubes for paints: Aluminium made collapsible tubes are widely used in packaging of paints across the globe. Superior in quality, these products are known for their durability and can be offered in different sizes, Plastic Collapsible.

Aluminium collapsible tubes: Also used in packaging of Fairness Cream Tubes, Sealant Tubes, Ophthalmic Tubes, Antiseptic Cream Tubes, Aluminium Collapsible Printed Tubes, Aluminium Collapsible Tubes, Ointment Tubes, Laminate Tubes.

6.5 TIN

Tin is a chemical element with the symbol Sn50. Tin has10 stable isotopes. Tin is obtained chiefly from the mineral cassiterite, where it occurs as tin dioxide, SnO_2. Tin is a soft, pliable, silvery-white metal. Tin is not easily oxidized and resists corrosion because an oxide film protects it. Tin resists corrosion from distilled sea and soft tap water, and can be attacked by strong acids, alkalis and acid salts.

Physical Characteristics

Malleable, ductile, brittle, highly crystalline silvery-white metal.

Allotropes

Major Allotropes

1. α-tin (gray tin)–α-tin has a diamond cubic crystal structure, similar to diamond, silicon or germanium. Gray tin has no metallic properties at all, is a dull-gray powdery material and has few uses.
2. β-tin (white tin)–White tin, or the β-form, is metallic, and is the stable one at room conditions or at higher temperatures.

Chemistry and Compounds

Tin resists corrosion from distilled, sea and soft tap water, but can be attacked by strong acids, alkalis, and acid salts. Tin can be highly polished and is used as a protective coat for other metals in order to prevent corrosion or other chemical action. Tin acts as a catalyst when oxygen is in solution and helps accelerate chemical attack. Sn is dissolved by HCl, HNO_3, H_2SO_4 and, more slowly, by organic acids (acetic, oxalic or citric acid) and also by strong alkali, like NaOH and KOH. Tin becomes a superconductor below 3.72 K.

Production: Tin is produced by reducing the ore with coal in a reverberatory furnace.

Advantage: Tin is very resistant to Chemical attack.

Disadvantage: Tin is more expensive metal than aluminium, lead and iron.

Applications: Tin is used in for can coating: tin-plated steel containers are widely used for food preservation. Tin alloys are employed in many ways: as solder for joining pipes or electric circuits, pewter, bell metal, and dental amalgams. The niobium-tin alloy is used for superconducting magnets, tin oxide is used for ceramics and in gas sensors (as it absorbs a gas its electrical conductivity increases and this can be monitored). Tin foil was once a common wrapping material for foods and drugs, now replaced by the use of aluminium foil.

Tin containers: Metal Tin Container, Square Tin Container, Food Container, Oil Container, Pesticide Containers, Liquid

Container, Blue Container, Giftable Tin Container, Long Metal Containers.

Tin cans: Ghee Tin, OTS Cans, OTS Cans for Pickings, Flatten Tin Cans.

Food tin cans: Fancy cans, Beverage cans, Milk can oil and Paint tin cans- Oil tin cans, Additive containers, Olive oil Containers, Spout tins, Double tight tins, Container for Chemicals, Insecticide containers, Containers for preservatives, Liquid product containers, Tight lid tin cans, Small tin containers.

Tin plated metal from can: Tin bonds readily to iron, and is used for coating lead or zinc and steel to prevent corrosion. Tin-plated steel containers are widely used for food preservation, and this forms a large part of the market for metallic tin. Window glass is most often made via floating molten glass on top of molten tin. Most metal pipes in a pipe organ are made of varying amounts of a tin/lead alloy, with 50%/50% being the most common. Tin foil was once a common wrapping material for foods and drugs.

Solder: A coil of lead-free solder wire. Such solders are primarily used for solders for joining pipes or electric circuits.

Organotin compounds: Organotin compounds have a relatively high toxicity, and for this they have been used for their biocidal effects in/as fungicides, pesticides, algacides, wood preservatives, and antifouling agents. Tributyltin oxide is used as a wood preservative.

Precautions: Tin plays no known natural biological role in humans, and possible health effects of tin are a subject of dispute. Tin itself is not toxic but most tin salts.

6.6 LEAD

Lead's symbol Pb is an abbreviation of its Latin name plumbum for soft metals. Lead is a dense, ductile, very soft, highly malleable, and bluish white metal. Lead is highly resistant to corrosion. Lead is used to contain corrosive liquids (e.g. sulphuric acid). Lead is the only metal in which there is zero Thomson effect. Lead is used in building construction, lead-acid batteries, bullets and shot, weights, and is part of solder, pewter, fusible alloys and radiation shields. Lead is a poisonous metal that can damage nervous connections (especially in young children) and cause blood and brain disorders.

Physical and Chemical Properties

1. *Appearance:* Small, white to blue-gray metallic shot or granules.
2. *Odour:* Odourless.
3. *Solubility:* Insoluble in water.
4. *Density:* 11.34
5. *% Volatiles by volume @ 21°C (70°F):* 0
6. *Boiling Point:* 1740°C (3164°F)
7. *Melting Point:* 327.5°C (622°F)
8. *Vapor Pressure (mm Hg):* 1.77 @ 1000°C (1832°F)

Sources and Production

Lead metal is described as being either primary or secondary. Primary lead is produced directly from mined lead ore. Secondary lead is produced from scrap lead products which have been recycled.

Handling and Storage

Keep in a tightly closed container, stored in a cool, dry, ventilated area. Protect against physical damage.

Health Effects

Lead is a poisonous metal that can damage nervous connections (especially in young children) and cause blood and brain disorders. Lead poisoning typically results from ingestion of food or water contaminated with lead; but may also occur after accidental ingestion of contaminated soil, dust or lead based paint.

Advantages

1. Lead is a soft metal.
2. Lowest cos of all the metal used in pharmaceutical packaging.

Disadvantages

1. Lead is a poisonous metal that can damage nervous connections (especially in young children) and cause blood and brain disorders.

2. Lead container always required internal lining of inert metal or plastic.

Applications

- Lead bricks are commonly used as radiation shielding.
- Lead is used for the ballast keel of sailboats.
- It is used in scuba diving weight belts.
- Roman lead water pipes with taps.
- Lead pipe in Roman baths.
- Lead is a major constituent of the lead-acid battery used extensively as a car battery.
- Lead is frequently used in polyvinyl chloride (PVC) plastic, which coats electrical cords.
- Lead is used as shielding from radiation (e.g. in X-ray rooms).
- Molten lead is used as a coolant (e.g. for lead cooled fast reactors).
- Lead is used as electrodes in the process of electrolysis.
- Lead is used in high voltage power cables as sheathing material to prevent water diffusion into insulation.
- Lead has many uses in the construction industry (e.g. lead sheets are used as architectural metals in roofing material, cladding, flashings, gutters and gutter joints, and on roof parapets).
- Lead is still widely used in statues and sculptures.
- Tetra-ethyl lead is used as an anti-knock additive for aviation fuel in piston driven aircraft.
- Due to its half-life of 22.2 years the radioactive isotope 210_{Pb} is used for dating material from marine sediment cores by radiometric methods.

Former Applications

- Lead pigments were used in lead paint for white as well as yellow, orange and red.
- Lead was the hot metal used in hot metal type setting.
- Lead was used for plumbing in Ancient Rome.
- Lead was used as a preservative for food and drink in Ancient Rome.
- Lead was used for shotgun pellets in the US.

- Lead as a component of the paint used on children's toys-now restricted in the United States and across Europe.
- Lead was used in car body filler.

Testing

Water contamination can be tested with commercially available kits. Analysis of lead in whole blood is the most common and accurate method of assessing lead exposure in human. Erythrocyte protoporphyrin (EP) tests can also be used to measure lead exposure, but are not as sensitive at low blood lead levels (<0.2 mg/L). Lead in blood reflects recent exposure. Bone lead measurements are an indicator of cumulative exposure. While measurements of urinary lead levels and hair have been used to assess lead exposure, they are not reliable.

6.7 STAINLESS STEEL

In metallurgy stainless steel, also known as inox steel or inox Stainless steel does not stain, corrode, or rust as easily as ordinary steel (it stains less, but it is not stain-proof). It is also called corrosion-resistant steel. Stainless steel differs from carbon steel by the amount of chromium present. Carbon steel rusts when exposed to air and moisture.

Properties

High oxidation-resistance in air at ambient temperature are normally achieved with additions of a minimum of 13% (by weight) chromium, and up to 26% is used for harsh environments. When stainless steel parts such as nuts and bolts are forced together, the oxide layer can be scraped off, causing the parts to weld together.

Applications

Stainless steel's resistance to corrosion and staining, low maintenance, relatively low cost, and familiar luster make it an ideal base material for a host of commercial applications. There are over 150 grades of stainless steel, of which fifteen are most common. The alloy is milled into coils, sheets, plates, bars, wire, and tubing to be used in cookware, cutlery, hardware, surgical instruments, major appliances, industrial equipment, and as an automotive and aerospace structural alloy and construction material in large buildings. Storage tanks and tankers used to transport orange juice and other food are often made of stainless steel, due to its corrosion resistance and antibacterial properties. This also influences its use in commercial kitchens and food processing plants, as it can be steam-cleaned, sterilized, and does not need painting or application of other surface finishes. Stainless steel is used for jewellery and watches. The most common stainless steel alloy used for this is 316 L. It can be re-finished by any jeweller and will not oxidize or turn black. Some automotive manufacturers use stainless steel as decorative highlights in their vehicles.

Recycling and Reuse

Stainless steel is 100% recyclable. An average stainless steel object is composed of about 60% recycled material of which ≈40% originates from end-of-life products and ≈60% comes from manufacturing processes.

Types of Stainless Steel

There are different types of stainless steels: when nickel is added, for instance, the austenite structure of iron is stabilized. This crystal structure makes such steels non-magnetic and less brittle at low temperatures. For greater hardness and strength, more carbon is added. When subjected to adequate heat treatment, these steels are used as razor blades, cutlery, tools, Pipes and fittings, etc.

Stainless Steel Grades

There are a number of different systems for grading stainless and other steels. The article on US SAE steel grades details a large number of grades with their properties.

Stainless Steel in 3D Printing

Some 3D printing providers have developed proprietary stainless steel sintering blends for use in rapid prototyping. Currently available grades do not vary in properties significantly.

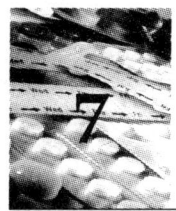

Blister and Strip Packaging

7.1 INTRODUCTION

Retail package in which a clear or opaque plastic or metal-foil seal holds the product (usually capsules, tablets, or other types of small items) against a sheet of card is called blister pack. And blister packaging is a method of packaging items in a clear plastic envelope or window that allows customers to view the contents prior to purchase.

A blister pack assembly of transparent sheet-sheet construction, said assembly comprising a bottom sheet that forms one halve of the envelope and a top sheet deformed to create a cavity in which an object may be contained or a blister pack is essentially a two layer sandwich of plastic with the upper layer deformed into a bubble in approximately the middle of the assembly to allow an object to be enclosed therein.

The term "blisters, blister packs, plastic blisters, custom plastic blisters, or blister packaging" are essentially generic terms which refer to the style, type and method of packaging. This type of packaging is created via the process of thermoforming. A "blister pack", or "blister packaging" consists of two distinct parts or halves. The "blister" portion of the package describes a clear plastic "bubble" or "shell" which has been designed to fit the intended product or products. The "seal" area of a blister is called the "flange". The other half of the "blister pack" consists of a paper or foil backing which contains a heat activated adhesive. This adhesive is activated by secondary sealing equipment and tooling through heat and pressure. During this process the product is "sealed" between the plastic blister and foil or paper backing creating a tamper evident, product encapsulated package.

Blister packaging is one of the most popular forms of packaging for both the pharmaceutical and retail environments. Its' popularity largely stems from the fact that it allows the product to be see, can be easily automated and is a relatively low cost packaging solution. Many pharmaceutical and drug manufacturers use a "form-fill and seal" blister application. This describes the process in which a machine will form the blister or blisters, fill the blisters with the intended product and then seal the product in the blister with either a paper or foil lid of some sort. The fact that this process is done on one machine and requires very little human involvement after start up makes "form-fill and seal" an ideal vehicle for the packaging of drugs and medication. There are however distinct limitations with regards to the blister size and design but again, when dealing with either medication or drugs "from-fill and seal" is still the best method for packaging these items.

The other method of blister packaging is generally best suited for small to high volume packaging of retail or consumer goods. This process allows for more flexibility with regards to the blister design and can accommodate larger and heavier objects than can a "form-fill and seal" operation. This type of blister packaging application does require secondary seal equipment and tooling, but change over from "job to job" is quicker and easier than with a "form-fill and seal" application.

One of the most prevalent forms of blister packaging, and also the most user-friendly, is found in single-dose strips of both over-the-counter (OTC) and prescription pharmaceuticals. The packs not only provide protection to the drugs themselves, but can be handy for the consumer in helping them make certain they have taken the correct dosage. These blister packs open quite easily, and do not require excessive ripping, tearing, cutting, or cursing.

7.2 BLISTER PACKAGE

- **Face seal blister:** Thermoformed PVC blister is heat sealed to the front of a blister card.
- **Trap blister:** Where a flange of the thermoformed blister is "trapped" between a front and a back blister card (or between a fold over card).

- **2 piece blister:** This is also referred to as a clamshell package where there is a front blister that matches up with a rear blister capturing a graphic card and the product in-between them. The two halves can then be snapped together or sealed around the perimeter using RF technology to secure the package.
- **Combination clamshell and blister:** This is a hinged clamshell that encapsulates the product and then snaps closed, but it has a flange around the perimeter of the clamshell that allows it to be heat sealed to a blister card. This style is especially beneficial for a product that requires a "recloseable" feature. In addition this option allows the product to be viewable from both sides of the blister card.

7.3 BLISTER DESIGN PARAMETERS

1. **Blister card size:** Blister card to be as small as possible as it will play a "cost" role in the sealing part of the process. Smaller is always better. Thickness or caliper of a standard style blister card is typically .021 points.
2. **Hang hole:** Every blister card has a die cut hang hole. This is not an additional cost and is required by most retailers.
3. **Foot:** This is a protrusion of plastic specifically designed at the base of the PVC rigid blister that would allow the final blister package to stand vertical on a store shelf. Blisters designed with a foot would still have a hang hole in the blister card.
4. **Minimum production runs:** Minimum run is 10K units.
5. **Artwork:** Art can be supplied on a disk. All art files. Recommendation of 4 colour plus any PMS colours for the front, but least expensive printing option is to have only 1 colour on the back of the card. This colour should be black. Many users prefer four colours on the back of the blister card but this could double the price of the card.
6. **Final pack-out options:** Blister packaged materials, should be packed into cartons that are shippable. Choices are master cartons (shippers), counter displays, POP displays, sidekick displays, PDQ displays, or club pack displays.

7.4 MATERIALS

1. Lidding Materials

The barrier and function demand for the blister package usually determine the lidding material. This is typically a foil structure that seals to the vinyl. The following materials offer properties that can aid in package stability, child resistance, tamper evidence and compliance. Lidding materials can be printed with product labelling or other related information.

Blister packaging material used mainly to "PTP" Medicinal hard aluminium foil and plastic film. Pharmaceutical aluminium foil is sealed in plastic film on the hard-sealing material, it hard for industrial use aluminium as a substrate, with non-toxic, corrosion-resistant, non-penetration, resistance heat, moisture, high-temperature sterilization may be blocking light and so on.

Medicinal aluminium foil material selection issues and principles: demand-side before the introduction of PTP aluminium foil, In the contract technical requirements for products must specify: the product name, size (width and thickness requirements), printing colour, aluminium foil roll arrangement of the direction and position of the text; aluminium foil structure, and adhesive coating weight, coating colour availability requirements, packaging requirements.

Aluminium Foil

Hard aluminium foil coated with heat seal lacquer- when sealed at an appropriate temperature, pressure and dwell time, it reduces the risk of reaction, spillage and leakage. It also protects drugs till the prescribed shelf life. The lidding material consists of support material like aluminium that has a printed primer on one side and a sealing agent like a heat-sealing lacquer on the other side. The sealing agent side faces the product and the forming films. And paper aluminium, paper/PET aluminium laminates, soft aluminium are also used as lidding material.

2. Forming Film Materials

Hard plastic sheet material is usually selected polyvinyl chloride (PVC), polyvinylidene chloride (PVDC), or composite materials. Their water, steam, light has good barrier properties.

To have the moisture and antioxidant requirements, or require a longer shelf-life of drugs can choose a hard PET film, PP rigid film.

Composite Hard films are: PVC and PVDC composite sheets (PVC/PVDC) or polyvinyl chloride and polyethylene and polyvinylidene chloride (PVC/PE/PVDC) composite films.

Oral, suppository medicines can choose PVC and polyethylene composite film (PVC/PE). Select Hard-chip pharmaceutical blister packaging materials.

PVC Film

The most commonly used blister film is polyvinyl chloride (PVC), which is considered to be a very forgiving material. Most materials to date have been PVC based. PVC scores high on properties like thermoforming, shape retention and sealing. PVC is an excellent thermoforming material providing good dimensional stability. When it is used as a forming film, it is called rigid PVC because it is almost free of softening agents-used for packing stable products.

PVDC Coated PVC Film

It is a primary packaging material for pharmaceutical applications for high moisture and oxygen sensitive products like capsules and vitamin tablets. PVdC coated PVC film has excellent barrier properties against: moisture, water vapour, and is used for packaging mid sensitive to sensitive products.

Cyclic Olefin Copolymer (COC)

Cyclic olefin copolymer (COC) offers exceptional cost and performance in pharmaceutical blister packaging. Not only does it provides long-term protection from water vapour, it thermoforms easily at low temperature, is exceptionally clear and has excellent stiffness. COC is used as the core layer in push-through packaging (PTP), either in five layer coextruded or three-layer laminated film structures. Outer layers can be made of polypropylene (PP), polyvinyl chloride (PVC) or polyvinylidene chloride-coated PVC. These materials can increase film impact strength and flexibility, add grease resistance and allow use of commonly available sealing systems. They also eliminate the need for lengthy trials, since they are approved for direct contact with pharmaceuticals.

Polypropylene (PP)

Polypropylene (PP), while rarely used, it is most difficult in terms of temperature ranges, shrinkage, and being unforgiving to new equipment. However, such problems do not appear to be the case with the newest blister film, cyclic olefin copolymer (COC), which is run with PP. In the structure, the COC is the core, and the PP is used like a film and has no structural function, and it has been perfectly processable, it does not crystallize. It is more or less an amorphous material.

If using cold-form foil, the process is a bit easier to predict because heat is not involved, and the materials are responding only to mechanical strain. Usually, the aluminium is laminated to two other materials, most often PVC and oriented polyamide (OPA), to resist cracking.

7.5 FORMATION

Principle Forming principle is either vacuum or compressed air thermoforming and plug assist for cold forming.

Types:
1. Thermoforming
2. Cold Forming

1. Thermoforming

The thermoforming process consists of heating a thermoplastic film to its softening temperature, then forcing the film against a cool forming mold by vacuum or pressure. The film is held against the mold surface and allowed to cool so that the plastic will retain the mold shape. The forming temperature of the sheet is one of the most critical processing parameters, and can be dependent on the cycle time. The core film temperature should reach 90 to 100°C, which corresponds to a pre-heating temperature of 110 to 130°C. It can be advantageous to reach higher temperatures with longer cycle times, rather than by increasing the plate temperatures to a level that causes sticking. Cooling temperature of the mold should be 10 to 20°C. Higher cooling temperatures can be used for deep forming or complex shapes. For thin-gauge thermoforming, the time to form and cool the sheet against the mold surface should generally equal the time to heat the sheet to the forming temperature.

Thermoforming Process

1. Principle of operation:
   - Thermoforming of the base web.
   - Filling the product.
   - Sealing the top web to the base film.
   - Cutting to finished shape.
   - Discharge of finishes packs.
2. Construction:
   - The chassis of the machine is made of anodized dural, the panels are produced in mild steel and all mechanical parts are treated against corrosion.
3. Thermoforming:
   - Male/Female forming.
   - The film is heated and blown into the shape of the mould by vacuumed and compressed air.
4. Loading:
   - This can automatically or manually carried out.
   - Manually filling of needle, syringe.
5. Sealing:
   - Is done by "Flat Sealing Plate".
   - Flat profile, regardless of the profile, a perfect seal is achieved by high even pressure at all points of the sealing area uniform temperature, accurate and adjustable temperature control.
6. Cutting:
   - The punch cutting tool is produced from hardened steel and incorporates edge cutting thereby eliminating centre wastage and ensure perfect alignment.
7. Discharge:
   - The finished packs are discharged from the machine on a collector to support the pack during cutting.
   - The waste film is automatically collected on other side.

8. Printing:
   - The thermoforming machine can be fitted with Ink Printer.
9. Operation:
   - The design of the thermo-forming machine is such that to obtain the best results, it is not necessary to have a skilled technician for its operation.

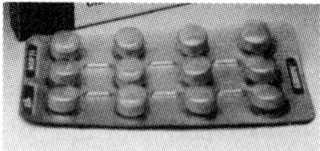

Fig. 7.1: Thermoform blisters

10. Chilled Water Plant
    - Thermoforming machine have an inbuilt chilled water plant and a separate unit is not required.

2. Cold Forming

Definition

Mechanical operation (such as bending, drawing, hammering, rolling) in which a metal shape is permanently deformed into a new shape, normally at room temperature. Cold forming increases the hardness and strength of the metal.

Cold forming is a process by which small, simple parts are produced. Unlike traditional metalworking processes, cold forming does not use heat. Instead, high pressure is applied to the metal blank in order to shape it. To be effective, this force must exceed the material's elastic limit. Because the process does not cut away material in order to form the metal part, cold forming is an efficient process that results in a minimum amount of waste product.

Cold headed fasteners have been formed by a similar process for over a century. During the cold forming process, a gripping die holds the cylindrical metal blank while an indented punch is used to form the metal into the desired shape. Today's cold formed parts are manufactured by automated equipment that can quickly produce parts that are consistent in shape.

Cold Forming Process

A laminated film in which a metal foil is sandwiched between two polymeric films is cold formed to define one or more blisters, and the base of the blister stamped with indicia, in two discrete stages. The blister is formed in the first stage using a standard technique of advancing a pin in a direction transverse relative to the plane of the film. According to the invention, once the blister forming stage is completed, indicia are stamped

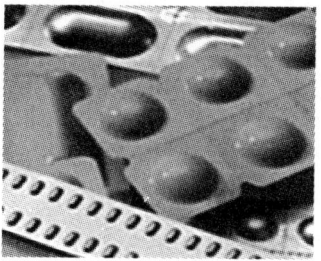

Fig. 7.2: Cold form blisters

into the base of the blister in the second stage by advancing a die from one side thereof to clamp the blister base against a mold held against the other side. The direction of the die and disposition of the die and mold may be selected such that the indicia project inwardly or outwardly from the blister base.

A method of forming a laminated film comprising a metal foil and a polymeric layer on either side of the foil with at least one blister.

In this process, an aluminium-based laminate film is simply pressed into a mold by stamp. Heat does not apply in cold forming.

The aluminium will be elongated.

This elongated aluminium sheet form a cavity and maintain a blister shape. During the formation of the blister the mold cavity is filled with an insert.

These blisters are called cold form foil (CFF) blisters. Finally it will be sealed with lidding material.

Advantages

Cold form blister packs offer an exceptional degree of protection to pharmaceutical products that may degrade through exposure to light, water vapour and other diffusing substances such as gases and odours.

All blister packs offer the advantages of convenience and improved patient compliance, as well as providing a finished, complete pack direct from the manufacturer to the end user.

In addition, suitably printed, they allow you a superb marketing opportunity to establish your brand identity in the patient's mind, improving the chances of your product gaining repeat purchase/prescription.

Disadvantages

The principle disadvantages of cold form Foil blisters are: the slower speed of production compared to thermoforming; the lack of transparency of the package and the larger size of the blister card (aluminium can not be formed with near 90 degree angles).

7.6 TYPES OF BLISTERS

1. Push Through Blister

Conventional blister packs are created by thermo-forming a web of plastic film, normally PVC, into pockets. These are filled with the pharmaceutical product, e.g. tablet or capsules and then sealed using heat and pressure. An important criterion for product and package development is to ensure that the dosage form (tablet or capsule) will not break when the patient pushes it out of the package.

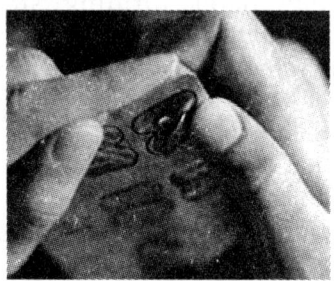

Fig. 7.3: Push through blister

Applications

Highly functional lidding foil that provides the best possible protection with a minimum of material. This foil is recommended for standard blister applications.

Function

Product can be accessed in a single step by simply pushing the blister's contents through the foil lid.

Benefits

- Strong seal to all blister materials, including PVC, PVdC, PP, PET, and cold-form blisters.
- Easy to push through.
- Total barrier to moisture, oxygen, and light means extended shelf life.
- Guaranteed to be pinhole-free for aluminium with a thickness of ≥ 20 μm.

- Attractive product appearance.
- Up to two-sided printing (in combination with exact front-to-back registration).
- FDA compliant

2. Peel Push Blister

Necessary steps to open the product:

1. Separate the individual blister cavity at the perforations.
2. Peel off the top layers (PET or PET/Paper at the designated place).
3. Push the pharmaceutical product through the foil.

Peel able lidding: Allows easy access to the product by simply peeling away the lid.

Child-resistant (CR): The combination of the appropriate blister bottom, lidding material and package design can.

Applications: Tablets, caplets, gel-caps-Powders-Diagnostics.

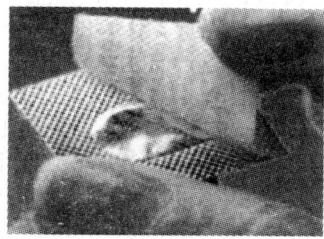

Fig. 7.4: Peel push blister

7.7 ADVANTAGES AND DISADVANTAGES OF BLISTER PACKAGING

Advantages

- Product is highly visible.
- Protects and holds the product securely (damage protection).
- Blister packs are very inexpensive to produce.
- Hanging slots for maximum display impact.
- Can be custom fit to help sell/promote products.
- Can have multiple products in a common blister.
- Many sizes available, from small unit-dose pills to large suit-case sized blisters.
- Allows products to be seen, but not touched.
- Hygienic storage conditions.
- Attractive design of blistercards using off-set printing.

The main advantages of blister packaging include a highly visible product, hanging slots for maximum display impact, product damage protection, hygienic storage conditions, attractive design of blistercards using off-set printing. It also included extended shelf life, due to protection against oxygen and humidity, that it provides for these medicinal tablets and capsules, compared to conventional packaging in bottles and containers. The aluminium foil is not supposed to be broken until just prior to the user ingesting the tablet or capsule.

Blister packs are widely used for medicinal and food supplement tablets and capsules, whereby these tablets or capsules are contained between a normally transparent, flexible plastic sheet, thermoformed so as to define a plurality of pockets, with each pocket being just large enough to receive the shape of the individual tablet or capsule, and a flat aluminium foil, heat sealed to said plastic sheet.

In the case of conventional bottles and containers, all of the tablets or capsules inside that bottle or container are exposed to external air and humidity every time that the cap is taken off in order to take out just one of these tablets or capsules.

The second advantage of blister packs is the convenience to the user of being able to carry around in his or her pocket or handbag just one flat and light blister card of tablets instead of having to carry the whole bulky and heavy bottle. The need to carry tablets on one's person applies to many tablets, such as headache, anti-histamine, contraceptive, antacid, anti-inflammatory and heart tablets, etc.

Disadvantage

- Blister packaging requires some type of a card to seal the blister to.
- Requires heat sealing the blister pack to the card.
- It suffers cost and non recyclability disadvantages.

The disadvantages include, for example, that the surfaces are often indented, which makes them difficult to grip, the sealing films are extremely thin (especially with pharmaceuticals), and the design surfaces used to display and present the products are very sensitive. Conventional mechanical, pneumatic, electrical grippers therefore usually reach their limits when it comes to handling products. A secure grip is often not guaranteed, especially in dynamic handling processes.

Polymeric blister films suffer from the disadvantage of being permeable, with the consequence that however well the individual blisters are sealed; there is always a potential storage problem if the contents of the blister must be protected from the surrounding atmosphere.

7.8 TYPES OF PROBLEMS/DEFECTS

Film Shrinkage

- Most Thermoforming films shrink somewhat during the thermoforming process.
- Concern is placed particularly on those films which shrink in an erratic manner.
- PCTFE films shrink more than PVC in the transmachine direction (TD). This shrinking both narrows the web and curls the film.
- Properly processed film may shrink 3–5% for copolymer and 1–3% for homopolymer PCTFE films.

Note: With all films, tension in the machine direction will result in loss of web width. Lessening the heat or increasing lines speeds will reduce the TD shrinkage in most films.

Film Curl

- Film Curl occurs when two or more films have different shrinkage rates.
- This most commonly occurs with PCTFE films that are laminated to PVC with a PE tie layer.
- Typical solutions to this difficulty are identical to reducing film shrinkage. Curl can also be reduced by duplex laminations and conversion to homopolymer materials.

Film Sticking

- May occur between the heating platens and/or to the forming mold.
- Most common with PVdC/PVC materials (PVdC-coating relatively tacky).
- Cleanliness and condition of heating platen surfaces important.
- Gap between platens should be uniform over entire area.

- Platens should be replaced or reconditioned periodically with a non-stick (e.g., Teflon) surface.
- Additional mold-cooling recommended for PVdC/PVC, but not for PCTFE laminations.
- Sticking may cause MD-stretching and web shrinkage.

Film Delamination

- PVC/PE/PCTFE – Adhesive is semi-activated during lamination, and is fully-activated upon application of heat during thermoforming.
- Adhesion strength increases remarkably during thermoforming.

Incomplete Blister Cavities

- Normally indicates insufficient heat to film.
- Is sometimes accompanied by milky-white areas within cavities.
- Is also seen with loss of forming air pressure (audible venting).
- Cavity formation may usually be improved by using more heat (higher temperatures and/or slower cycle speeds).
- Striations may be caused by excessive heat used on PCTFE laminations.
- The actual temperature of the heating plates needs to be calibrated against the read-out on the controller.

Poor Lid Stock Sealing

- Sealing temperature indicates heat applied to coating on aluminium foil-based lidstock.
- Sealing temperature normally identical for PVC, PVdC/PVC and PCTFE/(PE)/PVC (PVC is generally product and lidstock contact layer).
- Sealing to correct side?
- Minimum heat-seal activation temperature.
- Sealing pressure.
- Cleanliness, condition and pattern of sealing platens is important.
- Alignment and flatness of platens is important.

Blister Card Curl

- Most common with PCTFE laminations (card curls toward PCTFE side).
- Same phenomenon as film curl.
- Same cause as TD web shrinkage: higher TD shrinkage rate of raw PCTFE film compared to PVC and PE films.
- Curl normally may be decreased by using less heat at heating-platen station (lower temperatures and/or faster cycle speeds).
- Curl may also be decreased by utilizing duplex PVC/PCTFE construction.

7.9 BLISTER PACKING MACHINE

Products packed: Tablets, Dragees, Snapfit Capsules, Soft Gelatin Capsules, etc.

Packing material: Base Film: PVC Opaque or Transparent (thermoformable) and non-toxic, PVC with PVDC coating, PVC with PE/PVDC.

Lidding material: Aluminium (hard) with heat-sealable lacquer or PVDC coating.

Operation: The machine is used to Form, Fill and Seal Pharmaceutical products like tablets, capsules, dragees, etc. in blister packs.

PVC base film web is drawn off from a reel and fed into the blister-forming unit where blisters are continuously formed. The web is then passed over the guide track where the product is filled into the blisters by a suitable automatic filling unit and led to the sealing unit. Aluminium foil is drawn off a

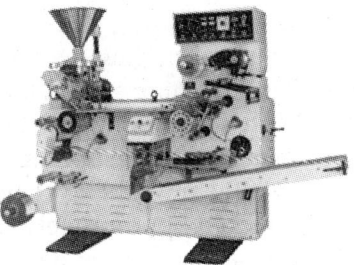

Fig. 7.5: Blister pack machine

separate reel and is fed to the sealing unit where it is sealed with the base web, thus sealing the product hermetically.

The filled and sealed web is then fed by an indexing mechanism into a pack punch unit where the packs are separated from the web. The web trim is sheared off to allow collection. The blister pack may either be collected in bins or be conveyed over a belt for further handling. The machine could also be linked to a cartoner.

Types of Blister Packing Machines

There are 2 main types of blister packing machine – the continuously operating line and the intermittently operating line. Here we outline the characteristics of both types.

1. Continuously Operating Lines

Advantage

The advantage of continuously operating machines, which are equipped with sealing rollers, is that they can achieve higher output.

Disadvantage

However, the heat-sealing process must be performed at higher temperatures; 200–300°C. This means that the packaging material is subjected to more stress and higher strains.

How Does it Operate?

With the following exceptions, the stations of the continuously operating machine function similarly to the stations of the intermittently operating machine:

- The unwinding station continuously supplies forming films and lidding materials.
- The stretching station follows the quality control station. With continuously operating machines, the eye-mark distances for the lidding material are sensed immediately after the unwinding station. Then the lidding material is stretched appropriately for the machine's speed.
- The sealing station on continuously operating machines is equipped with sealing rollers. The sealing temperatures range between 200 and 300°C.

In the course of this process, the lidding material is continuously sealed onto the forming film for the goods to be packaged.

2. Intermittently Operating Lines

Advantage

The major advantage of intermittently operating systems is that they work with sealing plates, and the sealing temperature can be relatively low: 140–200°C. Sealing with plates permits the use of larger widths of forming films and lidding materials because a more constant sealing effect can be expected.

Disadvantage

Intermittent processes tend to have slower operation, therefore slower output. Intermittent equipment also tends to require more maintenance because of the stop-and-start nature of the operation.

How Does it Operate?

The essential parts and functions of the intermittently operating packaging machine are outlined below:

- The unwinding station supplies the forming films and the lidding material at a rate corresponding to the speed of the packaging machine.

- The heating station raises the temperature of the plastic forming films to a level suitable for deep drawing. Forming films containing the PVC support material are heated to 120–140°C. PP forming films are heated to 140–150°C. Form films containing aluminium are not heated before the forming process.

- The forming station forms plastic films using either compressed air or die plates. Films containing aluminium are formed with mechanical forming tools only.

- The cooling station cools PP films after the forming process. There is no need to cool laminates containing PVC or aluminium.

- The feeding machine can be linked with the pockets, or the goods to be packaged can simply be swept into the pockets.

- The feeding machine can be linked with the pockets, or the goods to be packaged can simply be swept into the pockets.

- The feeding machine can be linked with the pockets, or the goods to be packaged can simply be swept into the pockets.
- The quality control station detects flaws that have occurred in the packaging process. After punching, these packages are rejected and scrapped.
- The sealing station heat seals the lidding material to the forming film that now contains the product.
- The cooling station is necessary with all forming films; PP forming films must be cooled longer than other types of film.
- The index station is a component only of machines that are controlled by a feeding mechanism. This device senses the eye-mark distances on the lidding material and thus governs the speed of the machine. This kind of control can operate satisfactorily only within very close eye-mark tolerances.
- The coding station marks the packages with a batch number.
- The perforating station makes a cross-shaped perforation along the sealing seams, which helps render the package child-proof.
- The punching station separates the packaging material into individual blisters.
- The cartoning station inserts the leaflet and the blister package into the surrounding carton or secondary package.
- The scales check the goods to be filled for the last time.
- The multi-packing machine packs the individual packages into bigger cartons.

Types of Blister Packing Process

Forming principle is either Vacuum or Compressed Air Thermoforming and Plug assist for Cold forming.

1. Vacuum based rotary thermoforming (Fig. 7.6)
2. Compressed air and Plug assist Platen forming (Fig. 7.7)

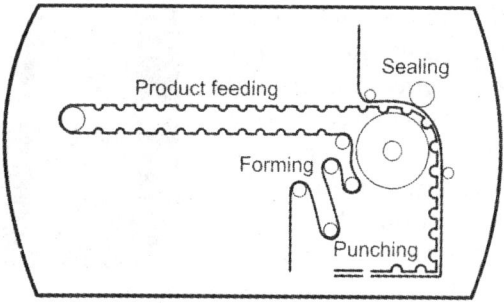

Fig. 7.6: Vacuum based rotary thermoforming

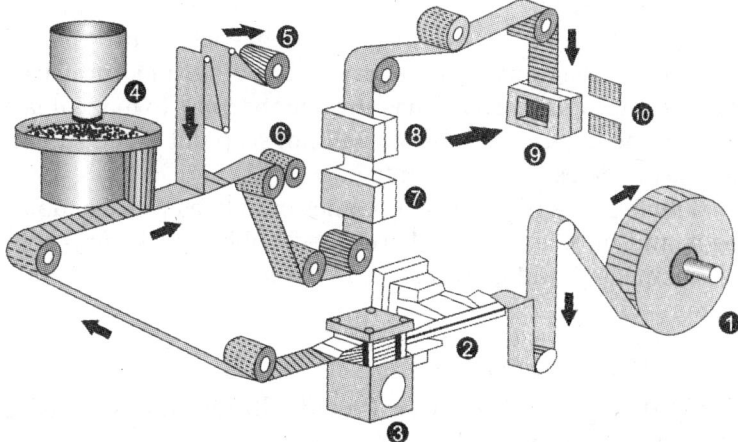

Fig. 7.7: Compressed air and plug assist platen forming: (1) Forming film rells, (2) Forming film preheating, (3) Pocket forming, (4) Auto feeding system (option), (5) Alu foil, (6) Sealing station, (7) Coding embossing, (8) Perforation, (9) Trimming and (10) Product

7.10 OTHER PACKAGES

1. Bubble Pack/Bubble Wrap

Flexible plastic sheeting containing numerous small air pockets, used in cushioning items during shipment. Also called bubble wrap. A transparent plastic blister used to package items of merchandise.

Bubble packaging is an extremely lightweight, durable packaging material that works well for wrapping items as well as filling the void in boxes. Bubble packaging absorbs shock to keep your fragile items safe. Its light weight also reduces shipping costs.

Bubble packaging comes in several different varieties. They usually vary in bubble size and barrier properties. Bubble packaging with small bubbles is generally used for small light items. Larger bubbles should be

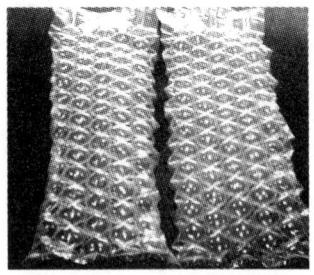

Fig. 7.8: Bubble pack/bubble wrap

used with larger and heavier items. The most economical bubble packaging has relatively weak barriers, which means the air will leak out over a shorter period of time. Industrial bubble packaging usually has stronger barriers to make it last longer and ensure that the air will not seep out when subject to heavy forces.

Bubble packaging normally comes in rolls, as well as bubble bags and bubble mailers. Perforated bubble packaging rolls save time and add convenience by eliminating the need for a cutter.

Bubble Packaging Benefits

Lightweight and effective: Provides better protection using less packaging materials.

Reduces damage: Cushioning material offers excellent protection for fragile items.

Reusable: Barriers trap air inside allowing bubble packaging to be reused.

Recyclable: Can be recycled.

2. Shrink Wrap

Shrink wrap is commonly used on commercial products where tamper-protection is a high priority, such as CDs or DVDs. After the item is wrapped, heat is applied to make the wrap shrink to fit. Because it creates such a tight seal and keeps moisture out, shrink wrap can also be used to package perishable food items.

3. Temper Resistant

Temper Resistance is resistance to tampering by either the normal users of a product, package, or system or others with physical access to it. There are many reasons for employing tamper resistance.

Tampering

Tampering involves the deliberate altering or adulteration of a product, package, or system. Solutions may involve all phases of product production, packaging, distribution, logistics, sale, and use. No single solution can be considered as "tamper proof". Often multiple levels of security need to be addressed to reduce the risk of tampering.

Safety

This prevents children and others who are careless or unaware of the dangers of opening the equipment from doing so and hurting themselves (from electrical shocks, burns or cuts, for example) or damaging the equipment.

Packaging

Layers of tamper resistance: carton with adhesive, shrink band, cap, innerseal.

Resistance to tampering can be built in or added to packaging. Examples include:

- Extra layers of packaging (no single layer or component is "tamper-proof").
- Packaging which requires tools to enter.
- Extra strong and secure packaging.
- Packages which cannot be resealed.
- Tamper-evident seals and features.

The tamper resistance of packaging can be evaluated by consultants and experts in the subject. Also, comparisons of various packages can be made by careful field testing of the lay public.

The blister pack has a reusable container mounted to a display card in a tamper resistant manner. The reusable container has a tray and a lid with the tray having frangible flanges thereon which are sealed to a presentation side of the display card. The lid has a deep channel which is received frictionally into the tray for securely closing the reusable container. Both the lid and the tray have enlarged finger engageable pull tabs for ease of opening the reusable container.

4. Helix Pack

Helix pack is an eco-friendly and low cost alternative to blister packaging. Blister packaging is well-known the world over. But it suffers cost and non-recyclability disadvantages. Traditionally, it is manufactured using individual product moulds and high grade PVC and this requires a significant investment in equipment and in energy during the manufacturing process.

The blister element is heat bonded to the backing card and as a result becomes contaminated with board fibres; this means it cannot be recycled.

Consumer has developed an alternative packaging system known as the helix pack which overcomes these disadvantages and adds further benefits. At the heart of the new design is a spiral (helix) cut sheet of material, which expands over the product, holding it securely against the backing card.

Benefits of Helix Pack Include

- Can be used in many different ways and it has a "one size fits" all capability.
- Unused packaging remains flat – reducing warehouse and transport demands.
- Increases production flexibility.
- Improves marketing by encouraging tactile shopping.
- Increases consumer appeal by its ease of opening.
- Allows a single item to be packed and shipped to a customer without in-line blister forming equipment – no tooling costs, no make-ready costs.
- Material savings up to 35% can be achieved, e.g. by using distortional elements in.
- Standard cardboard cartons.

Most importantly, the helix pack can be manufactured in such a way that all elements can be cleanly separated allowing them to be recycled in line with the European Packaging Waste Legislation: **Reduce – Reuse – Recycle**.

Helix pack has been awarded "Millennium Product" status by the UK Design Council and has been granted patents in the UK, Europe and the USA. On behalf of our client—the designer of the helix pack – we are now seeking a commercial packaging manufacturing partner who, with sufficient foresight and market reach, will be able to take on the design (for example, under a licensing agreement) and fully commercialise the product internationally.

7.11 STRIP PACKS—HIGH BARRIER LAMINATES

Strip packaging is just one of the quality packaging solutions for the packaging of tablets and capsules. Strip packaging is the form of unit dose packaging that is commonly used for the tablets, caplets, capsules or other relatively infrangible unit dosage forms. Strip packs are also known as high barrier laminates. In strip packaging individually enclosed elements arranged either in a single row or in at least two essentially parallel rows, and either the first or second sheet or both sheets are preferably opaque or dark-tinted.

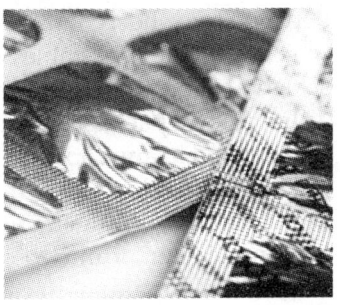

Fig. 7.9: Aluminium foil strip pack

This type of laminates will protect the product from moisture, light and oxygen whether the product is a tablet, effervescent tablet, and pill or transdermal therapy. Protection is provided from the time of manufacture all the way to the end-user. The package billboard can be printed very efficiently to generate strong product recognition and reinforce the required regulatory information. Besides product protection and marketing advantages, materials are designed to allow for optimal handling and maximum through put with conventional or custom packaging equipment.

"Strip package" or "strip packaging" formed by a method in which planar webs are brought together and sealed around the elements to be packaged. Thus, the strip package or packaging is based on two flexible sheets or foils which can be run as vertical webs on existing strip packaging machinery, and which contain no pre-formed blisters (whether they be cold-formed or thermo-formed) to which the said elements are fed to be packaged, and which are subsequently "lidded".

The flexible sheets on which the present strip packaging is based both together (and essentially equally) enclose the elements to be packaged, and the necessary accommodation of the elements is afforded by any necessary stretching of the material of each sheet as sealing takes place, not by any pre-forming operation. The packaged elements are enveloped between two sheets, one of which is burstable and the other of which is neither burstable not tearable, and which together are sealed around them to form a pocket enclosing each element.

In the strip package, the individually enclosed elements may be arranged in any convenient manner which (at the same time) generally affords a strip configuration. Thus, the elements may be in an in-line arrangement or staggered, and may be disposed in a single row, or in two or more rows, which generally will be essentially parallel to each other.

Strip packaging may be particularly appropriate for pharmaceutical products, it can also be used for other products where safety of young children is a factor. So that the package may meet current regulations, for example, as in the UK, the first and second sheet materials are preferably opaque. However, in some instances the use of dark-tinted material may be acceptable. In either event, the tinting or opacity may be provided by printing, or by the incorporation of one or more dyes, or more preferably one or more pigments, for example, a white pigment. Alternatively, a material which in itself is opaque such as one comprising a metal foil, may be selected.

Properties

- High barrier material for long shelf life
- Packaging of effervescent tablets, pills

- All laminate constructions are designed to run on high-speed packaging line.
- Strip packs can provide a cost effective, yet safe option for solid dose packaging.

Applications
- Effervescent Tablets
- Caplets
- Tablets
- Capsules

Advantages/Benefits
Some of the benefits associated with selecting strip packaging as primary packaging solution include:
- Strip packaging is an economical way to package small products and to prepare them for distribution.
- Strip packages will protect the product from moisture, light and oxygen.
- In addition to providing an efficient way to package products, strip packaging protects your products primarily from dirt and from being dropped or getting lost.
- Strip packaging keeps products free from contamination and it keeps small pills and tablets organized and separated until the moment they are ready to be consumed by customers.
- customer can use the product in a familiar, safe, and convenient way.

7.12 STRIP PACKAGING PROCESS
A method of manufacturing a strip package, which method comprises continuously feeding a web of first sheet material and a web of second sheet material, to a packaging station where they are disposed essentially vertically, feeding a plurality of elements to be packaged between the webs at the said station, sealing together the webs to form pockets around and to enclose the elements as one or more rows between the

webs and, if necessary or desired, sub-dividing the sealed webs into strip packages.

In strip package the two sheets include paper or metal foil, the first sheet preferably comprising a laminate of paper and a tear-resistant plastics material, together with an adhesive layer, or a metal foil laminated with a tear-resistant plastics material and including an adhesive layer, and the second sheet preferably comprising a laminate of paper and a plastics material which can provide adhesion and any necessary strength, or a metal foil having a layer of plastics material which can provide the necessary adhesion.

Wherein the first sheet comprises a laminate of paper, biaxially oriented nylon, and a low density polyethylene or vinyl adhesive, or a laminate of aluminium foil, polypropylene, and a low density polyethylene or vinyl adhesive, and/or the second sheet comprises a laminate of paper and a low density polyethylene or vinyl adhesive, or aluminium foil and a low density polyethylene or vinyl adhesive.

When the webs are chosen so that they can be adhered together by heat sealing and the webs are brought together under heat and pressure.

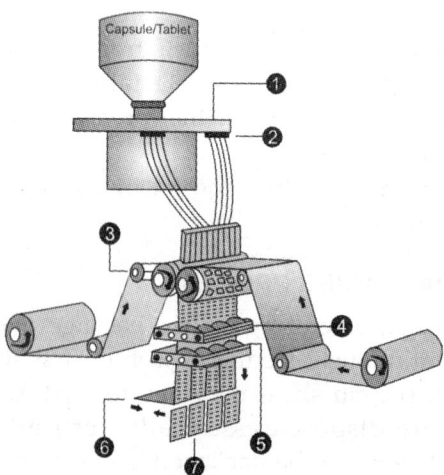

Fig. 7.10: Strip packaging: 1. Hopper, 2. Disc plate, 3. Heated crimping rollers, 4 and 5. Brush shaft, 6. Cut-off knife and 7. Strip packs

7.13 PACKAGING MATERIALS

The materials for the two sheets of the strip package may be chosen from a number of available packaging materials such as paper, metal foil and plastics materials. However, in order to meet the stringent requirements which in practice apply say to the packaging of pharmaceuticals in unit dosage form, the materials will preferably comprise laminated materials.

In particular, the first and second sheets may be provided as materials comprising a plurality of plies laminated together and preferably selected as follows:

First sheet: The first sheet preferably comprises one of the following materials, namely:

1. A laminate of paper, e.g. glassine, and a tear resistant, e.g. biaxially orientated plastics material such as a polyamide or polyester, together with an adhesive layer, preferably a heat-sealable adhesive layer. For example, a laminate of paper, e.g. glassine, biaxially orientated nylon, and a polyethylene, e.g. a low density polyethylene, or vinyl adhesive, or.

2. Metal, e.g. aluminium foil – typically soft foil laminated with a tear-resistant plastics material, such as polypropylene, and including an adhesive layer, preferably comprising a heat-sealable adhesive, for example, a polyethylene, e.g. a low density polyethylene, or vinyl adhesive.

Second sheet: The second sheet is preferably one which requires a push-through force of at least about 70 Newton, for example, about 75 Newton, before rupture takes place.

Given that additional criterion the second sheet preferably comprises one of the following materials, namely:

1. A laminate of paper, e.g. glassine, and a layer of plastics or other material which can provide adhesive (preferably heat-sealable adhesive) properties and any necessary strength properties, such as a polyethylene, e.g. a low density polyethylene, or vinyl adhesive. For example, a laminate of glassine and low density polyethylene; or.

2. Metal, e.g. aluminium foil – typically soft foil again provided with a layer of plastics or other material which

can provide the necessary adhesion, preferably heat adhesion, for example, a layer of a polyethylene, e.g. a low density polyethylene, or vinyl adhesive.

It will be understood, of course, that the two sheets chosen in any particular instance must have compatible adhesive properties within the limits of the chosen method of manufacture. Furthermore, they should preferably for convenience have a common adhesive material.

As described above the webs are preferably chosen so that they can be adhered together by heat sealing, i.e. by the application of heat and pressure, as the webs are brought together.

Sealant: PE, Surlyn, Coextrusion.

Choice of Drug Packaging Composite Film

Pharmaceutical companies the choice of drug packaging composite film, must be made by pharmaceutical properties (moisture, oxidation, Medicine Smell reservations, etc.) and shelf life is determined primarily on the basis of quality characteristics of pharmaceutical requirements, combined with characteristics of composite products choose to use, the following Medical composite membrane provides several features for reference:

a. *General composite membrane:* Composite structure of polyester with aluminium foil and polyethylene (PET/AL/PE), is characterized by a good printing adaptability, good for drugs gas, the moisture barrier.

b. *Medicinal easy tear strip composite films:* Composite structure in cellophane and polyethylene and aluminium foil compound (PT/PE/AL/PE). Characteristics are: easy to tear with a good, user-friendly access to products to consumers. Good gas, vapor barrier to ensure that the contents a longer shelf life. Applicable to effervescent agent, Paint, tablet capsules and other pharmaceutical packaging.

c. *Paper plastic composite films:* Composite structure to paper and polyethylene and aluminium foil composite (paper/PE/AL/PE), characterized by: a good printing and good stiffness. The gas or water has good barrier properties can ensure a longer shelf life medicines.

7.14 PROPERTIES OF MATERIALS

Strip packaging film has a certain tensile strength and elongation, suitable for a variety of shapes and sizes of the drugs, and packaged close to built-in medicine, not easy to produce rupture and wrinkles. At present, more widespread use of the aluminium-plastic composite film, such as cellophane and aluminium foil and polyethylene (PT/AL/PE), polyester and aluminium foil and polyethylene (PET/AL/PE), or aluminium foil and plastic film in order to stick compounding or extrusion laminated composite mixture made from the grass-roots, printing layer, barrier layer, sealing layer, grass-roots outside, including the sealing layer, barrier layer, printing layer in the middle. Base materials require excellent mechanical properties, good glossy print, transparency, good barrier properties, safe non-toxic, and no sealing ability. Typical materials are polyester (PET), cellophane (PT), and with a PVDC coated cellophane. Barrier layer should be good on gas and moisture barrier properties, not by bacteria and microorganisms, excellent mechanical properties, there is a certain elongation, cold and heat, safe non-toxic material is a typical soft aluminium foil. However, this soft aluminium foil opaque, itself does not rust, shading and strong. If the bar needs to be transparent packaging films, they have to make use of PVDC barrier layer materials.

PVDC barrier layer materials to make its most important feature is the gas, water vapor barrier properties superior. Sealing layer is the inner membrane strips, good sealing, while chemical stability and safety and health of the general use of low-density polyethylene material.

Advantages

The strip packaging may be used to package any element which is relatively infrangible. A strip package offers a higher level of resistance to being opened by children than current strip packages.

They can be produced by employing planar webs of two dissimilar materials to enclose the elements to be packaged, and thus to form the strip package, one material being highly tear resistant and the other sufficiently frangible to release a tablet or like packaged element when pressure is applied to the material via the tablet or the like. A child-resistant strip package, comprises a plurality of packaged elements each individually enclosed between a first sheet comprising a material which is tear resistant and which will not easily permit release of an element by tearing or application of pressure, and a second sheet adhered thereto and comprising a material which retains the elements but which is sufficiently frangible to permit release of an element by application of finger pressure to the element through the first sheet.

The strip packaging may be particularly appropriate for pharmaceutical products, it can also be used for other products where safety of young children is a factor. However, the invention particularly provides strip packaging for relatively infrangible pharmaceutical or like unit dosage forms such as tablets, caplets, capsules and the like.

7.15 CHILD-RESISTANT STRIP PACKAGE

Child-resistant packaging or C-R packaging is special packaging used to reduce the risk of children ingesting dangerous items. This is often accomplished by the use of a special safety cap. It is required by regulation for prescription drugs, over-the-counter medications, pesticides, and household chemicals. In some jurisdictions, unit packaging such as blister packs is also regulated for child safety.

A child-resistant strip package comprises a plurality of packaged elements each individually enclosed between a first sheet comprising a material which is tear resistant and which will not easily permit release of an element by tearing or application of pressure, and a second sheet adhered thereto and comprising a material which retains the elements but which is sufficiently frangible to permit release of an element by application of finger pressure to the element through the first sheet.

The package is manufactured by a method comprising continuously feeding a web of said first sheet material and a web of said second sheet material to a packaging station. There the webs are disposed essentially vertically and a plurality of elements to be packaged are fed between the webs. The webs are then sealed together to form pockets around and to enclose the elements as one or more rows between the webs.

Wherein the elements to be packed are tablets, caplets, capsules or other relatively infrangible unit dosage forms and including a multiplicity of individually enclosed elements arranged either in a single row or in at least two essentially parallel rows, and either the first or second sheet or both sheets are preferably opaque or dark-tinted. The first and second sheets are adhered together except where they form pockets around the elements. Wherein the first and second sheets are chosen so that they can be adhered together by heat and pressure sealing. The overall minimum width of any band of adherence between the sheets is at least about 5 mm. where the second sheet is one which requires a push-through force of at least about 70 Newton before rupture takes place.

Advantages

Strip packaging offers a higher level of resistance to being opened by children than current strip packages. Within a normal home environment most of the current forms of strip and blister packaging offer a high degree of protection against abuse by children. Strip packaging is also used for relatively infrangible pharmaceutical or like unit dosage forms such as tablets, caplets, capsules and the like.

. These forms of packaging afford less frequent cases of child-poisoning than conventional reclosable packs such as bottles.

A new type of strip package affords increased child-resistant properties and which, at the same time, can be used by adults without difficulty. In that respect, the unidirectional press- or push-through characteristics of the package (which typically may present the same overall appearance from both sides) can be conveyed to the adult user either in instructions printed on the package and/or in separate instructions on a package insert or on another associated packaging item.

The mode of opening the package of the invention differs from that of the conventional form of strip packaging in that with the present package there is a much higher level of resistance to tearing from the side-effectively amounting to a complete resistance to tearing by both young children and most adults-coupled with an intelligence element associated with the pressor push-through technique necessary to achieve opening.

Furthermore, when a tab of second sheet material is provided by a first opening, adjacent pockets generally cannot easily be opened subsequently by pulling the tab of second sheet material across the package.

Disadvantages

In forming the package, it is desirable that no perforations should be introduced into the package. As will be appreciated, any perforations could considerably reduce the level of its resistance to being opened by children, because any initiated cut or tear such as might be introduced by perforation could make the package susceptible of opening by further tearing. However, since the package permits the removal of individual elements through the second sheet by application of finger pressure, the presence of perforations, for example, to permit individually packaged elements to be torn away from the remainder of the package, is in any event not required.

Also, in practice, these forms of packaging afford less frequent cases of child-poisoning than conventional reclosable packs such as bottles. The disadvantage of reclosable packs lies in the fact that many people do not reclose them properly or refuse to accept packs with a child-resistant closure, thus offering a potentially greater hazard with a much larger and readily available number of tablets or the like than is ever presented by a strip or blister pack. In addition, there is the added factor of the interest shown by children to an audible sound or rattle, e.g. when a bottle is shaken, which is much less important for a strip or blister pack because such packs are less audibly interesting.

Nevertheless, we believe there is a potential need for a **new approach** to strip packaging in particular, which will permit of an even greater protection against abuse by children, and which at the same time can:

1. Permit the packaging to be run on existing machinery with little or no change to machine performance criteria.
2. Afford a commercially acceptable increase in material costs.

3. Present a greater obstacle to ingress by young children than most forms of packaging in current use.

4. Permit the packaging to be acceptable in a practical performance sense to the adult user. In particular, the package should be such as is openable without recourse to implements such as scissors while still offering the desired higher level of resistance to being opened by children.

7.16 STRIP SEALING MACHINE

- Suitable for high speed sealing of coated or uncoated tablets, capsules, lozenges, etc. of any shape or size in aluminium foils, polythene, cellophane or any other heat sealing material.
- *Feeding:* Fully automatic vibrator with hopper.
- *Chutes:* 2, 4, 6, 8 or 10 tracks to suite for application.
- *Sealing Rollers:* High precision carbon steel rollers, machined knurled, heat treated for minimum wear and tear, fitted with high quality heating elements.
- *Cutting Mechanism:* Horizontal and vertical cutting as required, achieved by steel knives fitted under the rollers and between the draw bushes.
- *Controls for Operation:* A Start – Stop switch is provided for the machine. A clutch for starting/Stopping the sealing rollers and a release mechanism for starting/stopping the feeding of tablets also provided. Rolls of the packing material are mounted on two shafts and knobs are fitted at the ends of the shafts for adjusting and positioning the rolls of the packing material in relation to the sealing rollers.
- *Speed Control:* By variable speed drive.

7.17 STRIP PACKING MACHINERY

Automatic high speed packing machine with a capacity up to 2500 tablets per minutes. In strip packing machine wide range of products can be packed automatically/semi-automatically. To operate the machine is very simple. The product is fed through hopper and feeding device flows to the heat sealing roller cavities, the desired laminated foil from the two rollers is drawn on the sealing rollers which packs and seals the products continuously. The sealed strip passes through the vertical and horizontal cutters to get desired strip sizes.

Application: Strip packing machine is extensively used to pack tablets, capsules, caplets, coated tablets, soft gelatin capsules. The same is also used to pack supari, tobacco, refills, battery cells, mats, bearings, oil seals, steel balls, chewing gum, toffees, etc.

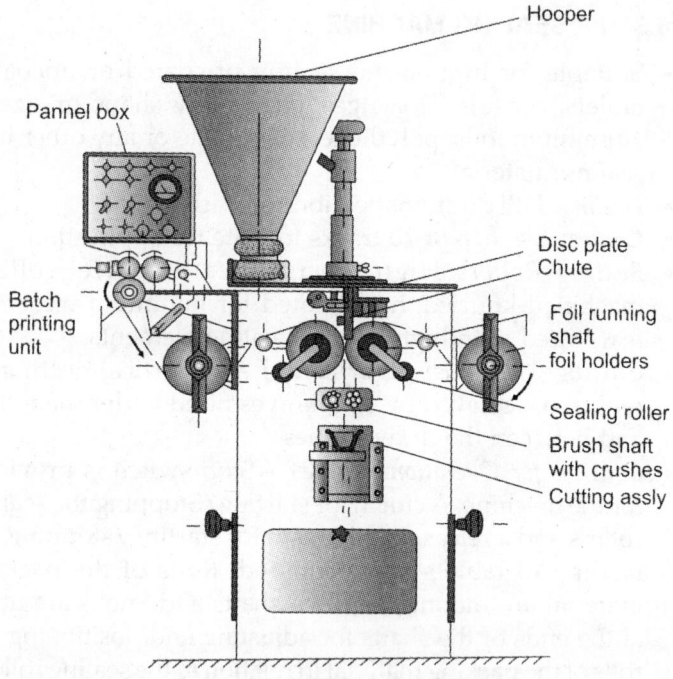

Fig. 7.11: Strip packaging machine

Features

- Suitable for most heat sealable foils like aluminium poly, glassine poly, paper poly, etc.
- All parts are standardised which ensures quick inter changeables.
- There are 5 different models, capacity ranging from 400 to 2500 tablets per minute.
- Trouble free smooth operation.

Strip Defoiler

This unit is ideal for recovery of tablets/capsules from rejected foils. The foils are fed in the machine where the tablets/capsules are separated. The machine has adjustable slitters, suitable for strip width of 45 to 90 mm, and is supplied with stainless steel tablet collecting tray, etc. All the shafts and rollers are made of stainless steel and the unit is driven by 0.25 hp, 3 phase motor.

7.18 MULTI-DOSE STRIP PACKAGING

Over the past decade many LTC pharmacies have adopted pharmacy automation technology that dispenses medications in multi-dose strip packaging (i.e. multiple medications for a patient and time in a single easy-to-open package). Because the packaging is easier to use when administering medications, many nursing facilities prefer it over traditional bingo cards. This fairly proven technology, which originated in the acute care/hospital market, also enables pharmacies to dispense medications in variable days supply. However, most LTC pharmacies have adopted 2–3, 3–4 and/or 7-day dispensing cycles. While shorter dispensing cycles significantly reduces medication waste, it does not completely eliminate it. Furthermore, since it provides very few benefits other than waste reduction, most pharmacies did not considered multi-dose strip packaging in the past.

Advantages

- Significantly reduces medication waste.
- Reduces nursing time spent administering meds.

Disadvantages

- Technology investment required.
- Does not reduce pharmacy fill or delivery costs.
- No mechanism (i.e. billing transaction) for shorter billing cycles with Part D.

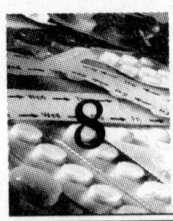

8 Ancillary Materials for Packaging

8.1 INTRODUCTION

In packaging, ancillaries cover a large group of products and play a vital role towards completeness of a package. Quantum and volume-wise, though ancillary materials have a smaller visible percentage of the total packages used, nevertheless, their absence or inadequacy may impair the performance of a package-functionally, aesthetically and statutorily. The ancillary materials along with the primary packaging materials provide product-package compatibility, product preservation and protection, containment, identification, consumer convenience and consumer protection. Some of the important ancillary materials, which are discussed here, include adhesives, printing inks, labels, caps and closures and reinforcement materials such as tapes and straps. In the case of packages, which come directly in contact with the pharmaceutical product, the safety aspects that apply to the primary package also apply to the ancillary materials. Typical examples are adhesives for laminates, printing inks for a pharmaceutical package/label, caps and closures for bottles and containers.

8.2 ADHESIVES

Adhesive bonding is the process of uniting materials with the aid of an adhesive, a substance capable of holding such materials together by surface attachment. Polymers are widely used as adhesives because of their versatility. The primary function of adhesives is to join parts together. Adhesives do this by transmitting stress from one member to another in a manner that distributes the stress much more uniformly than can be achieved with conventional mechanical fasteners.

Classification of Adhesives

Adhesives are broadly classified into:
- Waterborne adhesives
- Wet glues
- Hot-melt adhesives
- Solvent-borne adhesives
- Solventless adhesives
- Pressure-sensitive adhesives
- Laminating adhesives for flexible packaging
- Adhesives for labels.

Waterborne Adhesives

This is the oldest, and still, by far, the largest volume class of adhesive used in packaging. These adhesives share the general advantages of ease and safety of handling, energy efficiency, low cost, and high strength. Waterborne adhesives can further be classified into two categories – natural and synthetic.

Wet Glues

Wet glue adhesive is defined as those labeling systems where the label is not pre-coated with adhesive, but the adhesive coating is 'wet' and is applied to the labelling machine immediately prior to the label being placed onto the substrate. The 'wetness' would usually be aqueous-based or hot melt applied, but there may still be some solvent based adhesives that have not yet been replaced due to environmental pressures. These 'wet' aqueous adhesives are usually 'natural', in that they are based largely on modified animal or vegetable materials, e.g. casein, starches, dextrose or cellulose.

Hot-melt Adhesives

The backbone of any hot-melt is a thermoplastic polymer. Although almost any thermoplastic can be used, and most have been, the most widely used material by far is the co-polymer of Ethylene and Vinyl Acetate (EVA). These copolymers have an excellent balance of molten stability, adhesion and toughness over a broad temperature range, as well as compatibility with many modifiers.

Hot-melt adhesives are a well-established method of adhesion. A hot-melt adhesive is claimed to reduce the bloom and does not peel off PET, PVC or glass containers. An unusual development in the hot melt adhesive area is the introduction of an entire family of water dispersible adhesives. These are actually polyester based hot-melt adhesives which, when repulped in alkaline or neutral environments are dissolved and dispersed.

Solvent-borne Adhesives

Solvented polyurethane adhesives are widely used in flexible packaging for the lamination of plastic films. These multilayer film constructions find application in bags, pouches, wraps for snack food, meat and cheese packs and boil-in-bag food pouches.

Solventless Adhesives

This is a technique originally designed for lamination, but which can also be used as a replacement for solvent or aqueous-based adhesive systems. The system is a two component polyether or polyester urethane system, applied at room temperature by smooth roller coating. This is useful for pharmaceutical and food application as no solvent is used.

Pressure-sensitive Adhesives

Several developments are recorded in this field of adhesives. One company has developed a kind of adhesive, which can be used on high-quality roll label materials and is as effective below freezing point as at room temperature. Similarly, one other adhesive is a pressure sensitive adhesive suitable for freezer cabinet applications, providing a good bond to polyethylene film and carton board at temperatures as low as –30°C which is useful for frozen food and food stored at lower temperatures. Also, a specific adhesive for direct application to unpacked fruits and vegetables is on trial in some supermarkets.

Laminating Adhesives for Flexible Packaging

Flexible packaging materials are used extensively for packaging of pharmaceutical products, food and wide range of other products. These packaging materials are made from basic substrates such as plastic films, aluminium foil and various types of paper. "Dry Adhesive Lamination" is a process that is very commonly used to produce laminated flexible packaging.

Adhesives for Labels

Glues and different adhesives for food and pharmaceutical labels have to be selected with proper care. The range of surfaces needing adhesives is altering, thereby stimulating adhesives formulators to produce new and exciting adhesives. It is important that adhesives are fully tested, not only for the usual adhesion to the substrate but also for the penetration of constituents of the adhesive formulation through the substrate into the product.

8.3 PAPER

Paper is a thin material mainly used for writing upon, printing upon or for packaging. It is produced by pressing together moist fibres, typically cellulose pulp derived from wood, rags or grasses, and drying them into flexible sheets. Paper is a versatile material with many uses. Whilst the most common is for writing and printing upon, it is also widely used as a packaging material, in many cleaning products, in a number of industrial and construction processes, and occasionally as a food ingredient, particularly in Asian cultures.

Chemical Pulping

The purpose of a chemical pulping process is to break down the chemical structure of lignin and render it soluble in the cooking liquor, so that it may be washed from the cellulose fibres. Paper made from chemical pulps are also known as wood-free papers. Not to be confused with tree-free paper.

Mechanical Pulping

There are two major mechanical pulps, thermo mechanical pulp (TMP) and groundwood pulp (GWP).

Deinked Pulp

Paper recycling processes can use either chemical or mechanical pulp. By mixing with water and applying mechanical action the hydrogen bonds in the paper can be broken and fibres separated again. Most recycled paper contains a proportion of virgin fibre in the interests of quality. Generally deinked pulp is of the same quality or lower than the collected paper it was made from.

There are three main classifications of recycled fibre:
- Mill broke or Internal mill waste
- Preconsumer waste
- Postconsumer waste

Recycled papers can be made from 100% recycled materials or blended with virgin pulp. They are (generally) not as strong nor as bright as papers made from virgin pulp.

Additives

Besides the fibres, pulps may contain fillers such as chalk or china clay, which improve the characteristics of the paper for printing or writing. Additives for sizing purposes may be mixed into the pulp and/or applied to the paper web later in the manufacturing process. The purpose of sizing is to establish the correct level of surface absorbency to suit the ink or paint.

Producing Paper

The pulp is feed to a paper machine where it is formed as a paper web and the water is removed from it by pressing and drying. Pressing the sheet removes the water by force. Once the water is forced from the sheet, felt (not to be confused with the traditional felt) is used to collect the water. When making paper by hand, a blotter sheet is used. Drying involves using air and or heat to remove water from the paper sheet.

Finishing

Paper at this point is *uncoated*. Coated paper has a thin layer of material such as calcium carbonate or china clay applied to one or both sides in order to create a surface more suitable for high-resolution halftone screens.

Some Paper Types Include

Bond paper, book paper, coated paper: Glossy and matte surface, cotton paper, electronic paper, wallpaper, waterproof paper, wax paper.

Tissue Paper

Tissue paper is used inside a container to fill empty space so that the packed items do not shift in transit. Fragile contents like glass or porcelain are often wrapped in tissue paper before being placed inside another type of protective container for shipping.

Applications

Paper can be produced with a wide variety of properties, depending on its intended use.

- **To represent a value:** Paper money, bank note, cheque, security, voucher and ticket.
- **For storing information:** Book, notebook, magazine, newspaper, art, zine, letter.
    - for personal use: diary, note to remind oneself, etc. for temporary personal use: scratch paper.
    - for communication to someone else.
- **For packaging:** Corrugated box, paper bag, envelope, wrapping tissue, Charta emporetica and wallpaper.
- **For cleaning:** Toilet paper, handkerchiefs, paper towels, facial tissue and cat litter.
- **For construction:** Papier-mâché, origami, paper planes, quilling, Paper honeycomb, used as a core material in composite materials, paper engineering, construction paper and clothing.
- **Other uses:** Emery paper, sandpaper, blotting paper, litmus paper, universal indicator paper, paper chromatography, electrical insulation paper and filter paper.

8.4 PAPERBOARD

Paperboard is (like paper) a 'vegetable-fibre web' formed from a water suspension. While there is no rigid differentiation between paper and paperboard, paperboard is generally thicker (usually over 0.25 mm or 10 points) than paper. According to ISO standards, paperboard is a paper with a basis weight (grammage) above 224 g/m², but there are exceptions. Paperboard can be single or multiply. Paperboard used for the manufacture of folding cartons and rigid set-up boxes is often called boxboard. Paperboards used for the manufacture of corrugated fibreboard are called containerboard. It can be easily cut and formed, is lightweight and is strong used in packaging. Another enduse would be graphic printing, such as book and magazine covers or postcards. Sometimes it is referred to as cardboard, which is a generic, lay term used to refer to any heavy paper pulp based board.

Production

Fibrous material is turned into pulp and bleached, to create one or more layers of board, which can be optionally coated for a better surface and/or improved visual appearance. Paperboard are produced on paper machines that can handle higher grammages and several plies.

Raw Materials

The above mentioned fibrous material can either come from fresh (virgin) sources (e.g. wood) or from recycled waste paper. Around 90% of virgin paper is made from wood pulp. Today paperboard packaging in general, and especially products from certified sustainable sources, are receiving new attention, as manufacturers dealing with environmental, health and regulatory issues look to renewable resources to meet increasing demand. It is now mandatory in many countries for paper-based packaging to be manufactured wholly or partially from recycled material.

- Hard wood
- Soft wood
- Recycled material
- *Others:* It is also possible to use the fibres of Straw, Hemp, Cotton, Flax

Pulping

Mainly two methods for extracting fibres from its source are used:

- **Mechanical Pulping** is a two stage process which results in a very high yield of wood fibres.
- **Chemical Pulping** uses chemical solutions to convert wood into pulp, yielding around 30% less than mechanical pulping.

Bleaching

Pulp used in the manufacture of paperboard can be bleached to decrease colour and increase purity.

There are three categories of bleaching methods:
- Bleaching by delignification using chlorine gas, which is a method that has been largely replaced by procedures which are gentler to the environment such as the use of oxygen as a replacement for the chlorine gas.
- Bleaching by oxidation using chemicals such as chlorine dioxide, hydrogen peroxide or sodium hypochlorite.
- Bleaching by reduction using chemicals such as sodium bisulphite.

Coating

In order to improve whiteness, smoothness and gloss of paperboard, one or more layers of coating is applied. Coatings are usually made up of:
- A pigment, which could be china clay, calcium carbonate or titanium dioxide.
- An adhesive or binder and water.

Additional components could be OBA (optical brightening agents).

Classifications

Based on the production process and the source of the pulp, different types of paperboard are produced. The common industry abbreviations are:
- **FBB/GC/UC (Folding Box Board)** is a virgin fibre board with a middle layer of mechanical (CTMP) pulp, which gives it a light yellow colour.

- **SBB/SBS (Solid Bleached Board)** is a virgin fibre board made purely from bleached chemical pulp, which is white throughout.
- **SUB/SUS (Solid Unbleached Board)** is a board made from unbleached chemical pulp (yellow) or recycled material (grey).
- **WLC (White Lined Chipboard)** is a board made from virgin and recycled material (grey).

Application

Paperboard is extensively used products with high demands for stiffness and printing results. It is used for such applications as food and pharmaceutical packaging, but also for graphics end uses like book covers and cards. Paperboard is a good material for making attractive, high quality boxes and cartons. Paperboard is particularly suitable as tasteless and odourless packaging for food, personal care products and pharmaceutical products, as well as for chocolate and confectionary boxes. Paperboard boxes and cartons offer a very good surface for printing, making them ideal as presentation packaging for tobacco and luxury goods. Since paperboard comes from a renewable resource, growing forests that absorb carbon dioxide and produce oxygen, it is highly sustainable with a low carbon footprint.

8.5 LEAFLETS

A leaflet that, by order of the Food and Drug Administration, must be placed inside the package of every prescription drug. The leaflet must include the trademark for the drug, its generic name, and its mechanism of action; state its indications, contraindications, warnings, precautions, adverse effects, and dosage forms and include instructions for the recommended dose, time and route of administration.

A leaflet is a written or pictorial message on a single sheet of paper. It has no standard size, shape, or format. In selecting the size, shape, and weight of the paper, the primary consideration is that the paper accommodates the message and be easy to distribute.

A label/leaflet assembly includes a support web with a release coating on which is placed an adhesive label with a leaflet secured on its front face. The leaflet has a front cover one end of which extends beyond the underlying panels of the leaflets. This end of the leaflet has a first part which is permanently joined to the main body of the front cover and which is releasable and re-sealable adherent to the label, and a second part which is permanently secured by an adhesive to the label and is connected to the first part and/or the main body of the front cover along one or more tear lines. Until opened the leaflet is held firmly sealed by the second part. When opened the leaflet is re-sealable, but the torn tear lines show that the leaflet has been opened. The assembly is thus tamper-evident.

Categories of Leaflets

Leaflets may be categorized as persuasive, informative, and directive.

Physical Characteristics of Leaflets

The major factors involved in selection of paper weights and leaflet sizes are:
- Message length.
- Artwork required.
- Delivery system to be used.
- Press capabilities.
- Purpose of the leaflet .

Advantages

The printed word has a high degree of acceptance, credibility, and prestige. Printed matter is unique in that it can be passed from person to person without distortion.

Disadvantages

A high illiteracy rate reduces the effectiveness and usefulness of the printed message. Printing operations require special, extensive, continuing logistical support. Dissemination is time-consuming and costly, requiring the use of special facilities and complex coordination.

Leaflet Use

Leaflets are developed for specific uses, such as standard, special situation, safe conduct, and news.

8.6 PACKAGE INSERTS

Package insert or product label is an essential feature of drug packaging. These inserts are present in most of the medicinal and pharmaceutical products as apiece of paper with information pertaining to that particular product. Ethically and legally speaking they should provide all

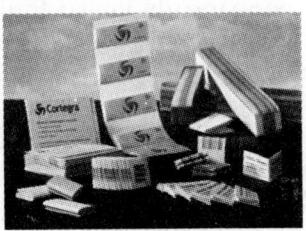

Fig. 8.1: Inserts and outserts

the necessary information of the drugs in correct and easily understandable form for safe and effective use. The information should be unbiased, should not hide anything and regularly updated. Often unread they have potential educational and even legal implications.

When customer get the prescription filled, they usually receive additional written information. This may be just a brief summary provided by the pharmacy, or you may receive a very detailed "package insert" filled with information provided by the drug manufacturer and approved by the US. Food and Drug Administration (FDA). Such package inserts are available for all prescription medications approved by the FDA. Similar information is available for nonprescription medicines and for some herbal medicines and dietary supplements as well. The information in a package insert is written in technical language. It is usually very long and can be difficult to understand. It is a good idea to look through it as it contains important information about the drug.

The package insert follows a standard format for every medication. After some identifying information such as the brand name and generic name of the product, the following sections appear:

- Description
- Microbiology and clinical pharmacology

- Indications and usage
- Contraindications
- Warnings
- Precautions
- Adverse reactions
- Over dosage
- Dosage and administration
- How supplied

Example-package inserts for some HIV drugs begin with "Box Warnings," which highlight especially serious (often life-threatening) adverse reactions that have been reported but are rare.

The package insert will most often use the generic name of the drug. Patients usually know a drug by its brand name, so this can be confusing.

Description

This section gives the chemical name of the drug and a diagram of its chemical make up. It tells whether it is in tablet form, capsules, liquid, or powder, and how it should be given – by mouth or by injection. It also lists all inactive ingredients such as fillers, artificial colours, or flavourings.

Microbiology and Clinical Pharmacology

For most people who are not health care professionals, a lot of the information in this section is difficult to understand. Basically, this section tells how the medicine works in the body to fight against disease. It also tells whether studies in different groups of people found any differences in how it works for treatment-experienced patients, treatment new patients, women, children, and elderly people.

Indications and Usage

This section lists the uses (indications) for which the drug has been FDA-approved. This section will also state if the drug can be used in treatment experienced patients, treatment new patients, or both.

Contraindications

This section describes situations when the drug should be used with caution or not at all. These are called contraindications. For instance, a medicine should not be prescribed for someone who has had an allergic reaction (hypersensitivity) to the same medication or one that is similar, or for someone who is taking another medicine that interacts with it in a harmful way. This section also may warn doctors not to prescribe the medicine for people with certain medical conditions because they are at greater risk of dangerous side effects. If you have a serious medical disorder, this is the place to find out whether it is likely to cause a problem if you take this medicine.

Warnings

This section discusses serious side effects that may occur in people who take this medicine. If especially severe or life-threatening problems have been found, there may be a "Box Warning" on the first page of the package insert. As the name suggests, this information is clearly displayed using capital letters surrounded by a black box so it will not be overlooked. Patient should pay attention to these warnings so they will recognize any symptoms that could suggest a serious problem, but you should not be overly alarmed. It is unlikely that they will experience any of the conditions covered by Box Warnings.

Precautions

The Precautions section tells how to use the medication most safely and effectively. It alerts the doctor about types of patients who need close observation and offers guidelines about any laboratory tests that should be performed before the medicine is taken or during the time it is in use (e.g. lab tests to monitor lipid levels or liver enzymes).

One of the most important parts of this section lists Drug Interactions-the effects that this medicine may have on other prescription or over-the-counter medicines patient may be taking. This section also might warn that you should not take this medicine with a particular food or other product (such as an antacid).

It is a good idea to look through this section to see if it lists any medicines or other products that patient use regularly. Be sure your doctor knows about all the medications you are taking (including over-the-counter, prescription, street drugs, and herbs), even if patient only use them occasionally.

The Precautions section also may tell what is known about the use of this medicine by nursing or pregnant mothers, children ("Pediatric Use") and older people ("Geriatric Use"). Sometimes it may just say that not enough information is available. This does not mean that it is unsafe in these groups of people, just that not enough research studies have been done.

Adverse Reactions

This section lists all the side effects that were reported in people who took this medicine while it was being tested. These effects are usually grouped according to the body system affected and perhaps also by how many people reported each one. It can be hard to sort out which of the side effects on these lists patient really need to be concerned about. These lists of "adverse events" can look frightening because they include so many problems, ranging from minor to life-threatening. The thing to remember is that this section lists everything that happened to hundreds or thousands of people (and sometimes also animals) regardless of whether it actually had any connection to the medicine.

Over Dosage

This section tells what the results of a large overdose of the medicine are likely to be and how they should be treated. This kind of information is mainly useful to medical personnel. If patient suspect an overdose of medication, you should contact a poison control center or emergency room right away.

Dosage and Administration

This section gives the recommended dosages of the medicine and may advise if the drug should be taken with or without food. If the medicine is indicated for more than one use (e.g. to treat HIV and hepatitis B), you may see separate sections for each use. Separate information also may be given about dosages for women above and below a certain weight, children, older people, or those with certain medical problems.

How Supplied

This section lists all the available forms of this medicine, including tablets or capsules of various doses and perhaps liquids, and powder. Each one is described by colour, shape, and markings, so patients can be sure of which one they are taking. When reading the package insert for Fuzeon, this section will take about how to reconstitute, or mix, the powdered drug with sterile water. This section also gives storage instructions. This is where patient find out whether to keep the drug in the refrigerator or not. It also tells whether pills may be damaged from heat, light, or moisture. Usually there is a recommendation against leaving the medicine out in temperatures over 30°C (86° F), for instance.

8.7 PACKAGE OUTSERTS

Package outserts are known as circulars, brochures, monographs and patient package inserts. An outsert is a four page card wrapped around and attached to the outside of a magazine or other publication. It is purpose is to advertise a product (such as a subscription and/or free gift) and also to act as a flag for the publication to distinguish it from other titles on newsstand shelves. The outsert was first used on Running Magazine in the UK in 1981. The effect is to draw the attention of the browser to the magazine. Research shows the outsert increases sales of the publication. The best performing outserts use a single, bright colour to contrast with the magazine cover. An additional use of the term outsert is a multi-folded, instruction sheet applied to the outside of a bottle or carton of a pharmaceutical product. The instruction sheets are rather large and the font of the text is small so as to provide all mandated information about the proper use of and warnings about the product. The equipment that applies the outsert is called an outserter or outserting machine.

8.8 FIBERBOARD

Fiberboard is a type of engineered wood product that is made out of wood fibres. Types of fibreboard (in order of increasing density) include particle board, medium-density fibreboard, and hardboard. Fiberboard is sometimes used as a synonym for particle board, but particle board usually refers to low-density fibreboard. Plywood is not a type of fibreboard, as it is made of thin sheets of wood, not wood fibres or particles. Fiberboard, particularly medium-density fibreboard (MDF), is heavily used in the furniture industry. For pieces that will be visible, a veneer of wood is often glued onto fibreboard to give it the appearance of conventional wood.

Advantages

- Environmentally friendly made from fibreboard 100% recyclable.
- Strong, durable and reliable.
- Reduced shipment costs.
- Lightweight less than half the weight of timber pallets-less than 10 kg.
- Efficiency and ease of handling.

Uses

In the packaging industry, fibreboard is often used to describe a tough kraft-based paperboard or corrugated fibreboard bor boxes. The shipping container is formed solely of corrugated fibreboard to meet United Nations regulations governing transport of hazardous materials and configured to pharmaceutical glass bottles. Fiberboard is used in the auto industry to create free-form shapes such as dashboards, rear parcel shelves, and inner door shells. These pieces are usually covered with a skin, foil, or fabric such as cloth, suede, leather, or polyvinyl chloride.

Different uses and applications include:
- Sound proofing/deadening.
- Structural sheathing.
- Low-slope roofing.
- Sound deadening flooring underlayment.

High density coated wood fibre is an ideal cover board, and the industry apparently agrees.

8.9 JUTE

Jute is a long, soft, shiny vegetable fibre that can be spun into coarse, strong threads. It is produced from plants in the genus Corchorus, family Tiliaceae. Jute is one of the most affordable natural fibres and is second only to cotton in amount produced and variety of uses. Jute fibres are composed primarily of the plant materials cellulose (major component of plant fibre) and lignin (major components of wood fibre). It is thus a ligno-cellulosic fibre that is partially a textile fibre and partially wood.

Types

1. White jute (*Corchorus capsularis*)
2. Tossa jute (*Corchorus olitorius*).

Production

Jute matting being used to prevent flood erosion while natural vegetation becomes established. For this purpose, a natural and biodegradable fibre is essential.

Uses

Fibre

Jute is the second most important vegetable fibre after cotton; not only for cultivation, but also for various uses. Jute is used chiefly to make cloth for wrapping bales of raw cotton, and to make sacks and coarse cloth. The fibres are also woven into curtains, chair coverings, carpets, area rugs, hessian cloth, and backing for linoleum. The fibres are used alone or blended with other types of fibres to make twine and rope. Jute butts, the coarse ends of the plants, are used to make inexpensive cloth. Traditionally jute was used in traditional textile machineries as textile fibres having cellulose (vegetable fibre content) and lignin (wood fibre content). Jute can be used to create a number of fabrics such as Hessian cloth, sacking, scrim, carpet backing cloth (CBC), and canvas. Jute bags are used for making fashion bags and promotional bags. Jute floor coverings consist of woven and tufted and piled carpets. Jute has many advantages as a home textile, either replacing cotton or blending with it. It is a strong, durable, colour and light-fast fibre. It is UV protection, sound and heat insulation, low thermal conduction and anti-static properties make it a wise choice in home décor.

Food

Jute leaves are consumed in various parts of the world. It is a popular vegetable in West Africa.

Other

Diversified byproducts from jute can be used in cosmetics, medicine, paints, and other products.

8.10 WOOD

Wood is an organic material, a natural composite of cellulose fibres (which are strong in tension) embedded in a matrix of lignin which resists compression. In the strict sense wood is produced as secondary xylem in the stems of trees (and other woody plants). In a living tree it transfers water and nutrients to the leaves and other growing tissues, and has a support function, enabling woody plants to reach large sizes or to stand up for themselves. Wood may also refer to other plant materials with comparable properties, and to material engineered from wood, or wood chips or fibre.

Hard and Soft Woods

It is common to classify wood as either softwood or hardwood. The wood from conifers (e.g. pine) is called softwood, and the wood from dicotyledons (usually broad-leaved trees, e.g. oak) is called hardwood. These names are a bit misleading, as hardwoods are not necessarily hard, and softwoods are not necessarily soft. The well-known balsa (a hardwood) is actually softer than any commercial softwood. Conversely, some softwoods are harder than many hardwoods.

Uses

Fuel: Wood has a long history of being used as fuel.

Construction: Wood can be cut into straight planks and made into a wood flooring.

Engineered wood: Wood used in construction includes products such as glued laminated timber (glulam), laminated veneer lumber (LVL), parallam and I-joists.

Next generation wood products: Further developments include new lignin glue applications, recyclable food packaging, rubber tire replacement applications, anti-bacterial medical agents, and high strength fabrics or composites.

Furniture and utensils: Wood has always been used extensively for furniture, including chairs and beds. Also for tool handles and cutlery, such as chopsticks, toothpicks, and other utensils, like the wooden spoon.

In the arts: Artists can use wood to create delicate sculptures.

Sports and recreational equipment: Many types of sports equipment are made of wood, or were constructed of wood in the past. For example, cricket bats are typically made of white willow. The baseball bats which are legal for use in Major League Baseball are frequently made of ash wood or hickory, and in recent years have been constructed from maple even though that wood is somewhat more fragile. In softball, however, bats are more commonly made of aluminium (this is especially true for fastpitch softball).

Medicine: In January 2010 Italian scientists announced that wood could be harnessed to become a bone substitute. It is likely to take at least five years until this technique will be applied for humans.

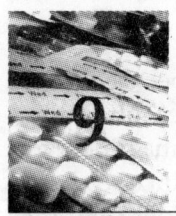

Natural and Synthetic Rubber

9.1 INTRODUCTION

Natural latex is found in the inner bark of many trees, especially those found in Brazil and the Far East. The white sticky sap of the milkweed is also a latex. Latex will turn into a rubbery mass within 12 hours after it is exposed to the air. The latex protects the tree or plant by covering the wound with a rubbery material like a bandage.

The rubber consists of polymeric chains which are joined in a network structure and have a high degree of flexibility. Upon application of a stress to a rubber material, such as stretching it, the polymer chain, which is randomly oriented, undergoes bond rotations allowing the chain to be extended or elongated. The fact that the chains are joined in a network allows for elastomeric recoverability since the cross-linked chains cannot irreversibly slide over one another. The changes in arrangement are not constrained by chain rigidity due to crystallization or high viscosity due to a glassy state. Since latex will solidify in air, a stabilizer is added to prevent polymerization if the latex is to be stored or shipped. The stabilizer is usually 0.5 to 1% ammonia. When the ammonia is removed by evaporation or by neutralization, the latex will solidify into rubber.

Natural Rubber

Latex being collected from a tapped rubber tree. Natural rubber is an elastomer (an elastic hydrocarbon polymer) that was originally derived from a milky colloidal suspension, or latex, found in the sap of some plants. The purified form of natural rubber is the chemical polyisoprene, which can also be produced synthetically. Natural rubber is used extensively in many applications and products, as is synthetic rubber.

Varieties

Source of natural rubber latex is the Para rubber tree (*Hevea brasiliensis*). Other plants containing latex include Gutta-Percha (*Palaquium gutta*), rubber fig (*Ficus elastica*), Panama rubber tree (*Castilla elastica*), spurges (*Euphorbia spp.*), lettuce, common dandelion (*Taraxacum officinale*), Russian dandelion (*Taraxacum kok-saghyz*), Scorzonera (*tau-saghyz*) and Guayule (Parthenium argentatum).

Properties

Rubber exhibits unique physical and chemical properties. Rubber's stress-strain behaviour exhibits the Mullins effect, the Payne effect, and is often modeled as hyperelastic. Rubber strain crystallizes. Owing to the presence of a double bond in each repeat unit, natural rubber is sensitive to ozone cracking.

Solvents

There are two main solvents for rubber: turpentine and naphtha (petroleum). An ammonia solution can be used to prevent the coagulation of raw latex.

Chemical Makeup

Latex is a natural polymer of isoprene (most often cis-1, 4-polyisoprene) – with a molecular weight of 100,000 to 1,000,000. Typically, a small percent (up to 5% of dry mass) of other materials, such as proteins, fatty acids, resins and inorganic materials (salts) are found in natural rubber. Polyisoprene is also created synthetically, producing what is sometimes referred to as "synthetic natural rubber".

Natural rubber is an elastomer and a thermoplastic. However, it should be noted that as the rubber is vulcanized, it will turn into a thermoset. Most rubber in everyday use is vulcanized to a point where it shares properties of both; i.e. if it is heated and cooled, it is degraded but not destroyed.

Elasticity

In most elastic materials, such as metals used in springs, the elastic behaviour is caused by bond distortions. When force is applied, bond lengths deviate from the (minimum energy) equilibrium and strain energy is stored electrostatically.

Vulcanization of rubber creates more disulfide bonds between chains, so it shortens each free section of chain. The result is that the chains tighten more quickly for a given length of strain, thereby increasing the elastic force constant and making rubber harder and less extendable.

In natural rubber, the following additives are added to change its physical and chemical properties:

1. Activators – Zinc oxide, stearic acid.
2. Fillers – Carbon black, lime stone.
3. Vulcanizing agent – Sulphur.
4. Lubricant – Talc, zinc stearate.
5. Pigments – Coal-tar, dyes, oxides and sulphides of antimony, cadmium, iron.
6. Softners – Mineral oils.
7. Antioxidants – Phenyl-p-naphthylamine.

Uses

The use of rubber is widespread, ranging from household to industrial products, entering the production stream at the intermediate stage or as final products. Tires and tubes are the largest consumers of rubber. The remaining 44% are taken up by the general rubber goods (GRG) sector, which includes all products except tires and tubes.

Textile Applications

Additionally, rubber produced as a fibre sometimes called elastic, has significant value for use in the textile industry because of its excellent elongation and recovery properties. For these purposes, manufactured rubber fibre is made as either an extruded round fibre or rectangular fibres that are cut into strips from extruded film. Because of its low dye acceptance, feel and appearance, the rubber fibre is either covered by yarn of another fibre or directly woven with other yarns into the fabric.

Vulcanization Natural rubber is often vulcanized, a process by which the rubber is heated and sulfur, peroxide or bisphenol are added to improve resilience and elasticity, and to prevent it from perishing. Vulcanization greatly improved the durability and utility of rubber from the 1830s on.

The development of vulcanization is most closely associated with Charles Goodyear in 1839. Carbon black is often used as an additive to rubber to improve its strength, especially in vehicle tires.

Allergic reactions: Some people have a serious latex allergy, and exposure to certain natural rubber latex products such as latex gloves can cause anaphylactic shock.

Synthetic Rubber

Synthetic rubber is any type of artificial elastomer, invariably a polymer. An elastomer is a material with the mechanical (or material) property that it can undergo much more elastic deformation under stress than most materials and still return to its previous size without permanent deformation. Synthetic rubber serves as a substitute for natural rubber in many cases, especially when improved material properties are required.

Uses

Nowadays synthetic rubber is used a great deal in printing textile. In this case it is called rubber paste. In most cases titanium dioxide is used with copolymerization and volatile matter in producing such synthetic rubber for textile use. Moreover this kind of preparation can be considered to be the pigment preparation based on titanium dioxide.

Comparison of Natural and Synthetic Rubber

Natural rubber coming from latex is mostly polymerized isoprene with a small percentage of impurities in it. This limits the range of properties available to it. Also, there are limitations on the proportions of cis and trans double bonds resulting from methods of polymerizing natural latex. This also limits the range of properties available to natural rubber, although addition of sulfur and vulcanization are used to improve the properties.

Synthetic rubber can be made from the polymerization of a variety of monomers including isoprene (2-methyl-1, 3-butadiene), 1,3-butadiene, chloroprene (2-chloro-1,3-butadiene) and isobutylene (methylpropene) with a small percentage of

Table 9.1: Common synthetic rubbers

ISO Standard Code	Technical Name	Common Names
BIIR	Bromo Isobutylene Isoprene	Bromobutyl
BR	Polybutadiene	Buna CB
CIIR	Chloro Isobutylene Isoprene	Chlorobutyl, Butyl
CR	Polychloroprene	Chloroprene, Neoprene
CSM	Chlorosulphonated Polyethylene	Hypalon
ECO	Epichlorohydrin	ECO, Epichlorohydrin, Epichlore, Epichloridrine
EP	Ethylene Propylene	
EPDM	Ethylene Propylene Diene Monomer	EPDM, Nordel
FKM	Fluoronated Hydrocarbon	Viton, Kalrez, Fluorel
FVQM	Fluoro Silicone	FVQM
HNBR	Hydrogenated Nitrile Butadiene	HNBR
IR	Polyisoprene	(Synthetic) Natural Rubber
IIR	Isobutylene Isoprene Butyl	Butyl
MVQ	Methyl Vinyl Silicone	Silicone Rubber
NBR	Acrylonitrile Butadiene	NBR, Nitrile rubber, Perbunan, Buna-N
PU	Polyurethane	PU, Polyurethane
SBR	Styrene Butadiene	SBR, Buna-S, GRS, Buna VSL, Buna SE
SEBS	Styrene Ethylene/ Butylene Styrene	SEBS Rubber
SI	Polysiloxane	Silicone Rubber
XNBR	Acrylonitrile Butadiene Carboxy Monomer	XNBR, Carboxylated Nitrile

isoprene for cross-linking. These and other monomers can be mixed in various desirable proportions to be copolymerized for a wide range of physical, mechanical, and chemical properties. The monomers can be produced pure and the addition of impurities or additives can be controlled by design to give optimal properties. Polymerization of pure monomers can be better controlled to give a desired proportion of cis and trans double bonds.

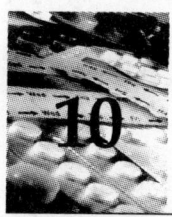

Closures and Liners

10.1 INTRODUCTION

A closure is a device which seals the container to exclude oxygen, carbon dioxide, moisture and prevents the loss of volatile substance. It is also used to close and open the mouth of container. It also prevent the leakage of the medicament during transportation. It also prevents deterioration of the product from the effect of environment and microorganisms.

The term a closure refers to caps and lid, because they provide the seal in many packaging systems, they are often critical components of packages. Closure is a sealing or covering device affixed to or on a container for the purpose of retaining the contents and preventing contamination thereof. Cap is a cover type of closure with external threads to engage external threads of containers or may be held by friction, air pressure, etc.

All forming processes result in some variation in the dimensions of the final product. When sealing is critical, packagers often depend on a closure to compensate for the manufacturing inaccuracies not only in the closure, but also in the container. To achieve a tight hermetic seal that is capable of protecting control of the closure itself, as well as provision of some resilient sealing surface which can deform to compensate for materials can be successfully used, thermoplastics are increasingly the material of choice for plastic closures, and injection is PP, HDPE, LDPE and PVC, in that order, Thermoset phenolics and urea used to be commonly used for closures, but have increasingly been replaced by thermoplastics. Thermoplastics have also replaced a large share of the metal closure market. Three major categories for plastic closures can be identified: friction, snap-on, and threaded.

Against external parts of opening. In today's aggressively competitive pharmaceutical packaging industry, at least three important demands are made of a closure:

- It must be absolutely reliable.
- It must aesthetically enhance the product it contains.
- It must be supplied at a competitive price.

These three criteria are critical in the drug and food market where the consequences of product contamination are often too monumental to think about. The innovations in caps and closures in all sectors have been considerable in recent years.

Requirements for Closures

Must be compatible with the product. Closures are made of metal, plastic or rubber bungs. Rubber bungs are used for parenterals that require multiple or single piercing for multiple use without any detachment of particles by fragmentation.

10.2 TYPES OF CLOSURES

Closures need a means of attaching to the container with sufficient security. Threads, lugs, hinges, locks, adhesives, etc are used.

Many closures need to have the ability to adjust to slight manufacturing variation in the container and the closure structure. Some closures are made of flexible material such as cork, rubber or plastic foam. Often an o-ring, or a closure liner (gasket made of pulp or foam cap liner) are used. Linerless closures often use a deformable plastic rim or structure to maintain the seal.

Secondary seals are common with sensitive products that may deteriorate or where extra security is needed. Foil or plastic innerseals are used on some bottles, Heat sealed lidding films are used on some tubs. External shrink bands, labels, and tapes are sometimes used outside the primary closure structure.

Friction Closure/Friction Fit

Some containers have a loose lid for a closure. Laboratory glassware often has ground glass joints that allow the pieces to be fitted together easily. An Interference fit or friction fit requires some force to close and open, providing additional security. Paint cans often have a friction fit plug.

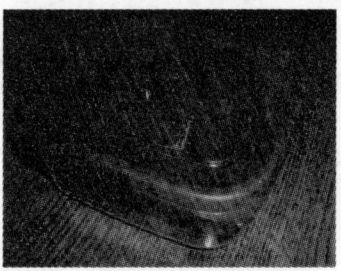

Fig. 10.1: Friction closure/friction fit

Friction closures have the simplest design. The closure is designed deform as it is pushed into the mouth of the container. The resilience of the material causes it to attempt to return to its original dimensions, providing a seal by the tight fit between the closure material and the container. Friction between the outside of the closure and the inside of the mouth of the container provides the force that resists removal of the closure. A cork oldest design of plastic friction closures is used for inexpensive bottles of champagne. It is hollow inside, and has a ridged outer surface.

Screw Top

A screw closure is a mechanical device which is screwed on and off of a threaded "finish" on a container. Either continuous threads (C-T) or lugs are used. Metal caps can be either preformed or in some instances, rolled on after application. Plastic caps may use several types of molded

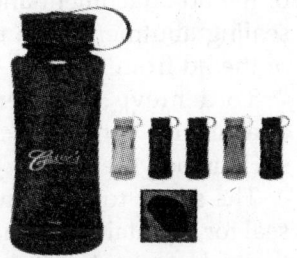

Fig. 10.2: Screw top

polymer. Some screw tops have multiple pieces. For example, a mason jar often has a lid with a built in rubbery seal and a separate threaded ring or band.

A screw top closure comprising a main portion formed of hard plastics material and a resilient member (the resilient member comprises a material member or rubber like in feel that is softer than the said hard plastic) attached to the main portion and projecting there from wherein the exterior surface of the resilient member is provided with projections in the form of dimples for improved grippability so that a person endeavoring to reseal a bottle with the closure can engage the resilient member and obtain an adequate purchase to apply the necessary torque to the closure to cause the closure to form a good seal with the bottle. Or in other words a screw top closure comprising a screw lid with internal threading and a separate lid attachment with external threading. The lid attachment is designed for application on the neck of a container to carry the removable lid, the lid attachment being in the form of an annular element with an upper part serving as support for the lid, and two concentric tubular flanges protruding downwardly therefrom. These flanges between them in downward direction define an open pocket for receipt of the neck of the container. The lid is provided with an inner tubular flange protruding downwardly from an upper portion thereof, the flange being insertable into the lid attachment and designed to be brought into sealing abutment under pressure against the inner tubular flange of the lid attachment at a lower portion thereof having reduced inner diameter in relation to the part of the flange located above such that the inner flange of the lid attachment and the inner flange of the lid remain in sealing abutment with each other during partial unscrewing of the lid from the neck of the container.

To achieve sufficient elasticity in the lid and the lid attachment, both these are made of yielding plastic material, such as polythene.

The screw top closure may suitably be used as an original seal for a container. To allow visual inspection to ascertain that the seal is unbroken it should be provided with suitable sealing members. According to the invention such sealing members may advantageously comprise a sealing ring joined by breakable bridges in a manner known per se to the lower part of the wall of the lid, said ring being designed to be separated from the lid when the lid is unscrewed from the lid attachment, due to the action of protrusions in the outer tubular flange of the lid attachment protruding into notches in the sealing ring.

Advantages

No chance of spoilage due to leakage, a good long-term barrier to oxygen, screw caps are easy to open, and close, requiring no special equipment.

Uses

Screw top closures are used for sealing jars of medicine. It is often vital that tablets or the like contained in such jars are not subjected to the action of moisture from the surrounding atmosphere. It is therefore desirable for the screw top closure to be such that it effectively prevents any penetration of moisture into the jar.

A good long-term barrier to oxygen, which can cause premature degradation of the wine. Glass stoppers are another option used by a number of wineries. As well as solving the potential cork taint problem, they are really quite attractive, and easy to open and re-seal. Their biggest negative is cost, hence they are not as widespread as other alternate closures.

Crown Cap

A metal cap that is clipped onto the open end of the neck of a bottle of sparkling wine in the bottle fermentation phase of méthode champenoise. The cap collects the unwanted yeast protein and other sediment that is then removed during disgorgement.

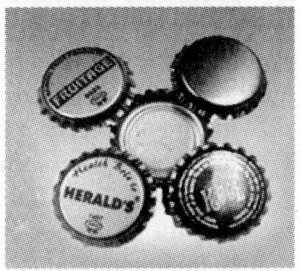

Fig. 10.3: Crown cap

The crown cork (also known as a crown cap or just a crown), the first form of bottle cap, was invented by William Painter in 1891 in Baltimore. The company making it was originally called the Bottle Seal Company, it changed its name with the almost immediate success of the crown cork to the Crown Cork and Seal Company. It still informally goes by that name, but is officially Crown Holdings. The Patent was granted in 1892, as US patent 468, 258. The crown cork was the first highly successful disposable product (it can be resealed but not easily). Crown corks are collected by people around the world who admire the variety of designs and relative ease of storage.

Uses

Beverage bottles are frequently closed with crown beverage caps. These are shallow metal caps that are crimped into locking position around the head of the bottle.

The Maxi Crown Cap

Maxi crown meets all requirements on a modern bottle closure for beer (or any other beverage to be consumed directly after opening): its sealing performance equals that of the crown cork (with respect to sealing speed, reliability, pressure holding, etc). In addition it is safe and it is easy to open.

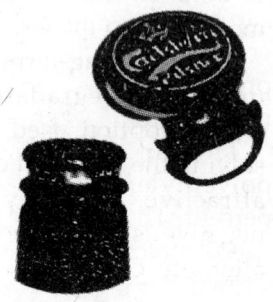

Maxi crown is safe: Modern consumer expectations include that any packaging use for food should be

Fig. 10.4: Maxi crown cap

tamper-proof, i.e. any previous attempts to open and reseal a package should be easily recognizable. Moreover, to an increasing extent, product liability laws have been issued to provide this protection for the consumer.

Maxi crown meets these expectations: It provides both one way bottles and refillable bottles–Glass, PEN and PET–with tamper proof sealings: once opened, the shell of a Maxi Crown cap is torn apart and cannot be used to reseal the bottle, granting the consumer and the filler a safe protection against tampering-and this with maintained sealing performance.

Maxi crown is easy to open: No opener is required: the cap is as easy to open as a can.

Description of the Cap

Maxi Crown is suitable for bottles. Maxi Crown is a three-piece cap consisting of a shell (made from semi-soft aluminium), a liner (made from low density polyethylene), and a ring (made from high density polyethylene). The design allows an economic utilization of materials with a minimum waste, thus providing optimal material costs.

The cap shell: The shell is punched and scored from pre-printed sheets of aluminium. Carefully arranged layout enables maximum use of the sheets. Waste becomes negligible.

The liner: Sealing to the bottle neck is made with a low density polyethylene (LDPE) molded liner, on request with scavenger effect added. The liner is shaped and applied to the cap by using a molding process which is standard as well for crown cork. The liner in Maxi Crown has a profile which provides a double sealing effect. It seals both the outside and inside or top of the bottle neck.

The ring: The pull ring is made from high density polyethylene (HDPE). The utilization of materials is 100 percent. The ring is formed and jointed to the shell in a high speed molding machine that is especially designed for Maxi Crown.

Décor print: Maxi Crown is punched from sheets of aluminium with standard offset printing. The same method has been used for aluminium screw caps for a long time. The printing can in principle comprise any number of colours, but is normally limited to four. The printing on aluminium allows very detailed décor with high finish.

Opening the Maxi Crown Cap

Maxi Crown is opened by hand without the use of tools or openers. The ring is pulled up over the cap top in the same way as a can is opened.

Snap on

Snap is any clasp or fastener that closes with a click. A snap-fit, or snap-on, closure is made of resilient materials and is designed to deform as it passes over a protruding feature on the container. Removal of the closure requires deformation again "snap" the closure back over the protruding feature, which is typically a retaining ring. When the closure is in place, some resilient part of the closure system that is in contact with the container remains deformed, and provides a seal as it attempts to return to its original dimensions, This category of closure is widely used, and a variety of designs exist. Examples

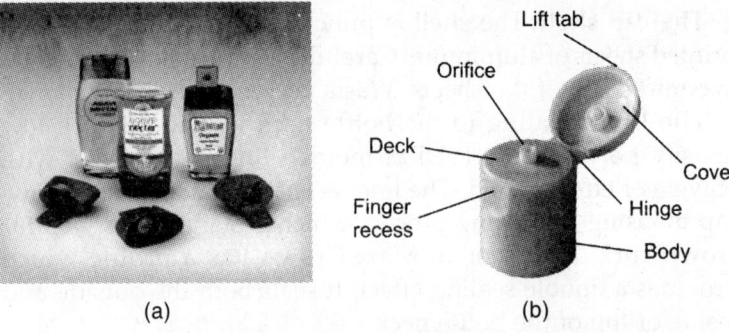

(a)   (b)

Fig. 10.5: Snap on cap

include plastic lids on coffee cans, as well as "line-up-the-arrows" child-resistant caps on medicine bottles. Some closures snap on. For opening, the top is designed to pry off or, break off, or have a built in dispenser. These caps are used in shampoo bottle, oil bottle sauce bottle, etc.

One of the major **advantages** of snap-fit closures is that they can be applied very quickly. A **disadvantage** is that they cannot be used for containers with internal pressures exceeding one atmosphere, since the pressure may act to snap the closures back off of the container.

Childproof, snap-on cap—A childproof safety screw cap and container having yieldable cap retainer means which are overcome, to effect cap removal, by a quarter-turn twist that produces a relatively large axial cap travel due to the provision of multiple screw thread elements thereon. The cap can be pushed straight on, accompanied by bypassing of the threads. The retainer means and the threads increase their interlock action if the cap is squeezed laterally, as by the act of a child applying its teeth to the cap. A shielding flange on the container defeats efforts to bite the cap under its bottom rim, and a bevelled top peripheral portion of the cap defeats its being gripped at the top, by the teeth.

Threaded Stopper

Threaded closures are applied by screwing them onto a container, and removed by screwing them off. They contain a set of threads that is designed to match the threads on the container. These threads are usually continuous, leading to the designation CT closure. Threaded closured are very versatile, and can be used for packages that contain internal pressure, such as carbonated beverages, as well as for vacuum packages and those at atmospheric pressure. Chile-resistant designs of several types are available, as well.

The amount of force required for application and removal of the closure is determined by how far the closure is rotated on the container. Removal torques are generally less than application torques, unless there has been some interaction between the liner and the contents, resulting in sealing the liner to the container. Removal torque typically declines with time for the first several days to a month or so after application, and then stabilizes. The change is caused by stress relaxation and creep in the liner, closure, and/or container. Recommended minimum removal torques are typically about half recommended minimum application torques. If an application torque is too low, the container may not be sealed adequately. On the other hand, if the application torque is too high, consumers may have difficulty removing the closure. It should also be noted that if application torques are too high, a variety of additional problems can result. The capping machinery may not be able to reliably the torque that is set. The forces involved may result in permanent deformation of the cap or the container, resulting In poor sealing, or even leakers. There may be excessive wear of the machinery, etc.

The sealing action is provided by deformation of a resilient surface that is either built into the closure design, or provided by a liner used in conjunction with the closure. As is the case with the other closure designs, the attempt of the resilient material to return to its original dimensions exerts force against the container and provides the seal. The liner may contain plastic as the product contact layer, plastic foam or paperboard for resilience and may also contain aluminium foil for barrier. Liners can be glued in place, but most often are held in place by being snapped behind a retaining ring built into the closure. Linerless closures are designed to provide a resilient sealing surface without requiring the use of a separate liner component. This resilient feature is molded into the closure itself. Usually the resilient feature is made of the same material as the rest of the closure and is produced during molding of the closure, providing resilience by a combination of its geometry and the nature of the plastic used fir the closure. In some cases, it is a distinct plastic material, with superior resilience characteristics, produced by a technique such as coinjection molding.

The size of CT closures (continuous threaded closures) is specified by the nominal outside dimension of the container opening in millimeters, plus a number that represents the style of finish. Both container and closure finishes are standardized so that, at least in theory, a closure of a given size and style should fit any bottle of that same size and style, from any manufacturer. US closure standards have been established by the closure Manufacturers Association, standards for glass bottles by the glass packaging institute, and for plastic bottles by the American society for testing and materials. Common closure diameters are 22–120 mm.

Critical dimensions for closure performance include T, the diameter of the root of the thread inside the closure; E, the inside diameter of the closure; H, the distance from the inside top of the closure to the bottom of the closure skirt; and S, the distance from the inside top of the closure to starting point of the thread.

1. Internal Threaded Stopper/Closure
2. External Threaded Screw Cap

Internal Threaded Stopper/Closure

The distinctive feature of this closure/finish combination is the continuous type threads which are found on the inside of the finish. The outside of the finish looks similar to other finishes of the era. There were two primary types of internal or inside threaded closures: hard rubber and glass.

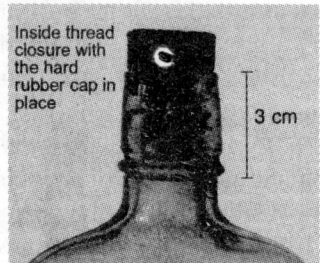

Inside thread closure with the hard rubber cap in place

3 cm

Fig. 10.6: Internal threaded closure

External Threaded Screw Cap

This ubiquitous finish/closure combination is distinguished by having some type of raised ridge or ridges on the outside surface of the finish that accepted an appropriately shaped cap which tightened and sealed the bottle when twisted. External thread finishes are so commonly used today that further explanation is probably not necessary; everyone is familiar with "screw-top" bottles.

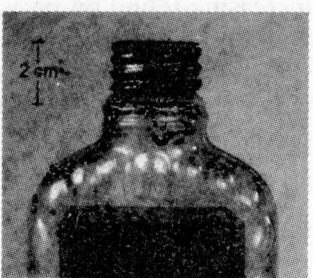

Fig. 10.7: External threaded screw cap

Specialty Closures

In addition to the basic design described above, a wide variety of special closure designs are available. Many of these are designed to provide a dispensing function, such as pumps, sprays, flips open caps, etc. They range in design from rather simple to extremely complex.

An important set of specialty closures are those that are designed to make packages child-resistant, difficult for young children to open. Child-resistant packaging, known as "special packaging" in the relevant regulations, is required on most prescription drugs, aspirin, and other over-the counter drugs, and on household chemicals that pose a serious risk to children if they are accidentally ingested. The regulations prescribe standards that must be met for packages to quality, and include the ability to successfully prevent opening by young children, while at the same time permitting opening by adults, including the elderly.

Some closures also are designed to provide temper-indicating features, typically, in closures, by incorporating some type of tear-off ring. Closure liners that are designed to release from the cap and seal to the bottle mouth can also be used to provide tamper-evidence. In the US, over the counter drug products are required by law to contain some tamper-evident feature, designed to alert consumers if a package has been opened and may have been tampered with. Such features are increasing found on packages for food and other products as well, although they are not required in these applications. Closures and liners, of course, are not the only way of providing tamper evidence. Other common mechanisms involving plastic packaging include shrink bands package necks and shrink warp around containers.

Fitments and Overcaps

Fitments are another set of devices associated with closures. These are components that are used in conjunction with a closure to provide some added utility by regulating the flow of product out of the package. A common example is the shaker-top on a spice jar. When dispensing device is built into the closure, instead of in a separate piece, the result is sometimes referred to as a fitment closure.

Overcaps, as the name indicates, are designed to be applied to over the closure. They may serve purely a decorative function, but most often they are designed to offer some protection to a dispensing closure so that it is not activated prematurely.

10.3 CLASSIFICATION OF CONTEMPORARY CLOSURES BY THEIR UTILITY

It is possible to place all closures into clean-cut categories where there is no overlap of functions.

Yet despite these limitations, a classification can provide focus for understanding contemporary closure trends. As defined by their utility the four classes of contemporary closures are – containment, convenience, control and special purpose.

1. **Containment closure:** Though all closures provide containment, a containment closure is here defined as an on-place cap whose primary function is to provide containment and access on vast production scales. CT caps (for general-purpose sealing), crowns and roll ons (for sealing of pressurised beverages), lug and press-on caps (for vacuum sealing of food) are within this class of containment closure.

2. **Convenience closure:** Closure development in recent years has been in response to consumer preferences for convenient access to the product. Convenience closures provide ready access to liquids, powders, flakes, and granules for products that are poured, squeezed, sprinkled, sprayed or pumped from their containers.

Some of the Convenience Closures used for Packaging

1. **Fixed-spout closures:** A spout is a tubular projection used to dispense liquid and solid materials. It may be fixed or movable and capable of dispensing a product in a wide ribbon/a fine bead depending on size and configuration of the orifice. Fixed spout caps incorporate a cylindrical or conical projection into the centre of a threaded or friction-fitting closure. Spouts on reusable containers are often sealed by a small sealer tip on the end of the spout.

2. **Movable-spout closures:** Also referred to as turret, swivel or toggle types, the movable spout concept features a hinged spout which can be flipped into operating position and reclosed with the thumb alone to provide one-handed access and reseal.

3. **Plug-orifice closures:** These closures first aided in the dispensing of personal-care and cosmetic products, and are now used in conjunction with multilayer high barrier plastic bottles for convenient dispensing of food products. The hinged-top designs represent the wave of the future in food packaging. The closure consists of a dispensing orifice incorporated into a screw-on base closure and plug, hinged within the top of the closure or moulded into a flip-up hinged cap.

4. **Tamper-evident closures:** Tamper-evident caps have been in use for years, though earlier they were referred to as "pilferproof caps". Today these metal and plastic caps provide visual evidence of seal disruption and are used for over-the-counter (OTC) drugs, beverages and food products. The two kinds of TE closures are "breakaway" or "tear band" closures used for pressurised and general sealing applications. The closure user can also

fulfil tamper-evident requirements through the use of inner seals, which cover the container mouth.

The two forms of tamper-evident caps are – mechanical breakaway and tear bands.

i. **Mechanical breakaway:** These are threaded caps with perforations along the lower part of the skirt which form a "break line" in the closure. When the closure is twisted for removal, the band, which is locked to the finish by crimping or rachets, separates from the closure along the break line.

   The cap is removed and the lower part of the skirt remains on the container neck. The breakaway cap can be efficiently applied, is highly visible, familiar to consumers and is durable enough to maintain its integrity throughout distribution. Metal closures of this type frequently crimp the band to the container neck for a friction hold. Variations in this type of TE closure include different band designs and methods of off-torque resistance.

ii. **Tear bands:** These types, frequently called tear tabs, employ a locked band to prevent cap removal. Access is accomplished by completely removing the band from the container. Frequently protruding tab is easy for the consumer to grasp and commence tearing. Many non threaded TE closures utilise this type of closure, such as the press-on friction fit closures found on milk containers. The closure is removed by tearing off the lower skirt, which overrides a bead on the container finish. Most of the removable-band types are made of plastic, usually polyethylene.

iii. **TE vacuum caps:** Marketing leverage, rather than legal mandate, accounts for the expansion of TE into food packaging and other products. These measures are not referred to as "tamper-evident" in label or closure communications, but are placed in a more positive light, such as "Freshness Sealed" or "Safety Sealed". The two major types of TE vacuum closures are vacuum button and vacuum tear-band caps. A popular TE option for food and pharmaceutical products packaged in glass containers under vacuum is the "button-top closure". These include lug versions used for jellies, sauces and juices and the threaded-seal version popular with the baby-food industry. A safety button, or coin-sized embossment on the top of the cap, pops-up as the jar is opened and its vacuum is lost. Accompanying this is the "pop" which serves as audible evidence of an undisrupted seal. When capped the embossed button is held down by vacuum pressure, providing the consumer with visual evidence that the container has not been opened. Another type, the "vacuum tear-band closure", is a two-component closure used for the packaging of nuts and condiments. It consists of a metal vacuum lid inserted into plastic tear-band closure skirt. Protrusions moulded into the plastic collar provide friction-fitting resealability for the container.

10.4 SPECIAL-PURPOSE CLOSURE

Special-purpose closures are those which are of specialized application or premium design. These include aesthetic closures, special-function closures, stoppers and overcaps.

- **Stoppers:** The wine and champagne industry is the largest user of stoppers. Cork stoppers are standardised by size and grades, the latter according to the degree of product vintage. Stoppers of natural rubber, synthetic silicone rubbers, and thermoplastic materials provide closure in some applications.
- **Overcaps:** The overcap is a secondary cap designed to protect the primary closure, dispenser, or fitment of a container. Metal or plastic overcap designs attach to the container by friction-fit or thread engagement, and are used to protect an aerosol and dispensing fitments.
- **Wire ties:** This type of closure is one of the two closures, which have emerged as the standards of the baking industry. Different models are used to attach to different types of bread and buns. This type of automatic bag-closing equipment is limited to about 60 packages per minute.

10.5 CLOSURE FUNCTIONS

A closure is an access-and-seal device attached to glass, plastic and metal containers. This includes tubes, vials, bottles, cans, jars, tumblers, jugs, pails, and drums. The closure works in conjunction with the container to fulfil various functions for Pharmaceutical products as are mentioned below:

- **Positive seal:** A packaged product is vulnerable to many forms of natural deterioration, including migration of water vapour, oxygen, carbon dioxide or contamination by microbes. The closure must provide an adequate seal until the contents are required for use. Usually this entails preventing escape of the contents and ingress of the external environment. Two closure methods provide containment and seal: friction-fitting closures - including snap-on and thread engagement closures - including plastic screw caps with continuous-thread or once at different interval. The degree of seal tightness, however, is dependent on the product packed, closure, container, and seal desired, the resiliency of liner, the flatness of the sealing surface and tightness or torque with which the closure is applied.

- **Access:** Contemporary closure design is shaped by the demands of pluralistic marketplace where strong consumer preferences for convenient access exist alongside legal mandates for access control. Many packages today are ergonomically designed systems capable of easy opening and dispensing and also affording critical access control. Closure technology has always sought to provide "a tight seal with easy access", but today's simultaneous demands for easy access and access control are the most polarised in the industry's history. In most instances it must be possible to open the container without difficulty and reseal it properly when only part of the contents is used at a time. Alternatively, of course, the closure may be provided with a dispensing device, such as a spout for oil container, which is operated without removal of the closure.

- **Control:** Concurrent to greater demand for convenience, often one-handed, access to a product, legal mandates and consumer preferences press for more access controls. These access controls are of two major types: tamper-evident and child-resistant. Regulated Tamper-Evident (TE) closures may be breakable caps of metal, plastic, or metal/plastic composites. In one variety, the closure itself is removable but a TE band remains with the neck of the bottle. In another, the TE band is torn off and discarded.

  Best example is of packaged drinking water. Another system incorporates a vacuum detection button on the closure. Other TE systems include paper, metal foil, or plastic inner seals affixed to the mouth of the container. Child-resistant closures (CRCs) are designed to inhibit access by children under the age of five. This is frequently accomplished through access mechanism involving a combination of coordinated steps, which are beyond a child's level of conceptual or motor skills development. Of these closures, 95% are made of plastic: the remaining 5% combine with plastic.

- **Product:** Closure Compatibility: The closure must not affect the contents of the container, nor be affected by them. It should be resistant to any climatic conditions likely to be encountered and it may need to withstand conditioning or processing treatment, such as pasteurization or sterilisation. The product/closure interaction is affected by the area of contact between the closure and the product and by the fact that many screw or snap-on closures may be fitted with internal wad or liner so that the closure material does not contact the contents. With narrow-necked bottles, the area of contact is very small in relation to the volume of the contents. Since migration is proportional to area of contact, the resultant hazard is small, with wide-mouth jars; of course, the area of contact can be quite appreciable.

- **Verbal and visual communications:** The closure is a focal point of the container. As such, it provides a highly visible position for communications, an integral aspect of today's packaging. Three communication forms include styling aesthetics, typography, and graphic symbols. Since the closure is handled and seen by the consumer every time the product is used, the audible, visual and tactile message (often subconscious) becomes very important to the packager.

- **Impact resistance:** The closure may also have to comply with certain performance requirements. Impact strength may often be a factor, for example, especially where conditions are severe, either on the filling line or in the distribution system. The closure may also have to be resistant to cracking and creep in order to withstand excess torque during screwing-on (as with screw caps) or other internal forces. Thermosets, such as phenol formaldehyde or urea formaldehyde are generally brittle but usually have excellent resistance to creep. HDPE has good impact resistance and is fairly rigid. Its creep resistance is limited, and this affects torque retention adversely. Of the other plastics commonly used for closures, high-impact polystyrene has good impact resistance and creep resistance. Polypropylene homo polymer gives a good overall spread of properties.

10.6 CLOSURE MATERIALS

In pharmaceutical industries, various types of materials are used for making closures. These materials are as follows:

- Cork closures
- Plastic closures
- Metal closures
- Glass closures
- Rubber closures

Cork Closures

Cork is obtained from the bark of oak tree. It is chemically inert and it does not give any colour and odour to the drug. Sometimes it reacts with the drug which can be prevented by giving the coat of wax on cork. The main disadvantages of cork closures are that there is chance of mould growth when they come in contact with aqueous solutions. Use of cork closures decreasing day by day. These have now been replaced by Plastic or rubber closures.

Plastic Closures

Plastic closures are now a days commonly used. They are unbreakable and light in weight. A liner is used in these closures. These closures must be tested for any extractable matter contained in them and for their incompatibility with content of container.

Moulded plastic closures are divided into two groups: thermoplastics (e.g. polyethylene, polypropylene and polystyrene) and thermosets (e.g. phenolic resins and urea components). Thermoplastic materials can be softened or recycled by heat; thermoset materials cannot be recycled once they are moulded.

- **Thermoplastics:** In general, thermoplastic closures offer the packager light weight, versatility of design, good chemical resistance to a wide range of products, and economical resins and manufacturing processes. Their relative flexibility is essential to contemporary closure design with its emphasis on convenience and control devices. Thermoplastics provide good application and removal torque. They maintain a good seal and tend to resist back-off. Unlike thermosets, thermoplastics can be pigmented in full-colour spectrum in strong, fade-resistant intensities. Most thermoplastic closures are produced by injection moulding, although some are made by thermoforming. Polypropylene and Polyethylene account for about 90% of all thermoplastic closures.

- **Polypropylene:** Polypropylene has unusual resistance to stress-cracking, an essential characteristic of hinged closures. In thin hinged sections, it has the remarkable property of strengthening with use. The homopolymer has limited impact resistance, but it can be modified for better performance. It has excellent resistance to acids, alkalies, oils and greases, and most solvents at normal temperature. It has the best heat resistance of all polyolefins, with a high melting point suitable for sterilised products, but it becomes brittle at low temperatures. Polypropylene has better printability than polyethylene but both are inferior to Polystyrene or thermosetting plastics in that respect. As a relatively rigid moulded material, it has outstanding emboss potential for closure communications.

- **Low density polyethylene:** LDPE is resilient and flexible. It is relatively tasteless and odourless, although some organoleptic problems are more prevalent with LDPE than with Polypropylene. It provides outstanding moisture protection, but it is not a good gas barrier. LDPE's economy as a closure material is provided by low-cost resins and relatively short injection-moulding cycle times. Though it is considered to have good resistance to stress cracking, problems may occur in the presence of certain chemicals. Communication embossments are good but limited by the softness of the material.

- **High density polyethylene:** Compared to LDPE, HDPE is stiffer, harder and more impermeable. It is tasteless, odourless and impact-resistant, but will stress-crack in the presence of some products unless it is specially formulated. Its heat resistance and barrier properties are superior to LDPE. HDPE resin is more expensive than LDPE, but it is still considered a relatively low-cost material. A particular drawback to HDPE closures is a potential for warpage and loss of torque.

- **Polystyrene:** Polystyrene is used for about 10% of the closures produced today. Polystyrene homopolymer is attacked by many chemicals, is very brittle, has relatively low heat resistance, and does not provide a good barrier against moisture or gases. Many of the disadvantages of polystyrene are overcome by rubber modification and/or copolymerization.

- **Thermosets:** Thermosets Phenolic and urea compounds have wide range of chemical compatibility and temperature tolerances. Some thermosets can sustain sub-zero temperature. Thermosets cannot provide the colour range or intensity of thermoplastics, but they accept vacuum metallising decoration in silver and gold with superior adhesion qualities. During the moulding process, thermosets undergo a permanent chemical change and cannot be reprocessed as thermoplastics can be. Thermoset closures are manufactured by compression moulding.

- **Phenolics:** Phenol-formaldehyde closures are hard and dense. They are the stiffest of all plastics, but are relatively brittle and low in impact strength. The properties of phenolics depend to a large extent upon the filler material used. Cotton and rag fibre additives increase the impact strength; asbestos and clay additives improve chemical resistance. Phenolics have excellent solvent resistance and heat resistance. Phenolics cost less than urea, and are easier to fabricate, but are limited in colour to black and brown unless decorated.

- **Urea:** Urea-formaldehyde is one of the oldest plastic packaging materials, first used in the early 1900s. The resin produces extremely hard, rigid closures with excellent dimensional stability, but is the most brittle. Urea compounds are odourless and tasteless, with good chemical resistance. They are not affected by organic solvents but are affected by alkalies and strong acids. They show good resistance to all types of oils and greases. They withstand high temperature without softening. Urea compounds are available in white and a wide range of colours, but with muted intensities compared to thermoplastics. Urea compounds, like phenolic resins, do not build up static electricity which leaves them free of dust. They are the most expensive of the plastic closure materials.

Metal

Metal caps, the strongest of closures, are used today for general, vacuum and pressurized applications. Tinplate and tin-free steel are used in the production of continuous thread, and vacuum press-on closures, lugs, overcaps and crown caps. The largest market for steel closures is vacuum packaging. Aluminium closures are primarily continuous thread caps and roll-on designs.

Glass

Glass closures are normally not used for pharmaceutical products. They are used in the stopper of the chemical reagent bottles in laboratories. Glass closures are ideal but they mostly slip during transportation and handling.

Rubber

Must be compatible with the product. Closures are made of metal, plastic or rubber bungs. Rubber bungs are used for parenterals that require multiple or single piercing for multiple use without any detachment of particles by fragmentation.

Properties of an Ideal Rubber Closures

   i. It should not absorb medicaments.
  ii. It should withstand the temperature and pressure of an autoclave.
 iii. It should be soft.
 iv. It should be impermeable to moisture and air.
  v. It should not release undesirable substance.
 vi. It should be enough elastic.

Advantages of Rubber Closures for Pharmaceutical Products

   i. The most important advantage of rubber closure is their self sealability after penetration with a needle.
  ii. They provide a hermetic seal to the container.
 iii. They provide adequate protection to the packed product from microbial contamination.
 iv. They are soft, elastic and easily fit on the container to give a perfect seal.
  v. They can withstand high temperature and pressure of autoclaving.
 vi. These are available in variety of composition so that a suitable material may be chosen depending on the compatibility of the product.

vii. These are available in a variety of colours and design and therefore aid in product identification.

Disadvantages of Rubber Closures

i. Permeability of air and moisture varies on the material depending on the material of construction and these are not completely impermeable.

ii. Additives used during the manufacture of rubber closures may leach out into the product and cause deterioration.

iii. Rubber closures may adsorb or absorb active medicaments as well as excipients like preservatives so as to render them ineffective.

iv. Compatibility of the closures with the product have to be evaluated on a product to product basis.

v. Certain rubber closures may show the problem with aging.

vi. Good quality rubber closures are comparatively expensive.

10.7 TYPES OF PLASTIC CLOSURES

Fin-lok	Beverage closure with mechanical tamper evident band.	NC-Flap	Two types of NC-Flap are available, one is One-piece liner less and the other has inner plug. Mechanical tamper evident band has flaps which engage with locking ring of the bottle finis.
Application	Soft drinks, Liquor		
Material	Polypropylene		
Seal	Plastic Mold Lining		
Size	Packing Liner		
Filling	28, 36, 38 mm	Application	Soft drinks, Condiment
Bottle	Flat, Hot-fill, CSD	Material	Polypropylene
		Seal	Linerless, Inner-plug
		Size	28 mm
		Filling	Hot-fill
		Bottle	PET bottle, Glass bottle

Uni-lok	One-piece linerless plastic beverage closure. It is designed for aseptic-filled beverages in PET bottles. It features high tamper evidence- ratchet band mechanism with dual threads.
Application	Water, Soft Drinks, Chemicals
Material	PP for Soft Drinks, PE for Chemicals
Seal	Linerless (for soft drinks) Packing liner for chemicals
Size	27 mm for Soft Drinks 25, 30,40 mm for chemicals
Filling	Aseptic, Flat
Bottle	PET bottle, Plastic bottle

NC-lok	Ratchet type of Tamper Evident band.
Application	Soft drinks
Material	Polypropylene
Seal	Plastic mold lining
Size	28 mm
Filling	Hot-fill
Bottle	Soft drinks

Pouch Spout Cap	Specially designed for food and beverage packed in pouches. The closure has tamper evident band and spout for drinking or pouring.
Application	Soft drinks, Condiments
Material	Polypropylene
Seal	Liner-less
Size	12, 21, 27 mm
Filling	Hot-fill, Flat
Bottle	Pouch

Sports Push-Pull Cap	Developed for beverage in the active scene. Convenience to drink and security of sealing forms in the design.
Application	Soft drinks
Material	Polyethylene, Polypropylene
Seal	Inner plug
Size	28 mm
Filling	Hot-fill
Bottle	PET bottle

AOV Cap	Heat shrink tamper evident band. Inner plug gives it convenient pouring with drain-back feature.
Application	Condiment
Material	Polyethylene
Seal	Linerless
Size	28 mm
Filling	Hot-fill
Bottle	Glass bottle

Pull Cap	Two piece tamper evident condiment cap. Tear off the pullring to break the seal. Upper body has thread and can reseal. Detachable type is also available.
Application	Liquid condiment
Material	Polyethylene
Seal	Linerless
Size	26, 32 mm
Filling	Flat, Hot-fill
Bottle	Glass bottle, PET bottle

Smooth Hinge Cap	No slits on the top panel, thus make the package hygienic. The lid opens widely with Adequate snapping. Various types and sizes of orifice are available.
Application	Desert toppings, Icing,
Material	Polypropylene
Seal	Linerless
Size	24, 25, 26, 27 mm
Filling	Flat
Bottle	Plastic bottle

Smooth Pull-Hinge Cap	One-piece condiment cap with snap open hinge and tear -off opening pouring mechanism. The closure is plugged on the bottle. This closure can be detached from the bottle
Application	Liquid condiment
Material	Polyethylene
Seal	Linerless
Size	26, 32 mm
Filling	Flat, Hot-fill
Bottle	Glass bottle, PET bottle

Side-score Cap	Tear-off the side score to break the seal and remove the closure from the bottle.
Application	Milk
Material	Polyethylene
Seal	Linerless
Size	37, 42 mm
Filling	Chilled filling
Bottle	Glass bottle, Plastic bottle

Push-pull Cap	Pull up the top knob to open and push it down to close.
Application	Sports drink, Kitchen detergent
Material	Polyethylene, Polypropylene
Seal	Linerless
Size	25, 30 mm
Filling	Flat
Bottle	PET bottle, Plastic bottle

10.8 SEALING SYSTEMS

Though often the smallest aspect of a package, the seal is responsible for keeping the entire concept intact. If the seal is not maintained by the closure, liner and container working together, the success of the product is at stake.

10.9 LINERS

A liner may be defined as any material that is inserted in a cap to effect a seal between the closure and container.

Today's lining material is either a single substance (usually paperboard or thermoplastic) or a composite material. Synthetic thermoplastic liners include foamed and solid plastics of varying densities. A composite

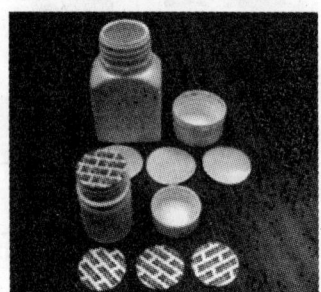

Fig. 10.8: Containers, closures and liners

lining material consists of a backing and a facing. The backing, usually made of cellulose or thermoplastic, is designed to provide the proper compressibility to affect the seal and proper resiliency force sealing. Facing materials, representing the side of a composite liner that comes into direct contact with the product are numerous, as are the variables of product chemistry which they must contend with. Generally, facing materials are thermoplastic-resin-coated papers, laminated papers of foil or film or multilayer types devised for special applications. Actually, it is the liner, which plays the vital role in the success or effectiveness of a closure in particular, and package performance in general. According to their composition, liners can be broadly classified into two groups, namely homogeneous and heterogeneous. As mentioned earlier, most closure liners contain two basic components – backing and facing. The backing provides compressibility, resiliency and re-sealability, and the facing provides mainly barrier protection and compatibility. In some liners, one component serves both functions, in some two-component liners are required.

10.10 CLOSURE LINER FUNCTIONS

The only part of a properly functioning closure and liner that comes in contact with the contents of the package is the face or facing of the liner. The threads or other parts of the closure perform no sealing function other than the mechanical one of maintaining intimate contact between the face of the liner and the glass sealing lip.

A properly functioning liner must fulfill three general requirements:

- When the face or facing is pressed against the container-sealing surface with normal closure pressure, it must provide a positive barrier against liquid leakage.
- It must provide an adequate barrier against escape of vapours of all components of the packaged product, and against entry of atmospheric moisture and gases.
- It must withstand constant contact with the product under all conditions of storage without appreciable chemical or physical change, and must contribute nothing deleterious to the products such as odour, flavour, toxicity, or unsatisfactory appearance.

10.11 CLASSIFICATION OF LINERS

Homogenous liners: These are available as a disc or as a ring of rubber/plastic. These are expensive and complicated. They are used for pharmaceuticals because they are uniform and can withstand high temperature sterilization.

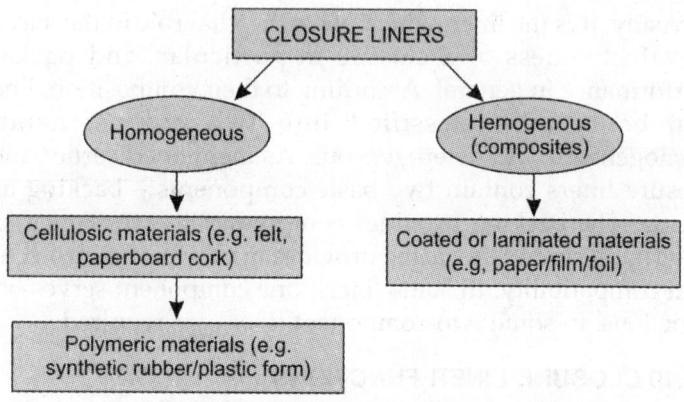

Fig. 10.9: Classification of closure liners

Heterogeneous liners: These are composed of layers of different materials chosen for specific requirements. They composed of two parts, facing and backing. Facing is in contact with the product and the backing provides the sealing properties.

10.12 SELECTION OF LINING MATERIAL

Different factors to be considered in the selection of liners:

The proper choice of a closure liner can often make the difference between the success and failure of a product. If the package integrity is not maintained due to improper selection of the closure liner, all other purposes are lost. Obtaining the proper sealing action is no simple matter and doing so at optimal cost requires a judicious evaluation of several variables.

• Product compatibility
• Secure macroseal
• Positive microseal

- Application and removal torque
- Other considerations

Besides the above, freedom from odour and taste contamination, heat resistance characteristics, appearance, and above all, the economies are to be considered for selecting an appropriate closure liner.

Usually the smallest component part of the package and usually overlooked is the selection of the cap liner. The liner must not alter or be altered by the product. It must withstand repeated applications and removals against the container surface while maintaining the integrity of the sealing surface.

Some information that may help in choosing the right liner from product

Material	Description	Applications
Poly-Vinyl	One mil poly vinyl fi lm bonded to one mil HDPE on a #30 white pulp paper backing. Superior to plain pulp paper because it provides excellent moisture barrier.	General purpose: Suitable for wide range of applications. Chemical resistance: Good for mild acids, alkalis, solvents, alcohols, oils and aqueous products; poor for active hydrocarbons and bleaches.
Poly-Seal®	Manufactured from LDPE. The unique cone design provides a wedge type seal that not only seals across the top but also across the inside diameter.	Unique problem solving type of liner. This liner is stress crack resistant and offers superior torque retention and excellent sealing characteristics. It is recommended that this liner be tested prior to use for leak seal.
Foamed Polyethylene	A one piece, three ply coextruded liner consisting of foamed and solid LDPE. The foam core is sandwiched with solid clear PE.	General Purpose: Broad applications base. Chemical resistance-good for acids, alkalis, solvents, alcohols, oils, household cosmetics and aqueous products. Poor for hydrocarbon solvents. Liner provides tight seal.

Contd...

Contd...

Pulp/Metal Foil	Aluminium foil bonded to pulp board.	Good barrier properties, good resistance to hydrocarbons, oils, ketones and alcohols. Not good for acids or alkalis.
Styrene-Butadiene Rubber (14B)	The white rubber lining material consists of homogeneous sulfur cured styrene-butadiene rubber (SBR). FDA Status complies with 21CFR 177.26, "Rubber articles intended for repeated use."	Excellent properties of resilience, resistant to moisture vapour. Satisfactory for most moderate chemicals. Not good for oils, strong acids and hydrocarbons. Autoclavable.
Styrene-butadiene rubber/ 0.005 PTEF	The white rubber/0.005" PTFE liner consists of virgin PTFE bonded to the white sulfur cured, styrene-butadiene rubber. Complies with the FDA 21CFR 177.1550.	Designed for the ultimate in product safety. PTFE provides totally inert inner seal and surface facing the sample or product. Autoclavable.
Teflon Faced Silicone Rubber	The liner consists of 0.005" thick Teflon bonded to 0.055" thick silicone rubber.	Ideal for low temperature storage applications. Teflon facing provides excellent chemical barrier. Autoclavable.
Teflon Faced Foamed Polyethylene	Teflon®-faced foamed polyethylene liner that offers the excellent chemical resistance of Teflon® with the compressibility and sealing properties of polyethylene foam.	Typical applications: analytical lab samples, high purity chemicals, strong acids, solvents. Excellent for environmental samples, pharmaceuticals and diagnostic reagents.

Note: Closures and liners are designed for a variety of applications. Product performance can vary depending on conditions. It is recommended that proper tests be performed to determine the best liner for the application.

10.13 OPTIONS FOR CLOSURE LINERS

The state-of-the-art in liner technology can best be described as 'crowded'. Available choices of liners currently number in the hundreds and new structures continue to appear. The salient features of some common liner materials are given below:

Backing Material Options

- **Pulpboard:** Widely used liner material. It costs less but compresses only 4 to 5% at a standard force (5lbs/sq inch or 0.775 kg/cm^2) with about 80% recovery.
- **Composite corksheet:** Manufactured from granulated cork binded with synthetic resin. It is more compressible, about 30% and recovers 90 to 95% of deflection. It is mostly used with a barrier film such as PVC to prevent permeability to gases and liquids. PVC faced cork liners, though widely used, have a tendency to shrink, thus falling out from the cap. Also, cork stock does not cut clean leading to dust. Other problems being delamination of PVC film due to poor adhesion between cork and PVC surface.
- **Rubber:** For serum vials and similar biological product containers, rubber liners are often used to maintain hermetic seal after sterilization. Certain chemicals such as hydrocarbons, oils, esters, and ketones attack and eventually dissolve rubber.
- **Plastic foams:** These offer the exception to all backing material limitations. The resiliency and compressibility of plastic foams can be varied to give enormous diversity of properties.

Facing Material Options

- **Paper coated with varnish or plastic resins:** These were the first liners and continue to be important, but with the introduction of superior materials their usage is likely to be restricted. Though varnish paper offers good resistance to heat and chemicals, low water vapour transmission and glossy appearance, they tend to be brittle and require additional wax coating for both microseal and macroseal. As for thermoplastic coatings on paper, the degree of performance is a shade lower as the coating is ordinarily thinner.

- **Aluminium foil:** It offers excellent barrier properties but with aqueous products, acids and alkalies, it corrodes quickly. If used with a liquid product, it should be coated with suitable material.
- **PVC film:** It is a good choice for resisting oil, grease, water or weak acids and alkalies. It should be avoided in use with organic solvents and essential oils. The water vapour transmission rate is marginal. It may be used with alcohol, provided it is confirmed that plasticisers are not extracted.
- **Polyester:** It is suitable for alcohols, most organic solvents, oil and grease. It should not be used with acids and alkalies. Water vapour transmission rate is marginal.
- **Polyethylene:** It stands up to solvents, strong acids and alkalies. Oil and grease resistance is adequate as is water vapour transmission rate. It is the most economically compatible facing material.

10.14 INNERSEALS

The innerseals afford TE protection by sealing the mouth of the container. Three common types of innerseals are inserted by closure manufacturers into the caps. A waxed-pulp backing and glassine innerseals are common within the food industry. After the filling operation, the container runs under a roller system which applies an adhesive to the lip of the container and then the cap is applied. Upon removal, the glassine adheres to the container while the pulp backing remains in the closure. Pressure-sensitive innerseals, generally foamed polystyrene, adhere to the lip upon application and require several hours to set. Heat-induction innerseals are plastic-coated aluminium foils, often adhered to a waxed pulp base liner.

10.15 LINERLESS CLOSURES

Plastic linerless closures provide a positive seal in certain circumstances, foregoing the need for intermediary materials and secondary liner-insertion operations. To many packagers, the cost savings provided by the linerless closure can be considerable. The seal of a linerless closure is achieved by moulded embossments forming diaphragms, plugs, beads, valve seats, deflecting seal membranes or rings which press upon, grasp, or buttress the sealing surfaces of the container. Over a dozen types of linerless closures are in common use, each designed to provide a seal at one or more critical sealing surface, the inside edge of the land surface or the outside edge of the land surface. Some form of land seal in conjunction with a valve or flange represents one type of effective linerless closure design. The land is typically the most consistent sealing surface. A land-seal ring can bite into plastic container finishes or deflect on glass finishes. An inner buttress can correct ovality problems in plastic containers by forcing such off-round finishes back into proper shape.

10.16 TYPES OF TAPES

Adhesive Tapes

An adhesive tape is composed of a backing element in a long strip upon which an adhesive is applied. Its function is to attach the carrier backing to some secondary surface. The attachment is made by activating the adhesive with solvent, heat or finger pressure. Tapes are used for holding, bundling, sealing, protecting, reinforcing, colour identification and box closing. Gummed tapes, stamps, etc are the most commonly known variety of solvent – activated tape, that is the adhesive is activated by wetting with water. For certain industrial application, an organic solvent activated adhesive is used. A second type of adhesive tape is the thermoplastic or heat activated variety. In this construction, the adhesive is made sticky by the use of heat and pressure. The most rapidly growing line of adhesive tapes is the pressure sensitive variety. This type of tape can be applied with hand pressure in the absence of solvent or heat and sticks aggressively to most common surfaces. Because of its extreme ease of application, it has gained wide acceptance.

Pressure Sensitive Tape

In such tapes, adhesives are composed of a rubbery type elastomer combined with a liquid or solid resin tackifier component. A mixture of resin may be used to provide a balance of properties. Pressure sensitive tape is used for closing boxes, combining packages, attaching packaging lists, colour coding, pallet unitizing, adding carrying handles, splicing, providing ease of package opening, protecting labels, reinforcing critical package components, holding documents, besides a variety of other jobs. There are hundreds of speciality tapes available for specific applications in packaging. The common theme is a backing material coated with an adhesive that adheres with a light touch without a need for activating solvent or heat.

Box-sealing Tape

The largest use of pressure-sensitive tape in packaging is the closure of regular slotted containers. A plastic film is coated on one side with a pressure sensitive adhesive. The film may have a release treatment on one side to allow easy removal of the tape from the roll during dispensing. Some film backings also are treated or coated on the adhesive side to increase the bond of the adhesive to the backing.

Filament Tapes

A second broad category of packaging tape is pressure sensitive filament tape, sometimes known as "strapping tape". Filament tape is typically made of a film backing (polyester or polypropylene) with reinforcing filaments embedded in the pressure-sensitive adhesive. The most common filament is fibre glass, which provides a high tensile strength with very little elongation. A few tapes have polyester or rayon filaments for extra impact or cut resistance.

Tapes are also available with integral polymeric filaments. The adhesive requirements for filament tapes are as critical as those of box-sealing tapes. Care should be taken to choose a tape with a balance of tack and shear-holding power.

Film Tapes

Polymeric films have found numerous applications as tape and label backings. The properties inherent in polymeric films (impermeability, thinness, smooth surface, good dielectric properties and inertness) are reserved for many electrical, packaging and decorative applications.

Example

Cellophane is the oldest transparent film tape.
PVC films are widely used as tape backings.

10.17 STRAPPING MATERIALS

Strapping is generally the last but a key step in the packaging operation. Strappings are normally used for reinforcing, baling, palletising, unitising, bundling and tying. It is very useful in brace shipments of goods during transit.

Types of Strapping Materials

Metallic

- Round Wires
- Steel Straps (Bands)

Non-metallic

- Polyester
- Nylon
- Polyolefin
- Rayon

General Uses of Strapping Materials

- Strap may be used to secure a handling base (skids, platforms, pallets, runners, spacers, etc.) to a unit to expedite handling or to secure other packaging materials (battens, stiffeners, wrappings, etc) in position.
- Strap may be used for local securement or within the transport vehicle. It is applied under tension to restrain or control for movement of loading and thus accommodating in-transit shocks or irregular movements.
- Straps also provide security against accidental loss or theft of the contents.
- Different packages can be colour coded with strapping for easy identification in warehouses.
- Strap functions best when all resultant forces act directly parallel in line with the direction of the strap.

10.18 EVALUATING CLOSURE LINERS

Customers are responsible for evaluating or testing to determine the suitability of closure design and closure liner material for their specific product and package requirements. Kenplas has no control over product formulations, package design, package handling and storage and cannot therefore assume any responsibility for customer's choice of closure or closure liner materials. The entire package including the closure should be tested and evaluated by the customer to confirm that the package is satisfactory for its intended use.

Caution

Particular care should be exercised in the selection of liners for child-resistant closure systems. Certain products can alter the effectiveness of child-resistant closure if exposed to the child-resistant mechanism or closure components. Therefore, in selecting a child-resistant closure liner, appropriate testing should be conducted to demonstrate that the package remains child-resistant and adult-effective throughout its expected shelf life and use.

10.19 STANDARD LINERS

Where possible, standard liners are suggested as first choice with nonstandard liner materials as alternate suggestions, providing that standard liners are compatible with the product and are competitive in price. The use of standard liners is advantageous to customers because these materials are generally in stock.

10.20 TACSEAL

Tacseal© is the Owens-Brockway designation for an inner-seal liner, which is positioned in the closure and applied over the orifice of the container when the closure is applied. A Tacseal© liner remains in place on the container when the closure is removed and forms a seal until lifted or broken. There are three primary methods of applying the Tacseal© liner, namely, by wet adhesives, heat activation, or pressure activation. The Tacseal© is an extra seal that can add protection for such factors as water vapor and volatile components and protection against contamination and leakage. Tacseal© liners are normally available in sizes through 89 mm CT closures.

Again, the customer has the responsibility to evaluate the inner-seal system to be used with the product, the container to be sealed, and the equipment used to close and/or activate the materials selected.

10.21 SOLUTIONS

Wax Coatings

Three wax treatments are available: Lubricant Finish (LF), Light Wax (LW) and Full Wax (FW). Each of these coatings is applied at different coating weights and uses different wax formulations.

Lubricant Finish (LF)

Lubricant finish treatment is used to reduce excessive removal torque buildup typical of vinyl and polyethylene-coated papers. Vinyl and polyethylene-coated papers have a tendency to cold flow and as such, may result in removal torque buildup. This characteristic is accentuated with time and temperature.

The "LF" coating of wax does not completely eliminate the buildup but does materially reduce its effects to a practical workable range. The "LF" coating is also used with Saran film. Saran film has a tendency to grab the glass-sealing surface during capping, thus causing erratic capping performance, which results in false application values. Closures that appear to be on tight are reduced to approximately zero removal, which has a slight impact on handling. To overcome this tendency and to ensure good application and removal torque performance, the "LF" coating of wax should be used on all Saran liners when product compatibility will allow.

In view of the above characteristics of vinyl and poly-ethylene-coated papers and Saran film, it is strongly suggested that the "LF" coating of wax be used on these liners at all times, particularly with molded plastic caps with glued-in liners, when product compatibility will allow.

Light Wax (LW)

Light wax treatment is generally used to improve the moisture vapor barrier characteristic of a given liner facing. The type of wax used for this treatment also acts as a lubricant in the same manners that "LF" coating of wax does for vinyl and polyethylene-coated papers and Saran films.

Full Wax (FW)

Full wax treatment is generally used on wide-mouth closures as a caulking agent. Many liner facings provide a less than satisfactory seal for wide-mouth containers. The larger the finish, the greater the tolerance in both container and finish. The inherent waves and dips of large finishes also contribute to this condition. For this reason, full wax treatment is generally suggested for closures 58 mm and larger.

The full wax treatment will also provide an additional moisture barrier and act as a lubricant similar to the "LW" and "LF" coating treatments.

10.22 LINER DESIGNATIONS

Abbreviations for duplex liners describe the liner starting with the backing material and working toward the facing. Everything to the left of the "slant" is related to the backing material, and everything to the right of the "slant" is concerned with the facing and its treatment, i.e.

P/SFLF

    P = Pulpboard
    SF = Saran Film
    LF = Lubricant Finish Wax Treatment

10.23 LINER DESCRIPTION

14B White Rubber

White vulcanized styrene-butadiene rubber.

F1410

Teflon/silicone rubber/polypropylene film.

F-217

Co-extruded material. Foamed low-density polyethylene core between two solid layers of low density polyethylene.

Teflon-F-217

Teflon film laminated on one side to a one-piece 3-ply co-extruded material. Foamed low density polyethylene between two solid layers of low density polyethylene.

Linerless

A closure which has been engineered to function in specific applications without the use of an additional liner.

P/AF

Aluminium foil laminated to paper and bonded to pulpboard.

P/Poly

Polyethylene film laminated to paper and bonded to pulpboard.

P/RVTLF

Vinyl coating applied to high density polyethylene coated paper laminated to pulpboard.

P/TF

Tin foil laminated to paper and bonded to pulpboard.

Plastisol

Vinyl chloride resin applied as a liquid and baked to a final form.

Polycone

Cone-shaped low density polyethylene liner

PY

Solid Polyethylene.

Teflon Discs

Solid virgin Teflon TFE .015".

Unlined

A closure without a liner.

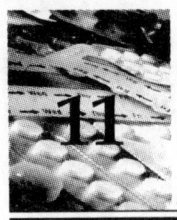

Corrugated Fiberboard Materials

11.1 INTRODUCTION

Corrugated Fiberboard (CFB) packaging is a versatile, economic, light, robust, recyclable, practical and yet dynamic form of packaging. Corrugated fiberboard packaging offers almost unlimited possible combinations of board types, flute sizes, paper weights, adhesive types, treatments and coatings. Corrugated fiberboard is routinely; custom designed to meet specific customer requirements. Corrugated Fiberboard is made from papers made up from cellulose fibres, which are virgin or recycled. This makes Corrugated Fiberboard a renewable natural resource.

Corrugated Board is made from a combination of two sheets of paper called liners glued to a corrugated inner medium called the fluting. These three layers of paper are assembled in a way which gives the overall structure a better strength than that of each distinct layer. Corrugated Fibre board boxes (CFB) are used for packing Fruits and Vegetables, automobile spare parts, Industrial goods, Pharmaceutical products, Paints, leather goods, textile garments, Food products, etc.

History

950BC	– The ancient Egyptians produced the first writing material by pasting together thin layers of plant stems.
100BC	– The Chinese created the first authentic paper from bamboo and mulberry fibers.
1400s AD	– Paper mills appeared in Spain, Italy, Germany and France.
1690	– The first sheet paper mill in North America was built near Philadelphia.

1767 – England wanted to regain their loss of colonial paper exports. They imposed the Stamp Act, which included a tax on all paper made in the colonies. Many consider this fuel for the American Revolution.

1803 – The first continuous papermaking machine was patented.

1854 – In England, the first pulp from wood was manufactured.

1856 – The first known corrugated material was patented for sweatband lining in tall hats of Victorian Englishmen.

1871 – Unlined corrugated first appeared as a packaging material for glass and kerosene lamp chimneys.

1874 – A liner was added to one side of the corrugated material to prevent the flutes from stretching.

1894 – Corrugated was slotted and cut to make the first boxes. Wells Fargo began using corrugated boxes for small freight shipments.

1903 – Corrugated was first approved as a valid shipping material and was used to ship cereals.

1909 – Rubber printing plates were developed which allowed for greater design creativity.

11.2 COMPONENTS OF CFB

Components of CFB: CFB has three components which are as follows:

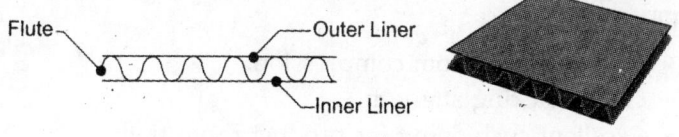

Fig. 11.1: Components of CFB

- Liner
- Fluting Medium
- Adhesive

1. Liner

Kraft paper of above 80 GSM to 250 GSM is used for making liner. Preferably outer most liner used for box should be of the maximum grammage.

Functions of Liner

i. Resist hazards like puncture, burst, abrasion, tear, etc.
ii. Properly hold the fluting medium when once combined.
iii. Resist moisture or water either outside or inside depending on the nature of product packed.
iv. Be amenable to printing.

Waterproof paper such as bitumen, sandwiched, poly-coated or wax coated are also used for liner.

2. Flutes

Types of Flutes

Flutes come in several standard shapes or flute profiles (A, B, C, E, F, etc.) A-flute was the first to be developed and is the largest common flute profile. B-flute was next and is much smaller. C-flute followed and is between A and B in size. E-flute is smaller than B and F-flute is smaller yet.

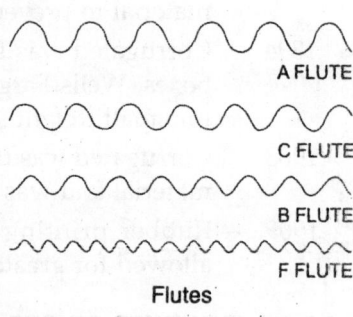

A FLUTE

C FLUTE

B FLUTE

F FLUTE

Flutes

Characteristics of Various Flute

A Flute

- High top to bottom compression.
- Good stacking strength.
- Excellent cushioning for product protection.

C Flute

- Good printing surface.
- Good top to bottom compression.
- Good resistance to flat crush.

B Flute

- High resistance to flat crush.
- Excellent printing surface.
- Scores and slots easily.
- Adapts well to automatic equipment.

E Flute

- High resistance to flat crush.
- Outstanding printing surface
- Mostly used for consumer goods shelf packaging.

F Flute

Good alternative to paperboard applications.

- Superior printing surface.
- High resistance to flat crush (Similar to E).
- Consumer goods shelf packaging (most applicable).

Functions of Fluting Medium

- Provides necessary cushioning desired.
- Provides rigidity to the board.
- Contributes to resistance to bending under stress particularly after converting into a box.
- The grammage of fluting medium may be in the region of 80–250 GSM.

3. Adhesive

While kraft paper is the main raw material for corrugated packaging industries, adhesive - as the second most important material has gained significance importance. Usually starch based adhesives are used for joining the outer liner (This has relation to printing) Sodium Silicate (near to natural) also is used. The silicate can give a rigid board but they can render the box brittle or lend to de-lamination depending upon the humidity.

11.3 TYPES OF CORRUGATED BOARD

Corrugated board consists of one or two outer plies, the flutes and, in multiply types of corrugated board, of 3 or more intermediate plies. Corrugated board is classified as follows according to the number of outer/intermediate plies and flutes:

1. Single face/2-ply corrugated board: Single face corrugated board consists of one ply of fluted paper, onto which paper or cardboard is glued.

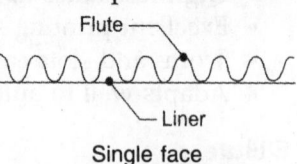

Single face

2. Single wall/3-ply corrugated board: Single wall (double face/3-Ply) corrugated board consists of one ply of fluted paper which is glued between two plies of paper or cardboard.

3. Double wall/5-ply corrugated board: Double wall/5-Ply corrugated board consists of two plies of fluted paper which are glued together by one ply of un-fluted paper or cardboard and the exposed outer surfaces of which are each covered with one ply of paper or cardboard.

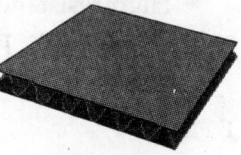

Single wall

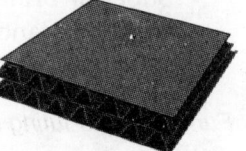

Double wall

4. Tri wall/7-ply corrugated board: Tri-wall corrugated board consists of three plies of fluted paper which are glued together by two plies of paper or cardboard and the outer surfaces of which are likewise each covered with one ply of paper or cardboard.

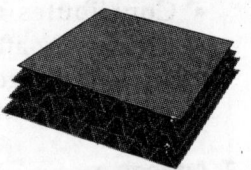

Tri wall

11.4 ADVANTAGES AND DISADVANTAGES

Advantages of CFB
- Effective cushioning material.
- Easy to fabricate.
- Easy to storing.
- Easy to disposal.
- More pilfer proof.
- No strapping necessary.
- Safe for human handling.
- Articles can be kept dust free after sealing.

- Could be specially made water resistance.
- Printing and advertising advantages.
- No self generating fungus.
- Desired in export market.
- Suitable for self service store display.

Disadvantages of CFB

- The base kraft paper not of desired standards.
- Road transport is not developed properly.
- Lack of Mechanical and Technical knowledge.
- Improper warehousing.
- Cargo handler resistance due to fear of damage.
- Failure to comply with dimensional specification.
- Supply of moist and damp material when hurry.
- De-lamination of layers.
- Use of unspecified adhesive and water proofing agents.

11.5 MANUFACTURING

Box Manufacturing

There are three steps involved in manufacturing of CFB box.

- **Slitting and scoring:** This operation trims the board to obtain proper dimension/size and creases the board for flap folding.
- **Slotting:** Slot is cut made in corrugated sheet usually to form flaps and thus permit folding.
- **Position of slot:** End of slot +/– 3 mm from center of flap score. Center of slot +/– 2 mm from center of panel score.

Joining is Done By

- Stitching (Staples)
- Gluing (usually plastic resin adhesive)
- Taping (Cloth or paper)

Strength obtained by gluing is good but stitching is common and less expensive. Depending upon the dimension of box there may be one, two or four joints.

11.6 BOX STRUCTURE

Corrugated fiberboard, or combined board, has two main components: the linerboard and the medium. Both are made of a special kind of heavy paper called containerboard. Linerboard is the flat facing that adheres to the medium. The medium is the wavy, fluted paper inbetween the liners.

The following illustrations demonstrate four types of combined board.

1. Single face: One medium is glued to one flat sheet of linerboard.

2. Single wall: The medium is between two sheets of linerboard. Also known as Double Face.

3. Double wall: Threesheets of linerboard with two mediums inbetween.

4. Triple wall: Four sheets of linerboard with three medium inbetween.

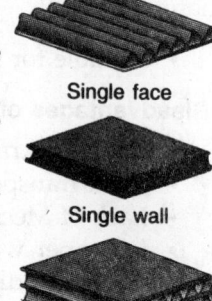

Single face

Single wall

Double wall

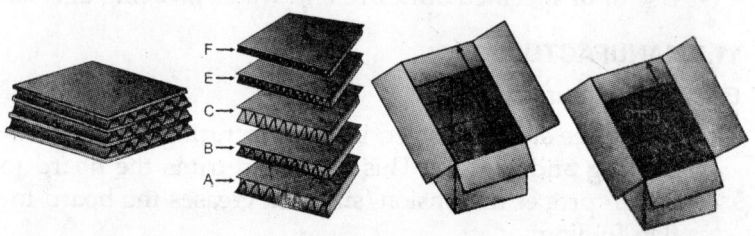

Triple wall

11.7 BOX DIMENSIONS

Dimensions are given in the sequence of length, width and depth. Internationally, the words length, breadth and height may be used to express these dimensions.

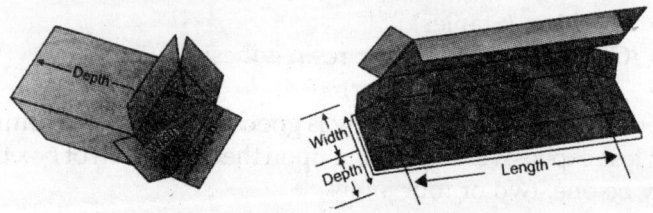

Box dimensions

Dimensions can be specified for either the inside or the outside of the box. Accurate inside dimensions must be determined to ensure the proper fit for the product being shipped or stored. At the same time, palletizing and distributing the boxes depends on the outside dimensions. The box manufacturer should be informed as to which dimension is most important to the customer.

11.8 TYPES OF BOX

Several designs of CFB boxes are commonly used in Packaging for Export goods. Some of the designs are as given below.

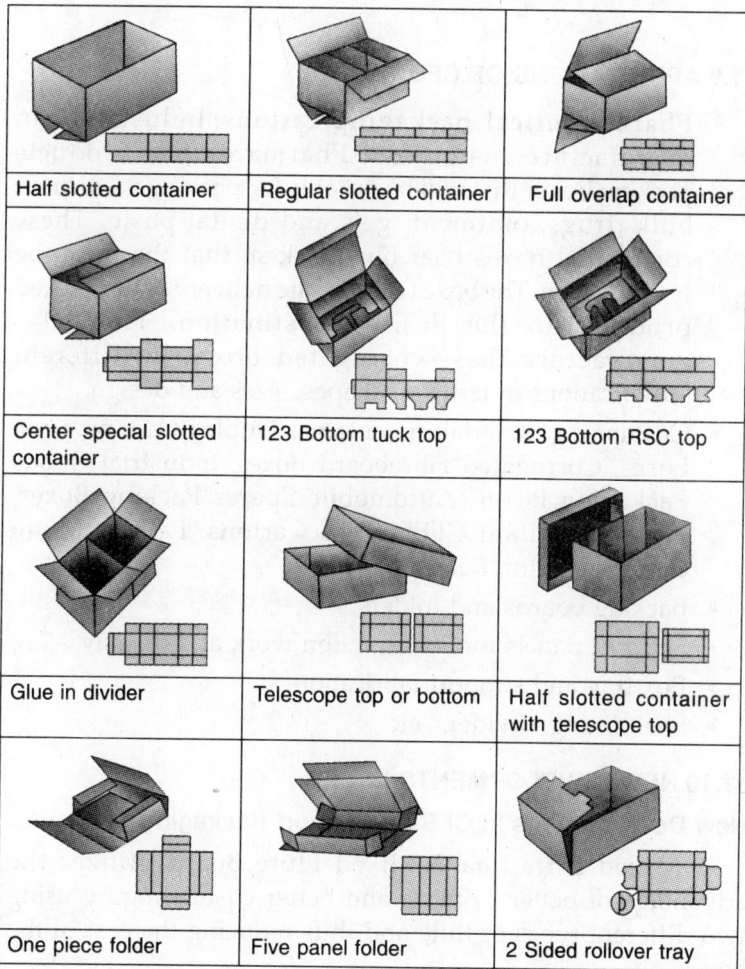

Half slotted container	Regular slotted container	Full overlap container
Center special slotted container	123 Bottom tuck top	123 Bottom RSC top
Glue in divider	Telescope top or bottom	Half slotted container with telescope top
One piece folder	Five panel folder	2 Sided rollover tray

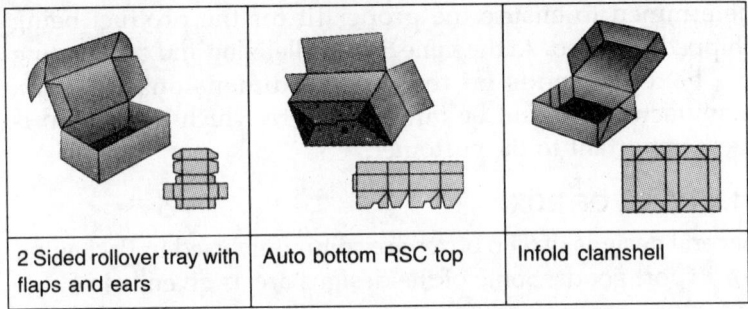

2 Sided rollover tray with flaps and ears	Auto bottom RSC top	Infold clamshell

11.9 APPLICATIONS OF CFB

- **Pharmaceutical packaging cartons:** Industries can manufacture customized Pharmaceutical Products packing boxes that will be durable for packing medicines, bulk drugs, ointment, gels and dental paste. These corrugated boxes bear our mark so that these can be trusted upon. The boxes ensure safe delivery of the packed products to the desired destination. They also manufacture these corrugated boxes in different specifications in terms of shapes, sizes and design.
- Cushioning material in container Duplex Cartons, Shoe Boxes, Corrugated Fibreboard Boxes, Industrial Goods Packaging Boxes, Automobile Spares Packing Boxes, Water Repellant CFB's, IMC Cartons, Pallets, Mono Cartons, Carton Packing Boxes.
- Backing boards and folders.
- Support panels for conservation work and display.
- Box tray and support fabrication.
- Shelf lining, dividers, etc.

11.10 NEW DEVELOPMENTS IN CFB

New Developments in CFBs for Export Packaging

1. Mixed flute board: Mixed Flute Board utilizes the advantage of better printing and better cushioning by using two different types of flute and thus reducing the cost of the box.

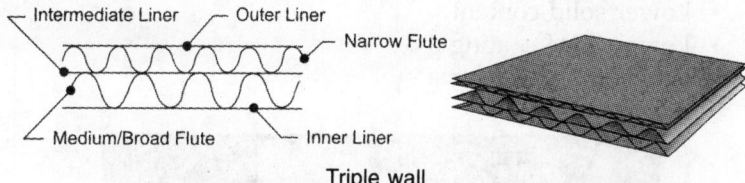

Triple wall

2. Duo arch board: Gives better strength by combining two flutes.

3. Paper IBC for liquids made from CFB: Paper IBC for Liquid is the ideal replacement for most drums, returnable totes and bottle-in-cage IBC. Carrying up to 1000 liters of liquid, replaces metal or plastic drums, reduces the filling and handling cost, provides efficient storage and transportation.

Duo arch board

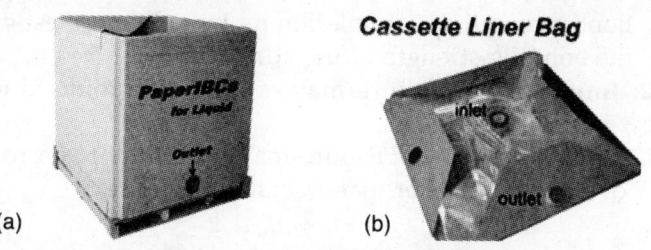

(a)   (b)

Fig. 11.2: Paper IBCs for liquid

Picture of Paper IBC for liquid is as shown in Fig. 11.2. These IBC's are collapsible and hence occupy very less volume during storage in the warehouses.

Paper IBC for liquid packaging for exports in ocean freight container is as shown in Fig. 11.3.

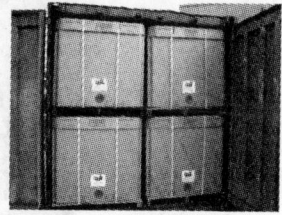

Fig. 11.3: Paper IBC

11.11 FAILURES IN THE CFB DURING EXPORT

1. Adhesive Failure: Adhesive failure in CFB during transport may result in delamination of the Flute and the Liner, which may occur due to:

- Lower solid content
- Lower GSM coating
- Poor quality adhesive

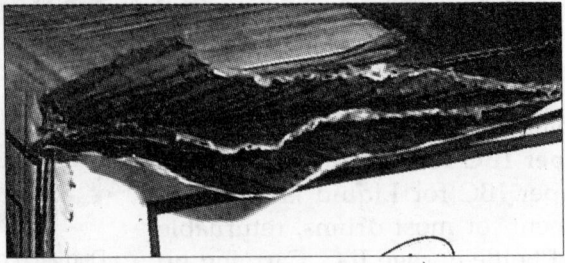

Fig. 11.4: Adhesive failure

Probable Solutions

- Stringent quality for adhesive.
- Bond strength determina-tion by pin adhesion test gives the bonding strength of the adhesive.

2. Joint failure: Failure may occur at the joints due to following reasons.

i. Stitching (Staples): Failure may occur due to corrosion of stapler and poor manufacturing practice.

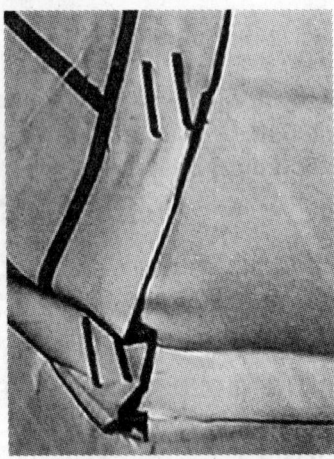

Fig. 11.5: Stitching (staples)

ii. Adhesive tape failure: Failure occurring due to poor shear properties of the adhesive tapes, or poor tensile property of tape.

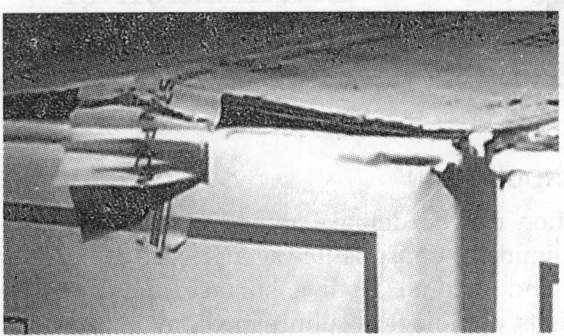

Fig. 11.6: Adhesive tape failure

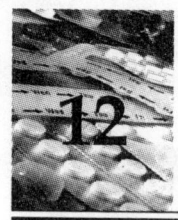

12 Sterilization of Packaging Materials

12.1 INTRODUCTION

Sterilization can be defined as any process that effectively kills or eliminates transmissible agents (such as fungi, bacteria, viruses and prions) from a surface, equipment, foods, medications, or biological culture medium. In practice sterility is achieved by exposure of the object to be sterilized to chemical or physical agent for a specified time. Various agents used as steriliants are: elevated temperature, ionizing radiation, chemical liquids or gases etc. The success of the process depends upon the choice of the method adopted for sterilization.

12.2 PHARMACEUTICAL IMPORTANCE OF STERILIZATION

Moist heat sterilization: Is the most efficient biocidal agent. In the pharmaceutical industry it is used for: Surgical dressings, Sheets, Surgical and diagnostic equipment, Containers, Closures, Aqueous injections, Ophthalmic preparations and Irrigation fluids etc.

Dry heat sterilization: Can only be used for thermo stable, moisture sensitive or moisture impermeable pharmaceutical and medicinal. These include products like; Dry powdered drugs, Suspensions of drug in non aqueous solvents, Oils, fats waxes, soft hard paraffin silicone, Oily injections, implants, ophthalmic ointments and ointment bases etc.

Gaseous sterilization: Is used for sterilizing thermolabile substances like; hormones, proteins, various heat sensitive drugs etc.

UV light: Is perhaps the most lethal component in ordinary sunlight used in sanitation of garments or utensils.

Gamma-rays: From Cobalt 60 are used to sterilize antibiotic, hormones, sutures, plastics and catheters etc.

Filtration sterilizations: Filtration is a method utilizing filters capable of screening out microorganisms. Filtration sterilizations are used in the treatment of heat sensitive injections and ophthalmic solutions, biological products, air and other gases for supply to aseptic areas. They are also used in industry as part of the venting systems on fomenters, centrifuges, autoclaves and freeze driers. Membrane filters are used for sterility testing.

12.3 PHYSICAL AND CHEMICAL FACTORS THAT AFFECT STERILIZATION

Several physical and chemical factors also influence sterilization procedures: temperature, pH, relative humidity and water hardness. For example, the activity of most sterilants increases as the temperature increases, but some exceptions exist. Furthermore, too great an increase in temperature causes the sterilants to degrade and weakens its germicidal activity and thus might produce a potential health hazard. An increase in pH improves the antimicrobial activity of some sterilants, but decreases the antimicrobial activity of others (e.g. phenols, hypochlorites and iodine). The pH influences the antimicrobial activity by altering the disinfectant molecule or the cell surface. Relative humidity is the single most important factor influencing the activity of gaseous disinfectants/sterilants, such as EtO, chlorine dioxide, and formaldehyde. Water hardness (i.e., high concentration of divalent cations) reduces the rate of kill of certain disinfectants because divalent cations (e.g., magnesium, calcium) in the hard water interact with the disinfectant to form insoluble precipitates.

12.4 TERMS COMMONLY USED

Survivor Curves

They are plots of the logarithm of the fraction of survivors (microorganisms that retain viability following a sterilization process) against the exposure time or dose.

Expression of Resistance

D-value

D-value is indicative of the resistance of any organism to a sterilizing agent. For radiation and heat treatment, D-value is the time taken at a fixed temperature or the radiation dose required to achieve a 90% reduction in viable count.

Z-value

Z-value represents the increase in temperature needed to reduce the D-value of an organism by 90%.

12.5 CLASSIFICATION OF STERILIZATION METHODS

1. **Physical Sterilization**
   A. **Heat (Thermal)**
      I. **Dry heat**
         • Hot air oven
         • Fleming
         • Incineration
         • Tyndallization
      II. **Moist heat (Autoclave)**
         • Below 100°C
         • At 100°C
         • Above 100°C
   B. **Radiation**
   C. **Filtration**

2. **Chemical Sterilization**
   A. **Gases**
   B. **Liquids**

1. Physical Sterilization

A. Heat Sterilization

Heat sterilization is the most widely used and reliable method of sterilization, involving destruction of enzymes and other essential cell constituents. The process is more effective in hydrated state where under conditions of high humidity, hydrolysis and denaturation occur, thus lower heat input is required. Under dry state, oxidative changes take place, and higher heat input is required.

This method of sterilization can be applied only to the thermostable products, but it can be used for moisture-sensitive materials for which dry heat (160–180°C) sterilization, and for moisture-resistant materials for which moist heat (121–134°C) sterilization is used.

The efficiency with which heat is able to inactivate microorganisms is dependent upon the degree of heat, the exposure time and the presence of water. The action of heat will be due to induction of lethal chemical events mediated through the action of water and oxygen. In the presence of water much lower temperature time exposures are required to kill microbe than in the absence of water. In this processes both dry and moist heat are used for sterilization.

I. Dry Heat Sterilization

Examples of dry heat sterilization are:
- Hot air oven
- Fleming
- Incineration
- Tyndallization

Dry heat can be used to sterilize items, but as the heat takes much longer to be transferred to the organism, both the time and the temperature must usually be increased, unless forced ventilation of the hot air is used. The standard setting for a hot air oven is at least two hours at 160°C (320°F). A rapid method heats air to 190°C (374°F) for 6 minutes for unwrapped objects and 12 minutes for wrapped objects(It employs higher temperatures in the range of 160–180°C and requires exposures time up to 2 hours, depending upon the temperature employed). The benefit of dry heat includes good penetrability and non-corrosive nature which makes it applicable for sterilizing glassware's and metal surgical instruments. It is also used for sterilizing non-aqueous thermostable liquids and thermostable powders. Dry heat destroys bacterial endotoxins (or pyrogens) which are difficult to eliminate by other means and this property makes it applicable for sterilizing glass bottles which are to be filled aseptically. Dry heat has the advantage that it can be used on powders and other heat-stable items that are adversely affected by steam.

Prions can be inactivated by immersion in sodium hydroxide (NaOH 0.09N) for two hours plus one hour autoclaving (121°C/250°F). Several investigators have shown complete (>7.4 logs) inactivation with this combined treatment. However, sodium hydroxide may corrode surgical instruments, especially at the elevated temperatures of the autoclave.

Glass bead sterilizer, once a common sterilization method employed in dental offices as well as biologic laboratories, is not approved by the U.S. Food and Drug Administration (FDA) and Centers for Disease Control and Prevention (CDC) to be used as inter-patients sterilizer since 1997.

Hot Air Oven

Dry heat sterilization is usually carried out in a hot air oven, which consists of the following:

- An insulated chamber surrounded by an outer case containing electric heaters.
- A fan
- Shelves
- Thermocouples
- Temperature sensor
- Door locking controls

Operation

- Articles to be sterilized are first wrapped or enclosed in containers of cardboard, paper or aluminium.

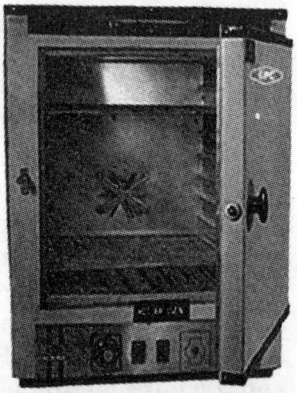

Fig. 12.1: Hot air oven

- Then, the materials are arranged to ensure uninterrupted air flow.
- Oven may be pre-heated for materials with poor heat conductivity.
- The temperature is allowed to fall to 40°C, prior to removal of sterilized material.

Flaming

Is done to loops and straight-wires in microbiology labs. Leaving the loop in the flame of a Bunsen burner or alcohol lamp until it glows red ensures that any infectious agent gets inactivated. This is commonly used for small metal or glass objects, but not for large objects. However, during the initial heating infectious material may be "sprayed" from the wire surface before it is killed, contaminating nearby surfaces and objects.

Incineration

Will also burn any organism to ash. It is used to sanitize medical and other biohazardous waste before it is discarded with non-hazardous waste.

Tindalization/Tyndallization

Named after John Tyndall is a lengthy process designed to reduce the level of activity of sporulating bacteria that are left by a simple boiling water method. The process involves boiling for a period (typically 20 minutes) at atmospheric pressure, cooling, incubating for a day, boiling, cooling, incubating for a day, boiling, cooling, incubating for a day, and finally boiling again. The three incubation periods are to allow heat-resistant spores surviving the previous boiling period to germinate to form the heat-sensitive vegetative (growing) stage, which can be killed by the next boiling step. This is effective because many spores are stimulated to grow by the heat shock. The procedure only works for media that can support bacterial growth - it will not sterilize plain water. Tindalization/tyndallization is ineffective against prions.

II. Moist Heat Sterilization

Moist heat may be used in three forms to achieve microbial inactivation.
1. Dry saturated steam – Autoclaving
2. Boiling water/steam at atmospheric pressure
3. Hot water below boiling point

Moist heat sterilization involves the use of steam in the range of 121–134°C. Steam under pressure is used to generate high temperature needed for sterilization. Saturated steam (steam in thermal equilibrium with water from which it is derived) acts as an effective sterilizing agent. Steam for sterilization can be either wet saturated steam (containing entrained water droplets) or dry saturated steam (no entrained water droplets).

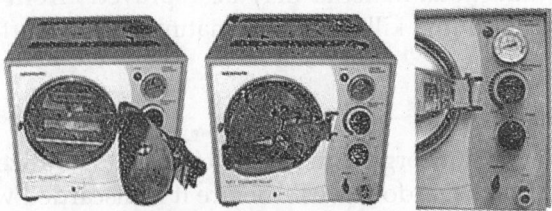

Fig. 12.2: Autoclave

Steam Thermal – Autoclave

A self-locking apparatus for the sterilization of material by means of steam under pressure. A widely-used method for heat sterilization is the autoclave, sometimes called a converter. Autoclaves use pressurized steam to destroy microorganisms, and are the most dependable systems available for the decontamination of laboratory waste and the sterilization of laboratory glassware, media, and reagents. For efficient heat transfer, steam must flush the air out of the autoclave chamber. Before using the autoclave, check the drain screen at the bottom

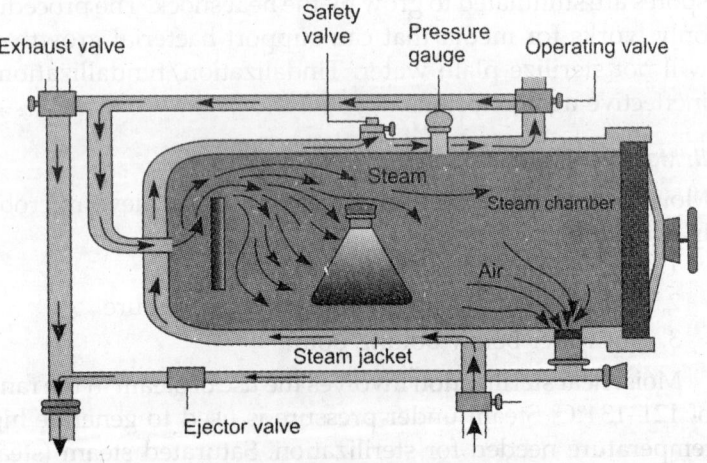

Fig. 12.3: An autoclave

of the chamber and clean if blocked. If the sieve is blocked with debris, a layer of air may form at the bottom of the autoclave, preventing efficient operation. Autoclaves should be tested periodically with biological indicators like cultures of *Bacillus stearothermophilus* to ensure proper function. This method of sterilization works well for many metal and glass items but is not acceptable for rubber, plastics and equipment that would be damaged by high temperatures.

Front-loading Autoclaves

Autoclaves, or steam sterilizers essentially consist of following:
- A cylindrical or rectangular chamber, with capacities ranging from 400 to 800 liters.
- Water heating system or steam generating system.
- Steam outlet and inlet valves.
- Single or double doors with locking mechanism.
- Thermometer or temperature gauge.
- Pressure gauges.

Operation

Autoclaves commonly use steam heated to 121–134°C (250–273°F). To achieve sterility, a holding time of at least 15 minutes at 121°C (250°F) or 3 minutes at 134°C (273°F) is required. For porous loads (dressings) sterilizers are generally operated at a minimum temperature of 134°C and for bottled fluid, sterilizers employing a minimum temperature of 121°C are used. Ensure that there should be sufficient water in the autoclave to produce the steam. The stages of operation of autoclaves include air removal, steam admission and sterilization cycle (includes heating up, holding/exposure, and cooling stages).

Proper autoclave treatment will inactivate all fungi, bacteria, viruses and also bacterial spores, which can be quite resistant. It will not necessarily eliminate all prions.

For prion elimination, various recommendations state 121–132°C (250–270°F) for 60 minutes or 134°C (273°F) for at least 18 minutes. The prion that causes the disease scrapie (strain 263K) is inactivated relatively quickly by such sterilization procedures; however, other strains of scrapie, as well as strains of CJD and BSE are more resistant.

B. Radiation Sterilization

Many types of radiation are used for sterilization like electromagnetic radiation (e.g. gamma rays and UV light), particulate radiation (e.g. accelerated electrons). The major target for these radiation is microbial DNA. Gamma rays and electrons cause ionization and free radical production while UV light causes excitation.

Radiation sterilization with high energy gamma rays or accelerated electrons has proven to be a useful method for the industrial sterilization of heat sensitive products. But some undesirable changes occur in irradiated products, an example is aqueous solution where radiolysis of water occurs.

Radiation sterilization is generally applied to articles in the dry state; including surgical instruments, sutures, prostheses, unit dose ointments, plastic syringes and dry pharmaceutical products. UV light, with its much lower energy, and poor penetrability finds uses in the sterilization of air, for surface sterilization of aseptic work areas, for treatment of manufacturing grade water, but is not suitable for sterilization of pharmaceutical dosage forms. Gamma rays are very penetrating and are commonly used for sterilization of disposable medical equipment, such as syringes, needles, cannulas and IV sets. Electron beam processing is also commonly used for medical device sterilization. X-rays, High-energy X-rays (bremsstrahlung) are a form of ionizing energy allowing to irradiate large packages and pallet loads of medical devices. Ultraviolet light irradiation (UV, from a germicidal lamp) is useful only for sterilization of surfaces and some transparent objects.

Gamma Ray Sterilizer

Gamma rays for sterilization are usually derived from cobalt-60 source, the isotope is held as pellets packed in metal rods, each rod carefully arranged within the source and containing 20 KCi of activity. This source is housed within a reinforced concrete building with 2 m thick walls. Articles being sterilized are passed through the irradiation chamber on a conveyor belt and move around the raised source.

Ultraviolet Irradiation

The optimum wavelength for UV sterilization is 260 nm. A mercury lamp giving peak emission at 254 nm is the suitable source of UV light in this region.

Application of Radiation Sterilization

Sterilization of Packaging Materials

The radiation stability of packaging and container materials must never be overlooked when considering radiation compatibility. Lists of radiation-compatible packaging materials are readily available. Treatment with gamma and electron radiation is becoming a common process for the sterilization of packages, mostly made of natural or synthetic plastics, used in the aseptic processing of foods and pharmaceuticals. The effect of irradiation on these materials is crucial for packaging engineering to understand the effects of these new treatments. Packaging material may be irradiated either prior to or after filling. The irradiation prior to filling is usually chosen for dairy products, processed food, beverages, pharmaceutical, and medical device industries in the United States, Europe, and Canada.

Sterilization of Rubber

A method sterilizing butyl rubber/styrene butadiene rubber (SBR) articles used in syringes or medical containers, comprising irradiating the butyl rubber/SBR elastomeric copolymer rubber article with gamma irradiation, wherein the SBR elastomeric copolymer comprises about 5% to about 50% of the rubber composition on a basis of total weight of the composition; and then exposing the irradiated rubber composition to a sterilizing gas for a time period sufficient to sterilize the rubber composition. The irradiated, sterilized rubber composition of the present invention is capable of maintaining superior performance standards with respect to sealability, recoverability from stress and elasticity.

C. Filtration Sterilization

Filtration process does not destroy but removes the micro-organisms. It is used for both the clarification and sterilization of liquids and gases as it is capable of preventing the passage of both viable and non viable particles.

The major mechanisms of filtration are sieving, adsorption and trapping within the matrix of the filter material. Sterilizing grade filters are used in the treatment of heat sensitive injections and ophthalmic solutions, biological products and air and other gases for supply to aseptic areas. They are also used in industry as part of the venting systems on fermentors, centrifuges, autoclaves and freeze driers. Membrane filters are used for sterility testing.

Application of filtration for sterilization of gases: HEPA (High efficiency particulate air) filters can remove up to 99.97% of particles >0.3 micrometer in diameter. Air is first passed through prefilters to remove larger particles and then passed through HEPA filters. The performance of HEPA filter is monitored by pressure differential and airflow rate measurements.

There are two types of filters used in filtration sterilization:

i. **Depth filters:** Consist of fibrous or granular materials so packed as to form twisted channels of minute dimensions. They are made of diatomaceous earth, unglazed porcelain filter, sintered glass or asbestos.

ii. **Membrane filters:** These are porous membrane about 0.1 mm thick, made of cellulose acetate, cellulose nitrate, polycarbonate, and polyvinylidene fluoride, or some other synthetic material. The membranes are supported on a frame and held in special holders. Fluids are made to transverse membranes by positive or negative pressure or by centrifugation.

Application of filtration for sterilization of liquids: Membrane filters of 0.22 micrometer nominal pore diameter are generally used, but sintered filters are used for corrosive liquids, viscous fluids and organic solvents. The factors which affects the performance of filter is the titre reduction value, which is the ratio of the number of organism challenging the filter under defined conditions to the number of organism penetrating it. The other factors are the depth of the membrane, its charge and the tortuosity of the channels. The merits, demerits and applications of different methods of sterilization are given in Table 12.1.

2. Chemical Sterilization

A. Gaseous Sterilization

The chemically reactive gases such as formaldehyde, (methanol, H.CHO) and ethylene oxide $(CH_2)_2O$ possess biocidal activity. Ethylene oxide is a colourless, odourless, and flammable gas. The mechanism of antimicrobial action of the two gases is assumed to be through alkylations of sulphydryl, amino, hydroxyl and carboxyl groups on proteins and amino groups of nucleic acids. The concentration ranges (weight of gas per unit chamber volume) are usually in range of 800–1200 mg/L for ethylene oxide and 15–100 mg/L for formaldehyde with operating temperatures of 45–63°C and 70–75°C respectively.

Both of these gases being alkylating agents are potentially mutagenic and carcinogenic. They also produce acute toxicity including irritation of the skin, conjunctiva and nasal mucosa.

1. Ethylene Oxide Sterilizer

Ethylene oxide (EO or EtO) gas is commonly used to sterilize objects sensitive to temperatures greater than 60°C such as plastics, optics and electrics. Ethylene oxide treatment is generally carried out between 30°C and 60°C with relative humidity above 30% and a gas concentration between 200 and 800 mg/L for at least three hours. Ethylene oxide penetrates well, moving through paper, cloth, and some plastic films and is highly effective. Ethylene oxide sterilizers are used to process sensitive instruments which cannot be adequately sterilized by other methods. EtO can kill all known viruses, bacteria and fungi, including bacterial spores and is satisfactory for most medical materials, even with repeated use. However, it is highly flammable, and requires a longer time to sterilize than any heat treatment. The process also requires a period of post-sterilization aeration to remove toxic residues. Ethylene oxide is the most common sterilization method, used for over 70% of total sterilizations, and for 50% of all disposable medical devices. The two most important ethylene oxide sterilization methods are: (1) the gas chamber method and (2) the microdose method.

Advantages of EtO Gas

1. Its compatibility with the product, material or substance being sterilized.
2. Acceptability of the packaging.
3. Penetration of the agent to remote areas that may contain viable microorganisms.
4. High level of lethal activity resulting in the need for only low quantities of the sterilizing agent.
5. Relatively inexpensive.
6. High degree of safety and low toxicity.
7. Simplicity.
8. Time required for the process; and
9. Adaptability to in-line processing.

Disadvantages of EtO Gas and Residue

One of its main disadvantages is the potential for toxic residues to be left in products and materials that have been sterilized. The three most common toxic residues of importance are ethylene oxide and two of its reaction products, ethylene chlorohydrin and ethylene glycol. For example, polyethylene retains 2 mg ethylene oxide per gram. In general sense, ethylene oxide toxicity is basically equivalent to that of ammonia; however, its additional reactivity and mutagenicity require that elaborate safety precautions to be taken with the use of this sterilizing agent. Ethylene oxide is a toxic gas, which irritates the mucosa, causing acute pulmonary edema in high concentrations. It has also shown adverse reproductive and transplacental effects. It can also contribute to chromosomal damage and cancer incidence.

Selection of Packaging Materials

For effective sterilization, selection of packaging material also plays important role apart from sterilization parameters. The

Table 12.1: Merits, demérits and applications of different methods of sterilization

Methods	Mechanism	Merits	Demerits	Applications
Heat sterilization	Destroys bacterial endotoxins	Most widely used and reliable method of sterilization, involving destruction of enzymes and other essential cell constituents.	Can be applied only to the thermostable products.	Dry heat is applicable for sterilizing glasswares and metal surgical instruments and moist heat is the most dependable method for decontamination of laboratory waste and the sterilization of laboratory glassware, media, and reagents.
Gaseous sterilization	Alkylation	Penetrating ability of gases.	Gases being alkylating agents are potentially mutagenic and carcinogenic.	Ethylene oxide gas has been used widely to process heat-sensitive devices.

Contd...

Contd...

Methods	Mechanism	Merits	Demerits	Applications
Radiation sterilization	Ionization of nucleic acids	It is a useful method for the industrial sterilization of heat sensitive products.	Undesirable changes occur in irradiated products, an example is aqueous solution where radiolysis of water occurs.	Radiation sterilization is generally applied to articles in the dry state; including surgical instruments, sutures, prostheses, unit dose ointments, plastics.
Filtration sterilization	Does not destroy but removes the microorganisms	It is used for both the clarification and sterilization of liquids and gases as it is capable of preventing the passage of both viable and non-viable particles.	Does not differentiate between viable and non viable particles.	This method is Sterilizing grade filters are used in the treatment of heat sensitive injections and ophthalmic solutions, biological products and air and other gases for supply to aseptic areas.

following are keys in selecting a suitable packaging material for gas sterilization: The packaging material must be permeable enough for ethylene oxide and moisture to enter the package (and air escape) and sterilize the contents within the desired cycle time: the penetration rate must be uniform. Productivity requirements make short cycles (high porosity) desirable. The packaging material must be impermeable to bacteria and other contaminants. The packaging material must not be deformed or porosity altered by pressure variations during vacuum cycles.

All plastic films used for wrapping should be evaluated on their ability to allow reasonable permeation of ethylene oxide gas, moisture, and air before and after sterilization. It has been observed that Medical Grade Paper on one side helps in faster aeration of EO Gas than laminate on both the sides. Permeability is one of the most important criteria. Not only must be sterilant be able to permeate the package, but the packaging material must have sufficient breathability to permit release of toxic residues (e.g. ethylene oxide residual gas). Additionally, the porosity and bond strength (the seal, or bond, between two packaging sub-strates) must be adequate enough to maintain package integrity.

For proper and safe EtO sterilization of medical devices, packaging materials and sterilization parameters go together. They need careful monitoring and selection. Ethylene oxide gas has been used widely to process heat-sensitive devices, but the aeration times needed at the end of the cycle to eliminate the gas made this method slow.

Low temperature steam formaldehyde (LTSF) sterilizer: An LTSF sterilizer operates with sub atmospheric pressure steam. At first, air is removed by evacuation and steam is admitted to the chamber.

2. Ozone

Ozone is used in industrial settings to sterilize water and air, as well as a disinfectant for surfaces. It has the benefit of being able to oxidize most organic matter. On the other hand, it is a toxic and unstable gas that must be produced on-site, so it is not practical to use in many settings. Ozone offers many advantages as a sterilant gas; ozone is a very efficient sterilant because of its strong oxidizing properties capable of destroying a wide range of pathogens, including prions without the need for handling hazardous chemicals since the ozone is generated within the sterilizer from medical grade oxygen.

B. Liquid Sterilization

1. Peracetic Acid Liquid Sterilization

Peracetic acid was found to be sporicidal at low concentrations. It was also found to be water soluble, and left no residue after rinsing. It was also shown to have no harmful health or environmental effects. It disrupts bonds in proteins and enzymes and may also interfere with cell membrane transportation through the rupture of cell walls and may oxidize essential enzymes and impair vital biochemical pathways.

In a low-temperature liquid chemical sterile processing system, several steps must be followed for effective sterilization:

1. Pre-cleaning of the devices is necessary because many devices have small connected lumens.
2. Leak testing is done to ensure there are no leaks that could allow fluid to enter/leak the ampoules/vials and cause damage.
3. The appropriate tray/container must then be selected and if the device has lumens, the appropriate connector attached.
4. The sterilant concentrate is provided in a sealed single-use cup and requires no pre-mixing or dilution.

The disadvantages of this method of sterilization are that the devices must be immersible, must fit in the appropriate tray and must be able to withstand the 55°C temperature the process uses.

2. Hydrogen Peroxide Sterilization

This method disperses a hydrogen peroxide solution in a vacuum chamber, creating a plasma cloud. This agent sterilizes by oxidizing key cellular components, which inactivates the microorganisms. The plasma cloud exists only while the energy source is turned on. When the energy source is turned off, water vapour and oxygen are formed, resulting in no toxic residues and harmful emissions.

There are five phases of the hydrogen peroxide processing cycle:

1. A vacuum phase creates a vacuum in the chamber and the pressure drops to less than one pound per square inch. This phase lasts about 20 minutes.

2. In the injection phase, the aqueous hydrogen peroxide is introduced into the vacuum chamber and is vapourized into a gas, which creates a rise in pressure due to the increase of molecules.

3. During the diffusion phase the hydrogen peroxide vapour spreads throughout the chamber and the increased pressure drives the sterilant into the packs, exposing the instrument surfaces to the sterilant and killing the microorganisms.

4. During the plasma phase the radiofrequency energy is applied, stripping the electrons from some of the molecules and producing a low-temperature plasma cloud. Following this reaction, the activated compounds lose their high energy and recombine to form oxygen and water.

5. The purpose of the venting phase is to introduce filtered air into the chamber and return the chamber to atmospheric pressure so that the door can be opened. It lasts about one minute.

Dry sterilization process (DSP): Uses hydrogen peroxide at a concentration of 30–35% under low pressure conditions. This process achieves bacterial reduction of $10^{-6}...10^{-8}$. The complete process cycle time is just 6 seconds, and the surface temperature is increased only 10–15°C (18 to 27°F). Originally designed for the sterilization of plastic bottles in the beverage industry, because of the high germ reduction and the slight temperature increase the dry sterilization process is also useful for medical and pharmaceutical applications.

3. Bleach

Chlorine bleach is another accepted liquid sterilizing agent. Household bleach consists of 5.25% sodium hypochlorite. It is usually diluted to 1/10 immediately before use. Bleach will kill many, but not all spores. It is also highly corrosive. Bleach decomposes over time when exposed to air, so fresh solutions should be made daily.

4. Glutaraldehyde and Formaldehyde

Glutaraldehyde and formaldehyde solutions (also used as fixatives) are accepted liquid sterilizing agents, provided that the immersion time is sufficiently long. To kill all spores in a clear liquid can take up to 12 hours with glutaraldehyde and even longer with formaldehyde. The presence of solid particles may lengthen the required period or render the treatment ineffective. Sterilization of blocks of tissue can take much longer, due to the time required for the fixative to penetrate. Glutaraldehyde and formaldehyde are volatile, and toxic by both skin contact and inhalation. Glutaraldehyde has a short shelf life (<2 weeks), and is expensive. Formaldehyde is less expensive and has a much longer shelf life if some methanol is added to inhibit polymerization to paraformaldehyde, but is much more volatile. Formaldehyde is also used as a gaseous sterilizing agent; in this case, it is prepared on-site by depolymerization of solid paraformaldehyde. Many vaccines, such as the original Salk polio vaccine, are sterilized with formaldehyde.

5. Phthalaldehyde

Ortho-phthalaldehyde (OPA) is a chemical sterilizing agent that received Food and Drug Administration (FDA) clearance in late 1999. Typically used in a 0.55% solution, OPA shows better mycobactericidal activity than glutaraldehyde. It also is effective against glutaraldehyde-resistant spores. OPA has superior stability, is less volatile, and does not irritate skin or eyes, and it acts more quickly than glutaraldehyde. On the other hand, it is more expensive, and will stain proteins (including skin) gray in colour.

Prions

Prions are highly resistant to chemical sterilization. Treatment with aldehydes (e.g., formaldehyde) has actually been shown to increase prion resistance. Hydrogen peroxide (3%) for one hour was shown to be ineffective, providing less than 3 logs (10^{-3}) reduction in contamination. Iodine, formaldehyde, glutaraldehyde and peracetic acid also fail this test (one hour treatment). Only chlorine, a phenolic compound, guanidinium thiocyanate, and sodium hydroxide (NaOH) reduce prion levels by more than 4 logs. Chlorine and NaOH are the most consistent agents for prions. Chlorine is too corrosive to use on certain objects. Sodium hydroxide has had many studies showing its effectiveness.

6. Silver

Silver ions and silver compounds show a toxic effect on some bacteria, viruses, algae and fungi, typical for heavy metals like lead or mercury, but without the high toxicity to humans that are normally associated with these other metals. Its germicidal effects kill many microbial organisms in vitro, but testing and standardization of silver products is yet difficult.

12.6 STERILIZATION OF PACKAGING MATERIALS

I. Sterilizing Glassware and Metal Instruments

Metal Instruments are best sterilized using a glass bead sterilizer, These sterilizers heat to approximately 275–350°C and will destroy bacterial and fungal spores that may be found on your instruments. The instruments simply need to be inserted into the heated glass beads for a period of 10 to 60 sec. The instruments should then be placed on a rack under the hood to cool until needed.

Metal instruments, glassware, aluminium foil, etc. can also be sterilized by exposure to hot dry air (130–170°C) for 2–4 hr in a hot-air oven. All items should be sealed before sterilization but not in paper, as it decomposes at 170°C. Autoclaving is not advisable for metal instruments because they may rust and become blunt under these conditions. Instruments that have been sterilized in hot dry air should be removed from their wrapping, dipped in 95% ethyl alcohol, and exposed to the heat of a flame. After an instrument has been used, it can again be dipped in ethyl alcohol, re-flamed, and then reused. This technique is called flame sterilization.

Safety is a major concern when using ethyl alcohol. Alcohol is flammable and if spilled near a flame will cause an instant flash fire. This problem is compounded in laminar flow hoods due to the strong air currents blown towards the worker. Fires commonly start when a flamed instrument is thrown back into the alcohol beaker. In case of fire do not panic. Limiting the supply of oxygen can easily put out fires. Autoclaving is a method of sterilizing with water vapour under pressure. Cotton plugs, gauze, labware, plastic caps, glassware, filters, pipettes, water, and nutrient media can all be sterilized by autoclaving. Nearly all microbes are killed by exposure to the super-heated steam of an autoclave for 10–15 minutes. All objects should be sterilized at 121°C and 15 psi for 15–20 min.

II. Sterilization of Plastics

The rising use of plastics in medical devices means that the capability of being sterilized is rapidly becoming a key selection criterion for any plastic to be used in a medical device.

Dry heat is not generally regarded as being suitable for plastics due to the low thermal transmission properties of plastics and the difficulty of insuring that all parts of the product have been exposed to the required temperature for an adequate time. Most plastics will degrade during prolonged dry heat sterilization.

Where autoclaving is to be used, the effect of multiple sterilization cycles needs to be considered to prevent cumulative effects of the treatment on the plastic. If the devices are to be packaged before autoclaving then the packaging material and packaging method needs to be carefully chosen.

Both gamma and E-beam sterilization use radiation and the effect on plastic materials is the same for both. Irradiation is very effective for fully packaged and sealed single-use items (most plastic films are effectively transparent to radiation) where only one radiation dose is required. Plastic devices subjected to irradiation sterilization will inevitably be affected by the radiation and the environment used during sterilization, and will experience changes in the polymer structure such as chain scission and cross-linking. These processes will lead to changes in the tensile strength, elongation at break and impact strength. The exact changes seen will depend both on the basic polymer and any additives used. The changes in mechanical properties may not be immediately apparent and there can be some time delay in their development.

The majority of plastics are unaffected by EtO sterilization treatment, but some can absorb EtO and these must be treated to eliminate any EtO before use. Some plastics are relatively permeable to EtO and the process can then be used to sterilize fully packaged articles by using thin packaging films, such as PE, that allow the EtO gas to enter the package and sterilize the contents. The packaging film must also be permeable to water vapour and air to be effective.

III. Sterilization of Container

In-container sterilization is the process of killing micro-organisms, that are present in all food, dairy and pharmaceutical products, by means of heating the product, that is in a hermetically sealed container (can, bottle, jar, pouch, etc.), to a predetermined lethal temperature and holding it for a specific amount of time. By doing so, the product becomes sterile and "shelf stable" and it will not be spoiled by living micro-organisms.

Surgical Containers

Deciding on the right sterilization method for the appropriate medical device has become very important. A lot of stress is laid on disinfecting the reusable devices. The sterilization is done either using Autoclaves, pressure steam sterilizes and chemical baths. Autoclaves and pressure steam sterilizers are the most preferred ones. There are plastic sterilization containers as well.

IV. Sterilization of Closures

A heat sterilization process for small, washed and bagged articles such as vial stoppers includes a conditioning or air removal phase prior to sterilization. During the air removal phase, a substantial majority of the liquid moisture is removed from the bagged articles by introducing brief periods of dry, warm air to the autoclave chamber. The air is introduced in short bursts at the point of greatest vacuum while pressure pulsing the chamber during the air removal phase. The air is heated and injected into the chamber through a supply valve which is rapidly opened and closed while the chamber is maintained within a preselected vacuum range between the pressure pulses. The result is a greatly reduced time for a complete sterilization and drying process.

V. Sterilize Bottles

A method of filling, sealing and sterilizing a pharmaceutical package including a polypropylene bottle containing a balanced salt solution includes the steps of filling each bottle to maximum capacity to exclude residual air, the introduction of a silicone rubber gasket into the bottle cap to absorb pressure and prevent leakage during a steam sterilization procedure, and the enclosure of the filled bottles in a blister pack before stream sterilizing. The blister packs have Tyvek™ closures and are placed blister-side-up during the sterilization process to eliminate deformation of the blister during sterilization. Maximum filling of the bottle with liquid and the substantial elimination of air prevents dimpling of the bottle.

12.7 TESTS FOR STERILITY

1. Media Used for Sterility Testing

Fluid Thioglycollate Medium (Medium 1) and Soybean-casein Digest Medium (Medium 2) are the two media generally used for tests for sterility.

Medium 1 (Fluid Thioglycollate Medium)

Composition

Pancreatic digest of casein	:	15.0 g
Yeast extract (water-soluble)	:	5.0 g

Glucose monohydrate/anhydrous	:	5.5 g/5.0 g
Sodium chloride	:	2.5 g
L-cystine	:	0.5 g
Sodium thioglycollate	:	0.5 g
0.1% Resazurin sodium solution (freshly prepared)	:	1.0 ml
Granulated agar (moisture not more than 15%)	:	0.75 g
Purified water	:	1000 ml
Polysorbate 80	:	5.0 ml
pH after sterilization (measured at room temperature)	:	7.1 ± 0.2

Method of preparation: The pancreatic digest of casein, yeast extract, glucose, sodium chloride, L-cystine, agar and water are mixed in the proportions given above and heat until dissolved. Sodium thioglycollate is dissolved in the solution. The specified quantity of Polysorbate 80 is added if this ingredient is to be included. If necessary, 1 M sodium hydroxide or 1 M hydrochloric acid is added so that after the solution is sterilized its pH will be 7.1 ± 0.2. If the solution is not clear, mixture is heated to boiling and filtered while hot through moistened filter paper. Resazurin sodium solution is added and mix.

Medium 2 (Soybean-casein Digest Medium)

Composition

Pancreatic digest of casein	:	17.0 g
Papain digest of soybean meal	:	3.0 g
Glucose monohydrate/anhydrous	:	2.5 g/2.3 g
Sodium chloride	:	5.0 g
Dipotassium hydrogen phosphate (K_2HPO_4)	:	2.5 g
Purified water	:	1000 ml
Polysorbate 80	:	5.0 ml
pH after sterilization (measured at room temperature)	:	7.3±0.2

Method of preparation: The ingredients are mixed in the proportions given above with slight warming. The solution is cooled to room temperature. The specified quantity of Polysorbate 80 is added if this ingredient is to be included. If necessary, sufficient 1 M sodium hydroxide or 1M hydrochloric acid so that after the solution is sterilized its pH will be 7.3 ± 0.2. If the solution is not clear it is filtered through moistened filter paper. Alternative media types may be appropriate where the nature of the product or method of manufacture can result in the presence of fastidious organisms (e.g. vaccines, blood products). Validation studies should indicate that alternative media are capable of supporting the growth of a wide range of micro-organisms in the presence of the product.

2. Methods

Tests for sterility are carried out by two methods:

   i. Membrane Filtration Method

   ii. Direct Transfer/Inoculation Method

The Membrane Filtration Method is used as the method of choice wherever feasible.

Method of Membrane Filtration

Procedure

The filter should be a membrane filter disc of cellulose esters or other suitable plastics, having a nominal average pore diameter not exceeding 0.45 µm. The membrane should be held firmly in a filtration unit which consists of a supporting base for the membrane, a receptacle for the fluid to be tested, a collecting reservoir for the filtered fluid, and the necessary tubes or connections. The apparatus is so designed that the solution to be filtered can be introduced and filtered under aseptic conditions. It permits the aseptic removal of the membrane for transfer to medium or it is suitable for carrying out the incubation after adding the medium to the apparatus itself.

Cellulose nitrate filters are recommended for aqueous, oily and weakly alcoholic solutions and cellulose acetate filters for strongly alcoholic solutions. The entire unit should be sterilized by appropriate means with the membrane filter and sterile airways in place. The method of sterilization should not be deleterious to the membrane, e.g. weaken it or change the nominal average pore diameter. The sterile airways should provide free access to the sterilizing agent. After sterilization, the apparatus should be free of leaks to the atmosphere except through the sterile airways.

Method of Direct Transfer

Procedures

1. Liquids and soluble or dispersible solids: Appropriate quantities of the preparation to be examined are added directly into Medium 1 and Medium 2. Approximately equal quantities of the preparation should be added to each vessel of medium. The test vessels of Medium 1 is incubated at 30–35°C and the vessels of Medium 2 is incubated at 20–25°C.

The volume of Medium 1 should be such that the air space above the medium in the container is minimized. The volume of Medium 2 should be such that sufficient air space is left above the medium to provide conditions that permit the growth of obligate aerobes. Unless otherwise prescribed, in no case should the volume of material under test be greater than 10% of the volume of the medium alone, i.e. 90% medium and 10% product. If a large volume of product is to be tested it may be preferable to use concentrated media, prepared so as to take the subsequent dilution into account. Where appropriate the concentrated medium may be added directly to the product in its container. Wherever possible solid articles such as devices should be tested by immersion in or filling with culture media. Immerse all parts of each article in sufficient medium contained in one vessel to completely cover all parts. The volume of Medium 1 should be such that the air space above the medium in the container is minimized. The volume of Medium 2 should be such that sufficient air space is left above the medium to provide conditions that permit the growth of obligate aerobes. Place half the articles into Medium 1 and the remaining half into Medium 2. Incubate the test vessels of Medium 1 at 30–35°C and the vessels of Medium 2 at 20–25°C.

2. **Ointments and oily preparations:** Ointments and oily preparations may be tested by the method of Direct Transfer if testing by the method of Membrane Filtration is not feasible, i.e. when a suitable solvent is not available.

12.8 INCUBATION AND EXAMINATION OF STERILITY TESTS

All test vessels of Medium 1 are incubated at 30–35°C. The vessels of Medium 2 are incubated at 20–25°C. All test and control vessels, other than the subcultured vessels referred to below, must be incubated for at least 14 days unless microbial contamination is detected at an earlier time.

If turbidity, precipitate, or other evidence of microbial growth during incubation is seen: the suspected growth is examined microscopically by Gram stain; attempts are made to grow single colonies using appropriate microbiological methods; colonies of each type of micro-organism present are examined for colonial morphology and cellular morphology by Gram stain; attempts are made to identify the isolates, as far as the genus, and preferably species.

12.9 INTERPRETATION OF THE TEST RESULTS

If microbial growth is not evident in any of the vessels inoculated with the product, the sample tested complies with the test for sterility, if microbial growth is evident the product does not comply with the test for sterility unless it can be clearly demonstrated that the test was invalid for causes unrelated to the product being examined. If the test is declared to be invalid it may be repeated with the same number of units as in the original test. If there is no evidence of growth in any vessels inoculated with the product during the repeat test the product passes the test for sterility. This interpretation applies even if growth occurs in negative product control vessels. If there is evidence of growth in the test vessels the product fails the test for sterility. Further testing is not permitted under any circumstances.

12.10 EVALUATION OF STERILIZATION METHOD

Sterile products possess several unique properties, such as freedom from microorganism, pyrogens, particulates and high standards of purity and quality. This ultimate goal in the manufacture of sterile products can be attained by evaluation of sterilization procedure. The sterilization processes are likely to be subjected to the most detailed and complex validation procedures.

The judgment of sterility has relied on official sterility test. A validated manufacturing procedure is one which has been proved to do what it purports to do. The proof of evaluation is obtained through the collection and evaluation of data, preferably beginning, from the process development phase and continuing through the production phase. Evaluation of processing includes equipment, process, personnel, material, etc.

The principle involve in the evaluation of sterilization process are:

   i. To build sterility into product.
  ii. Perform a maximum level of probability.
 iii. Establish specification and performance characteristic.
  iv. To provide greater assurance of support of the result.
   v. Specific methodology, process and equipment.
  vi. Final product testing using validated analytical method.
 vii. Verification, calibration and maintenance of equipment used in the processes.

Evaluation of sterilization methods are done to ensure that the product produce by design process should be of best quality. The process control and finished product testing alone are not sufficient to assure product quality. When testing a specified portion of the total product and if the specified portion passes the test of sterility, it cannot assure that the total product is sterile.

Evaluation of sterilization methods provides a high degree of assurance which indicates a specific process will consistently produce a product that will meets it predetermined specifications and quality assurance. So this action proves that any procedure, process, equipment, material activity or system actually leads to the expected result and produce quality product. This concept of evaluation has been expended to encompass a wide range of activities from analytical methods used for quality control of drug substance and drug products.

The purpose of evaluation of any material equipment is achieved by means of a validation protocol which details the test to be carried out; frequency of testing and results expected that is the acceptance criteria.

12.11 PROCESS OF MICROBIAL DESTRUCTION

Microbial destruction methods such as heat, chemical and radiation sterilization are used. Upon exposure of such treatment, microorganisms die according to logarithmic relationship between concentration or population of the living cells and the time exposure or radiation dose. The relationship between microbial population and time may be linear or non linear.

The D value or time required or dose required for one log reduction in microbial population may be calculated from these plots.

D Value

It is the rate of killing of micro organism. It determines the time required to reduce the microbial population by one decimal point, i.e. it is the time required for 90% reduction in the microbial population. Hence the time or dose it takes to reduce thousand microbial cells to hundred cells is the D value.

D value is important in the validation of sterilization process for several reasons:

i. It is specific for each microorganism in environment subjected to specific sterilizing agent or condition.
ii. The knowledge of D value at different temperature in heat sterilization is necessary for the calculation of Z value.
iii. The D value is used in the calculation of biological factor F.
iv. Extra-polation of D value predicts number of log reduction of microbial population.

D value is affected by several parameters which are as follows:

i. The type of microorganism used as biological indicator.
ii. The formulation component and characteristics.
iii. The surface on which the microorganism is exposed.
iv. The temperature, gas concentration and radiation dose

D Value is Determined By

i. *Survival curve method:* The survival curve method is based on plotting the log number of the surviving organism verses independent variable such as time, gas concentration or radiation dose.

ii. *Fraction negative method:* In this method, sample containing similar spore population are treated in an identical environment and the number of sample still showing microbial growth after treatment and incubation are determined.

Data obtained by survival curve method are plotted semi logarithmically. Data points are connected by least square analysis.

Log N = a + bt.

Where N is number of surviving organism, t is time, a is y intercept and b is slope of line as determined by linear regression.

D value is the reciprocal of linear slope.

D = 1/b.

Z Value

This term is exclusively used in the validation of heat sterilization process. The Z value is the reciprocal of slope resulting from the plot of the logarithm of D value verses the temperature at which the D value was obtained. The Z value may be defined as the temperature required for one log reduction in the D value.

The accepted standard (Z value) for steam sterilization of Bacillus stearothermophilus spores and dried heat sterilization for Bacillus subtilis are 10°C and 22°C respectively. These plots are important because one can determine D value of the indicator microorganism at any temperature of interest. The magnitude of slope indicates the relative degree of lethality as temperature is increased or decreased.

F Value

The F value measures equivalent time, not clock time that a monitored article is exposed to the desired temperature, e.g. 121°C.

F value is calculated from following equation.

$$F= \Delta t\Sigma 10^{(T-To)/Z}$$

Where; Δt is the time interval for the measurement of product temperature t.

T is reference temperature.

To is 121°C for steam sterilization.

12.12 EVALUATION AND IN PROCESS MONITORING OF STERILIZATION PROCEDURES

1. Dry Heat Sterilization

Physical Indicator

In this process temperature record chart is made of each sterilization cycle with dry heat sterilization. This chart forms the batch documentation and is compared against a master temperature records. The temperature should be taken as the coolest part of the loaded sterilizer, further information on heat distribution and penetration within sterilizer can be gained by the use of thermocouple place at selected site in the chamber or injected into test packs or bottles.

Chemical Indicator

It is based on the ability of heat to alter the chemical or physical characteristics of variety of chemical substances. This change should take place only when satisfactory condition for sterilization prevails. Thus conforming that sterilization cycle has been successfully completed. Chemical indicators generally under go melting or colour change.

Biological Indicator

The biological indicators are the standardized bacterial spore preparations which are usually in the form of suspension in water or culture medium or of spore dried on paper or plastic carriers, they are placed in sterilizer.

After the sterilization process the aqueous suspension/spores are on carriers are aseptically transferred to an appropriate nutrient medium, which is then incubated and occasionally seen for the growth. Clostridium species is generally used for dry heat sterilization indicator (Table 12.2).

Table 12.2: Dry heat sterilization

Indicators	Sterilization methods	Principle	Device	Parameter monitored
Physical	Dry heat	Temperature recording charts	Temperature recording charts	Temperature
Chemical	Dry heat	Temperature sensitive coloured solution	Browne's tube	Temperature, Time
		Temperature sensitive chemical	A temperature sensitive white wax concealing a black marked	Temperature
Biological	Dry heat	Temperature sensitive microbes	*Bacillus subtilis*	D value

2. Moist Heat Sterilization

Physical Indicator

In this process temperature record chart is made of each sterilization cycle with dry heat sterilization. This chart of the batch documentation is compared against a master temperature records. The temperature should be taken as the coolest part of the loaded sterilizer, further information on heat distribution and penetration within sterilizer can be gained by the use of thermocouple place at selected site in the chamber or injected into test packs or bottles.

Chemical Indicator

It is based on the ability of heat to alter the chemical or physical characteristics of variety of chemical substances. This change should take place only when satisfactory condition for sterilization prevails. Thus conforming that sterilization cycle has been successfully completed chemical indicator generally under go melting or colour change.

Biological Indicator

Spores of *B. stearothermophilus* in sealed ampoules of culture medium are used for moist heat sterilization monitoring and these may be incubated directly at 55°C, thus may eliminate the need of aseptic transfer (Table 12.3).

Aseptic transfer is also avoided by use of self contained units where the spores strip and the nutrient medium are present in the same device ready for mixing after use.

The bacterial spores should have following qualities:

  i. It should be non pathogenic.
 ii. Should posses above average resistant to the particular sterilization process.

Table 12.3: Moist heat sterilization

Indicators	Sterilization methods	Principle	Device	Parameter monitored
Physical	Moist heat	Temperature recording charts	Temperature recording charts	Temperature
Chemical	Moist heat	Temperature sensitive coloured solution	Browne's tube	Temperature, Time
		Steam sensitive chemical	A device which is impregnated into a carrier material	Saturated steam
Biological	Moist heat	Temperature sensitive microbes	*Bacillus stearothermophilus*	D value

3. Gaseous Sterilization

Physical Indicator

Gas concentration is measured independently of pressure rise, often by reference to weight of gas used.

Chemical Indicator

The chemical indicator used here are Royach Sacket, the indicator paper impregnated with reactive chemical which undergoes a distinct colour change on reaction. Chemical indicators are valuable monitors of the condition prevailing at the coolest of most in accessible part of a sterilizer.

Biological Indicator

As with chemical indicator they are usually packed in dummy packs located at strategic sites in the sterilizer. Alternatively for gaseous sterilization, these may also be placed in tubular helix device. The species of bacteria generally used for gaseous sterilization are *B.subtilis var.niger* and *B.subtilis var.golbigii*.

One of the longstanding criticisms of biological indicator is that the incubation period required is very long in order to find satisfactory results (Table 12.4).

Table 12.4: Gaseous sterilization

Indicators	Sterilization methods	Principle	Device	Parameter monitored
Physical	Gaseous	Temperature recording charts	Temperature recording charts	Temperature
Chemical	Gaseous	Reactive chemical	Indicator paper impregnated with reactive chemical	Gas concentration, Temperature, Time
		Capillary principle	Based on same migration along wick principle	Gas concentration, Temperature, Time
		Steam sensitive chemical	A temperature sensitive white wax concealing a black marked	Temperature
Biological	Gaseous	Temperature sensitive microbes	*Bacillus subtilis*	D value

4. Radiation Sterilization

Physical Indicator

In radiation sterilization a plastic or perspex dosimeter which gradually darkens in proportion to the radiation it absorbs give an accurate measure of the radiation dose and is considered to be the best technique currently available for the radiation sterilization process.

Chemical Indicator

Chemical dosimeter acidified with cerric ammonium sulphate or cerric sulphate solution. These responds to irradiation by dose change in the applied density. Those are considered best and accurately measure relation dose.

Biological Indicator

These are consist of standardized bacterial spore preparation which are usually in the form of suspension in water or culture medium or of spore dried on paper or plastic carriers, they are placed in sterilizer.

After the sterilization process the aqueous suspension/spores are on carriers are aseptic ally transferred to an appropriate nutrient medium, which is then incubated and periodically observed for the growth. *Clostridium* species is generally used for dry heat sterilization indicator (Table 12.5).

Table 12.5: Radiation sterilization

Indicators	Sterilization methods	Principle	Device	Parameter monitored
Physical	Radiation	Recording charts	Recording charts	Radiation dose
Chemical	Radiation	Radio chromic chemicals	Plastic device impregnated with radio sensitive chemicals which undergo colour changes at relative low radiation doses	Only indicate exposure to radiation
		Dosimeter device	Acidified ferric ammonium sulphate solutions responds to irradiation by dose related changes in their optical density	Accurately measures radiation doses
Biological	Radiation	Radiation sensitive microbes	*Bacillus pumilus*	D value

5. Filtration Sterilization

Physical Indicator

Sterilizing filters are subjected to a bubble point pressure test. This is a technique for determining the pore size of a filter, and may also be used to check the integrity of certain types of filters. The principle of the test is that the wetted filter in its assembled unit is subjected to an increasing air or nitrogen gas pressure difference. The pressure difference recorded when the first bubble of gas breaks away from the filter is related to maximum pore size. When the gas pressure is further increased slowly there is general eruption of bubble over the entire surface. The pressure difference here is related to the mean pore size. Pressure difference below the expected value would signify a damage or faulty filter (Table12.5).

Biological Indicator

Filtration sterilization require a different approach from biological monitoring, the test effectively measure in the ability of a filter to produce a sterile filtrate from a culture of suitable organism S.marcesence, a small gram-negative rod shape bacterium. B.diminuta used as a biological indicator having a dimension 0.5 micrometer and 0.3 micrometer respectively has been used for filters of 0.45 micrometer and 0.22 micrometer. The extent of the passage of this organism through membrane filter is enhanced by increasing the filtration pressure. Thus successful sterile filtration depends markedly on the challenge condition. Such test are used as the part of filter manufacture characterization and quality assurance process, and users initial validation procedure. They are not employed as a test of filter performance in use (Table 12.6).

Table 12.6: Filtration sterilization

Indicators	Sterilization methods	Principle	Device	Parameter monitored
Physical	Filtration sterilization	Forcibly passing of solution through the membrane	Bubble point pressure test	Pressure
Chemical	Filtration sterilization	Retention of bacteria	*P. diminuta*	Size of microorganism

Examples of Materials Sterilized by Different Methods

Different techniques which are used for the sterilization of different materials are discussed in the tabular form (Table 12.7).

Table12.7: List of materials sterilized by different methods

Materials		Methods of sterilization/preferred methods
Injections	**Intravenous infusions** a. Isotonic solution of sodium chloride Glucose b. Blood products and Plasma substitutes, e.g. Dextran and degraded gelatin.	Filtration sterilization Terminal sterilization a. Autoclaving for thermostables. b. Radiation for thermolabiles.
	Intravenous Additives e.g. Potassium chloride, lignocaine, heparin, certain vitamins, antibiotics.	Physical methods(Freeze Thaw Method).
	Total Parenteral Nutrition (TPN)	Filtration sterilization
	Small Volume Injections e.g. **Vaccines:** Influenza vaccines, vaccinea, polio vaccines, rabies vaccines.	Radiation sterilization (using gamma radiation)
	Antibiotics: Benzyl penicillin, streptomycin sulphate, zinc bacitracin, polymixin sulphate, dihydrostreptomycin sulphate.	Radiation sterilization (using gamma radiation)
	Vitamins: Ascorbic acid, Vitamin A, Vitamin E.	Radiation sterilization (using gamma radiation)
	Freeze Dried Products: Few hormones, several vitamins, vaccines.	Filtration sterilization
	Miscellaneous: Diazepam Inj., Insulin Inj., Promethazine HCl Inj.	Radiation sterilization (using gamma radiation)
Non-injectable sterile fluids	Non-injectable waters	Filtration sterilization/Terminally sterilization by autoclaving
	Urological irrigation solution	
	Peritoneal dialysis and haemodialysis solution	
	Inhaler solution	

Contd...

Contd...

Materials		Methods of sterilization/preferred methods
Opthalmic Preparation	Eye drops, e.g. Chloramphenicol eye drops, timolol eye drops, pilocarpin eye drops, brominidine eye drops, Atropine eye.	Thermostables by autoclaving at 121°C for 15 minutes. Thermolabiles by filtration sterilization
	Thermostables by autoclaving at 121°C for 15 minutes. Thermolabiles by filtration sterilization	Thermostables by autoclaving at 121°C for 15 minutes Thermolabiles by filtration sterilization
	Eye ointment, e.g. simple eye ointment BP	Dry heat sterilization at 160°C for 2 hours
	Contact lens solutions, e.g. wetting solution, cleansing solution, soaking solutions	Thermostables by autoclaving at 121°C for 15 minutes and thermolabiles by filtration sterilization
Dressing's	Chlorhexidine gauze dressing	Any combination of dry heat, ethylene oxide and gamma radiation
	Framycetin gauze dressing	
	Knitted viscous primary dressing	
	Paraffin gauze dressing	
	Perforated film absorbent dressing	
	Polyurethane foam dressing	
	Semi permeable adhesive dressing	
	Sodium fusidate gauze dressing	
	Absorbent cotton wool	Any methods
	Elastic adhesive dressing	Ethylene oxide or gamma radiation
	Plastic wound dressing	Ethylene oxide or gamma radiation
	Absorbent cotton gauze	Any methods
	Gauze pads	Any methods
	Adhésive viscose wadding	Any methods

Contd...

Contd...

Materials		Methods of sterilization/preferred methods
Implants	Steroid implants Hormonal implants	Dry heat sterilization
Absorbable Haemostate	Oxidized cellulose	Gaseous sterilization (using ethylene oxide and formaldehyde
	Absorbable gelatin foam	Dry heat sterilization at 150°C for 1 hour
	Human fibrin foam	Dry heat sterilization at 130°C for 3 hours
	Calcium alginate	Moist heat sterilization by autoclaving
Surgical Ligatures and Sutures	Catgut	Dry heat sterilization at 160°C for 2 hours/ gamma radiation
	Non-absorbable type, e.g. nylons, silk and polypropylene	Moist heat sterilization (Autoclaving)/gamma radiation
Equipment and Instruments	Syringes (glass) Syringes(glass),dismantled Syringes (disposable) Needles (all metal) Needle (disposable)	Dry heat using gamma radiation
	Metal instruments	Dry heat
	Disposable instruments rubber gloves administration sets	Gamma radiation
	Respiratory parts	Dry heat sterilization
	Dialysis machines Fragile heat sensitive equipment	Chemical sterilization using formalin and ethylene oxides
Miscellaneous	Dry bulk drugs	Dry heat sterilization
	Porcelain	Dry heat sterilization
	Food products	Radiation sterilization or gaseous sterilization
	Culture medium	
	Mouths of culture tubes and bottles	Dry heat sterilization
	Air sterilization in hospitals, manufacturing house, schools, etc.	Radiation sterilization

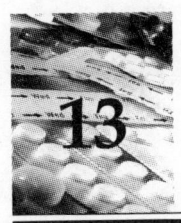

13 Packaging of Parenterals, Ophthalmics and Aerosols

13.1 INTRODUCTION

Parenteral products are products that are administered to the body by injection. Because this route of administration bypasses the normal body defence mechanisms, it is essential that these products are prepared with a higher degree of care and skills than utilised in preparing conventional oral or topical products. Parenteral preparations are sterile, pyrogen-free liquids (solutions, emulsions, or suspensions) or solid dosage forms containing one or more active ingredients, packaged in either single-dose or multi-dose containers. They are intended for administration by injection, infusion, or implantation into the body.

13.2 PACKAGING OF STERILE PHARMACEUTICALS

A. Parenterals
B. Ophthalmics

A. Parenterals
Parenteral Product Packaging

The packaging process of a parenteral product, usually in close conjunction with parenteral container processing.

1. Parenteral Drug Product: A sterile solution intended for administration by injection, internal irrigation, or for use in dialysis procedures.

Classification
I. According to the Volume
1. Large volume parenteral: A parenteral product packaged in a volume of 100 ml or more.

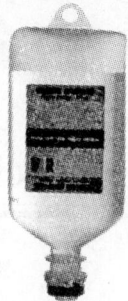

Fig. 13.1: Large volume parenteral

2. Small volume parenteral: A parenteral drug product packaged in a volume of less than 100 ml.

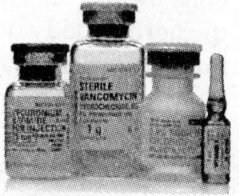

Fig. 13.2: Small volume parenteral

II. According to the Dose

1. Single dose preparations: The British Pharmacopoeia (BP) 1998 define single dose preparations as:

The volume of the injection in a single dose container is sufficient to permit the withdrawal and administration of the nominal dose using a normal technique.

The single dose container may be:
  i. Glass ampoules
 ii. Prefilled syringes
iii. Cartidges

2. Multiple dose preparations (BP 2004): Multidose preparations are multidose aqueous injections which contain a suitable antimicrobial preservative at an appropriate concentration except when the preparation itself has adequate antimicrobial properties.
  i. Vials
 ii. Large volume glass bottles
iii. Flexible plastic bottles.

2. Formulation of Parenteral Products

Sterile formulations must meet a number of special criteria such as:

    i. Sterility
   ii. Particulate material
  iii. Pyrogen free
  iv. Stability
   v. pH
  vi. Osmotic pressure

During the formulation of parenteral products, the following factors are critical:

    i. The vehicle in which the drug is dissolved or dispersed.
   ii. Volume (dose) of the injection
  iii. Adjustment to isotonicity
  iv. Adjustment of pH
   v. Stabilizers
  vi. Preservatives
 vii. Adjustment of specific gravity (for spinal anesthesia)
viii. Concentration units

The formulation of injections is not different to the formulation of products by other routes except for certain requirements which parenteral products must satisfy. The major ones are limits to the level of pyrogen present and of particulate matter. For formulation of injections, the injection route dictates the volume of the formulation. Hence the solubility of the drug in the selected vehicle is critical in the formulation. The preferred vehicle is water as it is well tolerated by the body, is easy to administer and has a large solvent capacity. Due to the wide variety of contaminants in mains water, water for injections must be used as the vehicle for parenteral products. 'Water for injections' (WFI) must be sterile and free from pyrogen.

Solutions for parenteral use and injections with a volume of 100 ml or more must comply with the BP test for the absence of particulate matter. Microns can be detected by visual inspection. Examples of such particulate materials are cellulose, glass, rubber cores, cloth or cotton fibres. Suitable filtration media for removal of particulate materials are sintered glass filters or membrane filters with a pore size of 0.45–1.2 µm.

As parenteral formulations are administered directly to tissues and systemic circulation, formulations prepared should not vary significantly from physiological pH, which is about 7.4. In certain cases however, acidic or alkaline solutions may be needed to solubilize drugs. The acceptable pH range is 3–10.5 for IV preparations and 4–9 for other routes. Buffers are included in injections to maintain the pH of the packaged product. However, the buffer used in the injection must allow the body fluids to change the product pH after injection. Acetate, citrate and phosphate buffers are commonly used in parenteral products.

The osmotic pressure of blood is approximately 300 mOsmol/L and ideally any sterile solution would be formulated to have the same osmolarity, e.g., 0.9% w/v Sodium Chloride IV solution has an osmolarity of 308 mOsmol/L and 5% w/v Dextrose iv solution has an osmolarity of 280 mOsmol/L. Intravenous solutions that have larger osmolarity values (hypertonic) or smaller osmolarity values (hypotonic) may cause damage to red blood cells, pain and tissue irritation. Parenteral solutions which are hypotonic need to be adjusted to isotonicity.

Osmolarity adjustment is made usually by using sodium chloride, glucose or mannitol using one of the following methods:
- The freezing point depression method
- Sodium chloride equivalent
- Molar concentrations
- Serum osmolarity.

Requirements for Specific Types of Parenteral Preparations

Injections

Injections are sterile, pyrogen-free solutions or dispersions (emulsions or suspensions) of one or more active ingredients in a suitable vehicle.

Whenever possible, an injection should be prepared using an aqueous vehicle. If necessary, suitable non-aqueous solvents are indicated in the individual monographs. Injections that are dispersions should remain sufficiently stable so that, after shaking, a homogeneous dose can be withdrawn.

The use of single-dose injections is to be preferred and is essential when the preparation is intended for administration by routes where, for medical reasons, an antimicrobial preservative is not acceptable, e.g. intracisternal, intrathecal.

Intravenous Infusions

Intravenous infusions are sterile, pyrogen-free aqueous solutions or emulsions with water as continuous phase, usually prepared to be isotonic. They are intended for administration in large volumes (usually 100 ml or more), and should not contain any antimicrobial preservatives.

On visual inspection, emulsions for intravenous injection should show no evidence of phase separation. The particle size of the dispersed phase should be controlled by the manufacturer.

Powders for Injections

Powders for injections are solid substances (including freeze-dried materials), distributed in their final containers and which, when shaken with the prescribed volume of the appropriate sterile liquid, rapidly form either clear and practically particle-free solutions or uniform suspensions. Powders for injections, after dissolution or suspension, comply with the requirements for injections or intravenous infusions, as appropriate.

Uniformity of Mass

Powders for injections (single-dose use) comply with the test for 5.2 Uniformity of mass for single-dose preparations, unless otherwise specified in the individual monograph.

Uniformity of Content

A requirement for compliance with the test for 5.1 Uniformity of content for single-dose preparations is specified in certain individual monographs where the active ingredient is less than 40 mg. In such cases, compliance with the test for 5.2 Uniformity of mass for single-dose preparations may not be required.

Implants

Implants are solid preparations containing one or more active ingredients. They are of a size and shape suitable for parenteral implantation, and provide release of the active ingredient(s) over an extended period of time. They are presented in individual sterile containers.

13.3 PACKAGING COMPONENTS

Packaging components for parenterals are:
Containers: Glass and plastic containers.
Closures: Rubber closures.

Characteristics of Packaging Materials

  i. They should not interact with any of the ingredients of parenteral preparations.
 ii. Container should protect the product from light, and microbial contamination.
iii. Glass container should be light amber colour to prevent the parenterals from light.
 iv. Glass container should be light colour to permit the inspection of the products.

1. Closures

Closures for parenteral preparation containers should be equipped with a firm seal to prevent entry of microorganisms and other contaminants while permitting the withdrawal of a part or the whole of the contents without removal of the closure. They should not be made of components that react with the contents, nor should they allow foreign substances to diffuse into the preparation. Plastic materials or elastomers of which the closure is composed should be sufficiently firm and elastic to allow the passage of a needle with the least possible shedding of particles. Closures for multidose containers should be sufficiently elastic to allow the puncture to reseal when the needle is withdrawn and protect the contents from airborne contamination. A tamper-evident container is fitted with a device that reveals clearly whether it has ever been opened.

2. Containers

Parenteral preparations are usually supplied in glass ampoules, bottles or vials, plastic bottles or bags, and prefilled syringes, which are coloured in the case of light-sensitive substances.

Except where otherwise indicated in individual monographs, these containers should be made from material that is sufficiently transparent to permit the visual inspection of the contents. They should not adversely affect the quality of the preparation, allow diffusion of any kind into or across the material of the container, or yield foreign substances into the preparation.

Plastic System Packaging for Liquid and Solid Medicines

This wide field ranges from eye droppers to nasal spray bottles and tablet containers and includes a wide spectrum of PET bottles. It is of additional interest because of its outstandingly diverse range of closure solutions, dosage systems and application aids, which mean that not only the plastic range but also glass packaging are increasingly independent of external suppliers. Now the new products with cross-system functionality included a series of PP28 caps with dosing cups. These tamper-evident closures with click-on dosing cups fit bottles and vials made of PE or PET as well as many which are made of moulded glass.

Glass Containers

Containers for parenteral products are produced from one of 3 types of glass or from one of a variety of plastic materials.

Types of Glass

Type I: Commonly known as neutral glass. It has a high resistance to hydrolysis and withstands autoclaving, weathering and solution of pH of up to 8.

Type II (sulphated glass): Containers may be treated with moist sulphur dioxide at high temperature to create a neutral surface film with high hydrolytic resistance. Lower resistance to autoclaving than for type I glass.

Type III (soda glass): This offers very little resistance to hydrolysis and should only be used for powders for reconstitution prior to injection and for non-aqueous preparations.

Type II and Type III glass containers should be used once only for parenteral preparations.

Types of Containers/Classification of Containers

- Single dose containers
- Multiple dose containers

Glass ampoules are the most commonly used single dose containers and can range from sizes of 1 to 50 ml. For aqueous solutions, neutral glass is used. After filling, glass ampoules are sealed by fusion of the glass and hence there is no danger of entry of micro-organisms. Amber glass ampoules are available for light sensitive products. Clear ampoules may be used provided that the ampoules are packaged in a light-resistant box.

Glass vials sealed by rubber closures are commonly used as multi-dose containers. The rubber closure is held in place by an aluminium sealing ring. The rubber closure permits the penetration of a syringe needle to allow the withdrawal of a dose of injection.

Single Dose Containers

A single dose container for parenterals are containing single dose. When they open once they cannot be resealed with assurance of sterility of product.

1. Ampoules

A small, hermetically sealed glass or plastic container, e.g. one containing medication for parenteral administration or semen for insemination. Called also ampoule.

An ampoule (also ampule or ampulla) is a small sealed vial which is used to contain and preserve a sample, usually a solid or liquid. Ampoules are commonly made of glass, although plastic ampoules do exist.

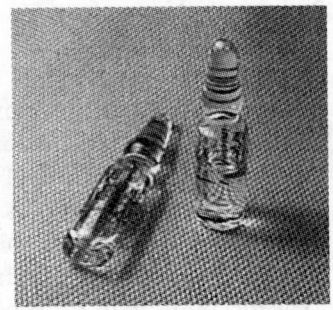

Fig. 13.3: Ampoules containing pharmaceutical products

Modern ampoules are most commonly used to contain pharmaceuticals and chemicals that must be protected from air and contaminants. They are hermetically sealed by melting the thin top with an open flame, and usually opened by snapping off the neck. If properly done, this last operation creates a clean break without any extra glass shards or slivers; but the liquid or solution may be filtered for greater assurance. The space above the chemical may be filled with an inert gas before sealing. The walls of glass ampoules are usually

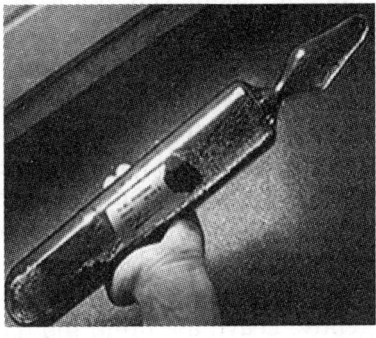

Fig. 13.4: A large ampoule containing 1.3 kg of high purity caesium

sufficiently strong to be brought into a glovebox without any difficulty.

Glass ampoules are more expensive than bottles and other simple containers, but there are many situations where their superior imperviousness to gases and liquids and all-glass interior surface are worth the extra cost. Examples of chemicals sold in ampoules are injectable pharmaceuticals, air-sensitive reagents like tetrakis(triphenylphosphine) palladium, hygroscopic materials like deuterated solvents and trifluoro-methanesulfonic acid, and analytical standards.

Ampoule Codes

Ampoules often have coloured rings of paint or enamel around their necks.

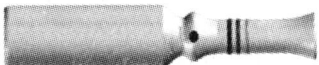

Fig. 13.5: Diagram of an ampoule showing colour-coded neck rings

Filling and Hand Sealing of Glass Ampoules

Ampoules must first be rinsed out using water for injections to remove any dust, particulate matter and/or glass fragments. Using a syringe, gently draw the volume required to be filled plus an excess volume. Invert the syringe to allow the air to rise towards the needle and push up the plunger to remove all air. Attach the membrane filter and needle to the syringe. Discard the first 0.5–1 ml of filtrate. Invert the ampoule over the needle and expel the required volume of liquid into the ampoule taking care not to splash the liquid into the neck of the ampoule.

Each ampoule must also contain a slight excess volume of product. This is necessary to allow the nominal injection volume to be drawn into a syringe.

Using a twin-jet burner, adjust the platform height and flame intensity. Try an empty ampoule first before sealing the products. Position the ampoule between the flames. Grip the end of the neck with a blunt-nosed forceps and when the glass is soft enough, pull off the top of the ampoule vertically and gently. Leave the tip in the flame for a second or two longer and then remove. The tip should now be smoothly and evenly rounded. Ampoules should have a reliable seal which can be readily leak tested. A good seal will not deteriorate during the lifetime of the product.

2. Pre-filled Syringe: The Future for Parenterals

The pre-fillable syringe is becoming the parenteral package and delivery method of choice, its popular among healthcare professionals and consumers.

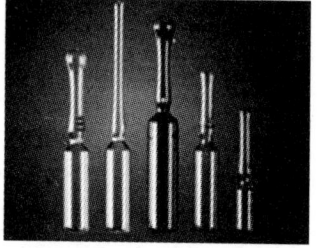

Fig. 13.6: Pre-filled syringe

The parenteral drug industry has grown in recent years with the development of new treatments and formulations to treat a wide range of acute and chronic conditions. In tandem with this growth has been increased sophistication of the packaging for parenteral drugs, including pre-filled syringes and disposable injection devices.

"The BD pharmaceutical systems UniJect™ device eliminates the need for any syringe and is tamper-evident and user friendly".

The market has moved in this direction for a number of reasons, including ease of drug administration, additional security, lower contamination risk and ease of injection by non-health professionals using pen or injectable devices.

A more ambiguous factor is cost. It has been estimated that the cost of pre-filled injection systems is 25% more than if the same drugs were packaged in conventional vials and ampoules. However, this seems not to be so much of a problem for premium medications such as biopharmaceuticals and anti-cancer drugs, where the price of the packaging is a small fraction of the overall cost.

Pre-filled Devices for Drug Administration

Pre-filled injection devices in cyclic olefin copolymer (COC) and cyclic olefin polymer (COP) are used in applications ranging from the very simple to the highly complex.

For example, the BD Pharmaceutical Systems UniJect™ device is a plastic tab with a small flexible bulb containing the injectable product, connected to a small sharp needle. Designed for use in developing-world immunisation and medication campaigns, the system eliminates the need for any syringe, is sterile, completely disposable, compact, tamper-evident and user friendly.

More complex is the Liquid Dry Injector, also from BD Pharmaceutical Systems. It is a two-part plastic pen injection device, where the active drug compound is contained as a lyophilised powder (typically because the drug would not be stable in solution).

When the patient is ready to administer their medication they push the two halves of the device together, mixing the lyophilised component with a diluent. They then attach a needle, adjust the dose using a graduated knob or dial, and inject, before disposing of the whole apparatus.

The advantage of this system is that the exact dose can be filled to the device, unlike conventional vials where 25% overfills are common due to the wastage in filling a syringe. Therefore, manufacturers can save valuable material (especially relevant for expensive biotech drugs) and the patient does not need to worry about dosing errors.

More complex still, the Plexis bone void-filling system, manufactured by Advanced Biomaterial Systems, is used in orthopedic procedures to inject medication into skeletal tissue under high pressure.

Suitable Drugs for Pre-filled Devices

Pre-filled devices are now used for more and more drugs, but the largest three sectors are antithrombotics, biopharmaceuticals and vaccines. Pre-filled systems are revolutionising self-administered medication for home use.

"The crucial reasons for pre-fillables' use are convenience and safety".

For some treatment regimes, such as the day-to-day administration of insulin to diabetic patients, pre-filled devices are ideal for convenience and safety.

There are some drugs which have to be kept as a lyophilised powder and only reconstituted a short time before administration; the pre-filled systems for this have the disadvantage of being more expensive, but score highly for simplicity and patient convenience.

For example, the leuprolide acetate treatment Lupron (which inhibits growth in some hormone-dependent tumours) is self-administered as a depot suspension using a pre-filled dual-chambered syringe, as described above.

Lyophilised drugs can sometimes be a more difficult proposition and do not always lend themselves so easily to a dual-chamber cartridge because of the volumes involved. For these, manufacturers are now starting to provide pre-filled diluent syringes for reconstitution.

Safe for Home Use

Pharmaceutical companies can make the use of pre-filled devices much easier by the development of liquid formulations. Copaxone from Teva is a multiple sclerosis (MS) treatment originally marketed as a lyophilised powder in vials for reconstitution by the patient, but now the drug is supplied in liquid form in a BD Hypak pre-filled syringe.

This is one of the most popular pre-filled devices on the market and is usually fitted with the Prevented safety device, which makes disposal in the home easier, with less risk of needle stick injury.

"For some treatment regimes, such as the administration of insulin to diabetic patients, pre-filled devices are ideal for convenience and safety".

This device is now also widely used for the packaging and administration of vaccines, since it means that companies can move away from the multi-dose vial that required the use of thimersol preservative to a single-dose, more secure pre-filled system, which does not.

Pre-filled devices of various designs and complexities are now an integral part of a large sector of the parenteral drugs market. Although they are more expensive and slower to manufacture, they provide much greater convenience for the home medication market and protect against incorrect formulation and overdosing.

With more biopharmaceuticals due to come on the market over the next few years, it is likely that pre-filled devices will become more prevalent. Their use solves many problems for the consumer/patient but can create difficulties for packaging designers. While pharmaceutical companies produce drugs, they also need to put them into an appropriate form and package them in such a way that they can be easily administered to or by the patient.

With the parenteral drug delivery system market projected to be worth over $30bn by 2007, one thing seems certain: parenteral drugs are here to stay, as are pre-filled devices and syringes – whatever form they take.

Glass vs Plastic

As pre-fillable syringes have grown in popularity, the choice of glass or plastic for their manufacture has become an important issue. Previously the majority of pre-filled syringes on the European and US markets were made of glass, which had superior barrier properties to plastics and did not leach out plasticisers and other undesirable compounds into the drug substance. However, the advent of cyclic olefin copolymer (COC) and cyclic olefin polymer (COP) has changed all this.

Some of the newer kinds of drugs, particularly biopharmaceuticals based on peptides and antibodies, have problems with glass. Glass can contain free alkali oxides and traces of metals, and it is possible that these can have a detrimental effect on product stability. Some of the new polymers have far fewer adsorption effects with proteins, and some actually make products more stable.

"It is estimated that pre-filled injection systems cost 25% more than conventional vials and ampoules".

A further problem with glass syringe devices is silicone and elastomer contamination of the product. Often a silicone lubricant is used to coat glass syringe plungers, which are typically made of elastomers. In pre-fillables, plastic plungers which use a fluoropolymer-coated stopper at their ends mean that a silicone- and elastomer-free alternative is available.

Nevertheless, while COC and COP-type materials are taking over from glass in the pre-fillables market, the polymers are not without their problems. Plastics are not yet well established in the parenterals market, and they will have to undergo extensive stability tests against each product and medium they are to be used with.

Plastic components cannot withstand the heat of the depyrogenation tunnels used for the traditional sterilisation of glass.

Furthermore, if manufacturers pre-sterilise the plastic parts they are more difficult to transfer to the filling line while keeping out contaminants. Other methods of sterilisation, such as gamma radiation, are being introduced for plastic components.

3. Cartridges

Cartridges are an ideal packaging for insulin and other drugs. They are used with pen or pump systems, auto-injectors and needle-free injectors. Highest precision and quality for all dimensional and functional aspects of the container are required to enable the functionality of these sophisticated drug delivery systems.

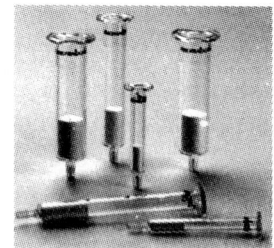

Fig. 13.7: Cartridges

Types

- Cartridges for pen system.
- Cartridges for pump system.
- Dual-chambered cartridges.
- Cartridges for auto-injector.
- Cartridges for needle-free injectors.
- Dental cartridges.

Multiple Dose Containers

A multiple dose container for parenterals is a hermetic container, which permits withdrawal of successive proportions of the contents without changing the strength, quality or purity of the remaining portion.

1. Glass Vials

A broad variety of vials from 1 ml to 100 ml with different neck finish designs, with or without blowback, for special requirements, industries also offer inside-coated vials for improved chemical stability, inertness and lyophilisation process.

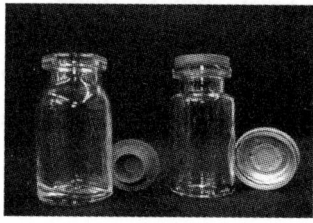

Fig. 13.8: Glass vials

Glass vials are filled using the same rinsing and filling procedure as for ampoules. In the case of vials containing a

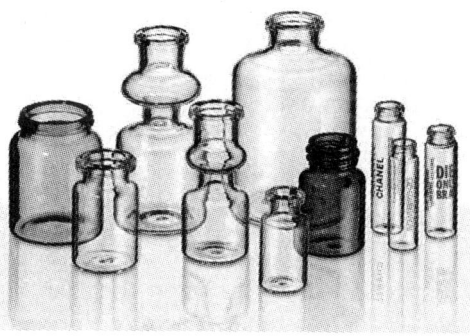

Fig. 13.9: Injection vials, screw-neck vials, tablet vials, dual chamber vials and perfume sample vials

fixed number of dose units, an excess volume is required to allow the stated number of doses to be withdrawn Vials are sealed using rubber closures, which are held in place by an aluminium sealing. A hand crimper is available in the laboratory to seal the rubber closures and aluminium sealing onto the vials.

Vials Made of Polymer

Vials made of cyclic olefin copolymer (COC) offer transparency comparable to glass. Due to excellent barrier properties, high chemical resistance and breakage resistance, this vial is an excellent alternative to glass, especially for emergency drugs, vaccines, diagnostic products and contrast media. Gamma irradiation is possible.

2. Large Volume Bottles

These bottles are used for filling large volume of solutions 100 ml or more. They are also rubber closures.

3. Flexible Plastic Bottles

These are the recent developments in the large volume parenteral packaging. These plastic containers are prepared from transparent PVC.

13.4 INSPECTION OF FILLED INJECTABLE PRODUCTS

Injection ampoules and vials should be checked for defects, cracks, chips, damage to the seals and closures. Injection solutions when examined under suitable conditions of visibility should be free from particles. BP 1998 Appendix XIII A and B describes tests for particulate contamination.

13.5 STORAGE AND LABELLING

Previously ampoules were labelled by use of paper labels. Presently this has been superseded by direct printing on the glass. For dispensing purposes in the practical lab, a paper label is used and should contain the following information.

- The strength expressed in terms of the amount of active ingredient in a suitable dose volume.

- The name and concentration of any added substance, e.g. antioxidant, anti-microbial preservative.
- Indication that a single dose preparation should be discarded after first use.
- Special labeling requirements for particular product, e.g. powders for reconstitution prior to use, concentrated solutions requiring dilutions prior to use.
- The date after which the preparation is not intended to be used (expiry date).
- The conditions under which the preparation should be stored.

Note: In practice, the expiry date should be determined for each product by conducting suitable stability studies. In hospital, sterile preparations are often given an expiry date of 1 week from date of manufacture/reconstitution.

13.6 UNITS OF CONCENTRATION

The concentration of the components in parenteral products may be expressed in various ways:

Percentage weight/volume: Examples include Magnesium sulphate injection 50%w/v, sodium chloride intravenous infusion 0.9% w/v.

Weight per unit volume: Examples include Atropine sulphate 600 µg/ml or ephedrine hydrochloride injection 30 mg/ml.

Millimoles per unit volume: Examples include Potassium chloride solution, strong (sterile) contains 2 mmol each of K^+ and Cl^- per ml; Calcium chloride injection BP contains 2.5 mmol of Ca^{2+} and 10 mmol of Cl^- in 5 ml.

13.7 PARENTERAL PACKAGING CONCERNS FOR DRUGS

Sources of Contamination

Extractables are the most common source of leachables contamination. An extractable is a chemical species, released from a container or component material, which has the potential to contaminate the pharmaceutical product. Extractables are generated by interaction between strong solvents and the package (including the glass vial and stopper) over time depending on temperature and extraction conditions.

A leachable is a chemical that has migrated from packaging or other components into the dosage form under normal conditions of use or during stability studies.

Mitigating the Risk from Rubber Closures

Fluorocarbon film coatings provide the best combination of protection from extractables from the stopper material while providing a high level of barrier protection for the drug product, therefore minimizing leachables.

When applied to stoppers, fluorocarbon films reduce adsorption of the drug onto the stopper, which is critical for maintaining the product's potency and shelf life. In addition, fluorocarbon films provide extra lubricity for proper vial seating, without the need for silicone oil. Fluoroelastomer films, which are made from inert materials, also reduce the possibility of extractables migrating from the rubber stopper into the biopharmaceutical product.

Strategies for Minimizing Risk

Drug developers who do not understand the impact of packaging on their biopharmaceutical products are courting an unnecessary level of regulatory and product-related risk. Problems often arise in this regard when a contract manufacturer tries to convince a sponsor that a particular stopper, vial, or other closure product is appropriate because it has been validated with the contractor's fill line. That is all well and good, and even necessary. However, stoppers need to be validated with the product first, and only then with the filling machinery. It is far more prudent, and in the long term much more cost-effective, to test and validate packaging within the context of the drug product.

Packaging Materials Associated with Parenteral Products

Components which are in contact with drug products and suitable for the pharmaceutical and medical device industries have a wide variety of applications and diverse functions. Plastic, elastomers, glass, metals, inks/coatings, adhesives and paper are the principle classes of materials used in CCS (container closure system) . Whether an individual component or combination of components are used in single-use devices, intermediate- or long-term storage applications, the material science must be understood to make informed decisions. The route of administration is a significant factor to determine the components to be evaluated, the amount of information needed to ensure patient safety and satisfy regulatory requirements. Inhalation, injectable, transdermal and ophthalmic dosage forms have a high degree of concern for package-product interaction and it is the regulatory expectation to assess leachables. Common CCS components used in different dosage forms. Other sources of potential leachables to be considered are drug product storage, process and filling equipment such as tanks, filters, reactors and disposable systems. Contamination from the CCS and equipment used in the manufacturing process for biologic protein products are of particular concern for contamination since leachables can have a negative impact to the patient as well as the protein products. A multi-component and multi-material CCS poses greater potential for package-dosage form interaction in conjunction with the affinity of migrants to the dosage form. The propensity for package interaction is related to the chemical constituents and nature of drug product matrices, i.e. solutions, emulsions, suspensions creams, solids, gels, aerosols, ointments. Leachables are a function of potential migrants (extractables) and their transport properties. There are scores of potential leachables to be considered because of migration, degradation and/or interaction. Plastics components will have many low molecular weight compounds that are not part of the polymer backbone which originate from polymer residuals, processing aids or performance additives. These are considered suspect leachables.

The Nature of Migrating Substances

Several different types of components can comprise a CCS which may be in contact with the drug product during various time intervals. The CCS components may be of a primary or secondary nature, and each component can be made of different polymers with a range of formulation ingredients. The release of these ingredients, when in direct contact with the drug product, can be the result of diffusion through the thickness of the package and at the package/drug product interface and through the product.

Developments in the Packaging of Parenterals

Bio-tech products are becoming more and more important because of their extraordinary pharmaceutical potential. Even today, 45% of new approvals are for drugs which contain biotechnological components. This trend will continue to strengthen in the future, in the next few years, 200 new approvals in total are expected world wide.

The active ingredients of bio-tech products are frequently too unstable to be incorporated into solid dose forms (typically tablets or capsules). Well over 90% of these products are therefore packaged as liquids in syringes, vials or ampoules. Since the products are substantially more expensive than other pharmaceuticals, they must be packed as securely as possible. Moreover, many products have to be transported at precisely controlled temperatures. Special 'cold chain logistics' must ensure that a product is maintained at the correct temperature from manufacture through distribution and storage to the point of dispensing.

Many pharmaceutical companies manufacture and market a wide range of products world wide. The different demands in the respective market and product segments therefore require a highly flexible packaging system that can handle a wide range of different items and at the same time provide optimal product protection. It is also always essential to guarantee efficient, low-cost packaging of small, medium and large lot sizes. Other requirements of a modern packaging system include item and code checks (vision systems), printing and checking of variable data, the shortest possible machine set-up times and compliance with GMP standards.

The Requirements of the Package

All packages must safeguard the product throughout its route from manufacture to final point of use. The package must also convey sufficient information that the product is used satisfactorily. Each package provides the vital link between manufacturer and consumer; it is an essential component of the product itself.

The pre-filled syringe is an example of a high-value product that must be safeguarded throughout a long shelf-life and yet be readily and accurately used whenever required. The proper selection of the package and the attention to its design will promote the benefits of the product in addition to fulfilling these fundamental functions. The syringe is not viable without a clever secondary package.

The package must enable rapid access to each of the pre-filled syringes it contains. The package must remain intact until the last of the syringes has been removed if that last syringe is to be safeguarded. The printing of the package will clearly present essential product information. Further features may confirm that the syringe is untouched until required for use.

A reclosable package can be retained for subsequent use without difficulty. If the package contains a course of treatment for a single patient, features to assist dosage compliance are appropriate. If the contents are to be used over an extended period, opening features that release only one syringe at a time can assist the user.

Concerning the logistics of distribution, costs are affected by the volume of package itself. Where the product must be held in a temperature controlled environment, it is particularly important to adopt a package of minimum volume relative to its contents. Minimising package volume also benefits storage immediately prior to use; for example in a hospital pharmacy.

Focus on Packaging Costs: Paperboard vs PVC

Inevitably, over the last few years, sober economic considerations have put the spotlight on packaging costs and on the packaging industry in general. It can be said some companies only take the costs of packaging materials into account, whilst others have a more holistic approach. This might also encompass investment costs and operating costs such as personnel, set-up times, the cost of format parts and last but not least the overall equipment efficiency.

A good example from Dividella is that they were able to demonstrate cost benefits in terms of the packaging material alone. The NeoTOP solution "wins out" against the PVC or PET blister and the attendant end load carton. The key principle is that the more product in the folding box, the greater the cost saving. One of the reasons for this is the low volume of the pack in comparison with the blister. One internal study by a Swiss pharmaceutical company has shown that savings of up to 30% in volume are possible using the NeoTOP concept for disposable syringes. If this is applied to the annual production of just one product, it corresponds to a considerable financial saving. If the product then has to be refrigerated until it gets to the patient, a smaller pack offers another major cost advantage.

Additional advantages can be identified. By opening the packaging from the top, the user immediately sees the entire contents. The leaflet or patient information insert can be extracted without any problem, can be read and replaced. The packaging is suitable for printing additional information on both internal and external panels. Needles or vials can also be integrated into the package without any problems. Evidence of prior opening is provided either by the opening mechanism itself or by means of relevant additional labels; the opening mechanism may offer re-closure if required.

However, looking at packaging costs alone is short-sighted, the even greater benefit lies on the machine side – or rather the process side.

- Only 1 installation instead of a thermoforming machine and a cartoning machine.
- No thermoforming process, that is a substantially lower energy consumption.
- Fewer personnel required.
- Change over between different formats in 30 minutes.
- Mono material packaging independent of changes in the price of oil.
- Higher machine efficiency.
- Flexibility in machine allocation.
- Retrofitting/conversion of installations is practical thanks to the machinery's modular construction.

It is a far-reaching strategic decision by managers in the pharmaceutical industry to opt for monomaterial solutions in preference to packages that combine a number of different materials. However, this decision will bring commercial advantages in the day-to-day packaging process and in terms of greater systems flexibility.

One thing is absolutely clear: Switching over existing products packaged in PVC involves considerable effort - this is without question.

According to Dr Manfred Zurkirch, Managing Director of Dividella AG, Switzerland, "In accordance with the customer request - that is our understanding of packaging flexibility. In order to live up to the high expectations of our customers, we have developed new modular transfer systems as a result of our long standing experiences in the field of product handling. These allow us to pack up to 800 syringes per minute. By the way, these packaging systems are not only suitable for syringes (with or without needle protection), but also for pens, injectors, inhalers and other similar devices".

Protection from Counterfeiting or Tampering

Dividella has been concerned with guaranteeing originality for many years and have introduced the simple expedient of applying a spot of hot-melt glue at critical points on the carton. If the carton has been opened, this is immediately apparent to the user — and it involves virtually no extra machine costs and has no effects at all on performance.

Biotechnology products in particular are complex to produce and are therefore expensive to manufacture. The risk of these products being counterfeited or manipulated is unfortunately omnipresent and is regularly encountered in some parts of the world. Whether a counterfeit product is used for cancer therapy or for analgesia, the consequences for the patient can be severe.

The co-operation between two Swiss companies, one a specialist folding carton business, the other a security printing specialist, has yielded a solution that can be rapidly implemented on existing packages. An invisible code for the pack, product and information on usage ensures the necessary security—and also allows "Track and Trace".

Energy and Environmental Considerations

Until very recently, it was almost frowned upon to refer to the energy and environmental aspects of a packaging concept. The argument frequently given was: "This topic has no resonance among our management... but personally I clearly see the advantage".

Today, if a manager in the pharmaceutical industry were to try to sweep this topic under the carpet, it would certainly not be advisable—for the following reasons.

- Energy costs are rising and very volatile—this variable cost is difficult to predict.
- Production costs (including packaging costs) are clearly a competitive advantage.
- Customers decide whether packaging is environmentally friendly.
- Costs of disposal are rising. Major consumers such as hospitals will exercise pressure.

Dividella's TopLoad packaging solutions are based on 100% mono material, namely cardboard; unlike the still more commonly used blister in sideload cartons involving plastics.

Production of the required raw materials like cardboard and plastic foils makes a substantial difference concerning, for instance, the airborne emissions that are associated therewith. Data provided by the Swiss Federal Institute of Technology shows that for a similarly sized package, the cardboard based TopLoad solution causes 3 to 5 times less CO_2 emissions than a blister in a box solution, depending on the kind of plastic that is chosen.

With methane, another gas that is believed to contribute to global warming, that ratio is even higher thus favouring the Dividella solutions.

Sustainability

The goal of sustainable packaging is to reduce environmental impact and the ecological footprint of a products package.

Eco-friendly packaging considerations go well beyond creating a recyclable package. Consideration must also be given to the amount of material used, the type of material, biodegradability, overall package volume and weight reduction to minimize transportation energy, printability of the material to eliminate separate labels, and even the amount of energy required for forming the package.

These "green" considerations are sometimes contrary to the unique needs of parenteral packaging features including increased product protection, increased billboard space for patient compliance, tamper evidence, and unit dose packaging trends.

A well designed green parenteral package starts with package material selection. Eco-friendly materials are derived from renewable resources, are easy to recycle, have relatively low energy requirements and are biodegradable.

Paper has the inherent advantage of coming from a renewable resource. Trees are considered a renewable resource because they can be replaced within a human life-time. Paper is also commonly recycled, and can be directly printed, thus reducing the need for separate labels. Paper packages are formed easily by folding using less energy than for plastic packages that must be heated before the forming process.

Laminated materials, commonly used in packaging, present challenges in recycling. Most must be physically separated before recycling, a process that is not always feasible.

One of the most important aspects of any sustainable package design is overall cost. The reality is that if any package design adds significant expense, it is doomed to failure. Overall cost can include package material (bulk or blanks), labour for forming, as well as shipping costs for inbound material and outbound finished products. Paperboard blanks can be shipped flat to minimize volume for inbound shipping, then formed, glued, and filled using automatic machinery. State-of-the-art Dividella machinery is capable of erecting cartons, gluing partitions, and filling products at high speeds. Machines with a high degree of flexibility can produce different package formats with quick changeovers and high Overall Equipment Efficiency (OEE). This further contributes to sustainability by reducing the overall plant floor space, resulting in less energy required for heating/cooling, and even construction and building materials.

Sustainable packaging is obtained by utilizing an engineered approach that addresses the entire packaging and product life cycle, not merely the package itself. Paper-based engineered packages can offer significant advantages in achieving an Eco-friendly and a high performance package while providing the least total cost of ownership.

13.8 PACKAGING OF OPHTHALMICS

A. Ophthalmics

Ophthalmic preparations are sterile, liquid, semi-solid or solid preparations intended for administration upon the eyeball and/or to the conjunctiva or to be inserted in the conjunctival sac. Several categories of eye preparations may be distinguished:

- Eye drops
- Eye lotions
- Semi-solid eye preparations
- Ophthalmic inserts

Characteristics of Ophthalmic Containers

1. They should preserve the sterility of the content.
2. Not extract out anything to the containers.
3. Not absorb anything from the contents.
4. Provide protection physical, chemical, microbial.
5. It should be easy to sterilized.
6. They should be easy to handle and storage.

I. Preparation of Eye Drops

Extemporaneous preparation of eye drops involves the following:

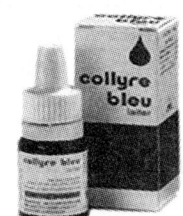

- Preparation of the solution
- Clarification
- Filling and sterilization

Fig. 13.10: Eye drops

Preparation of the Solution

The aqueous eye drop vehicle containing any necessary preservative, antioxidant, stabilizer, tonicity modifier, viscosity modifier or buffer should be prepared first. Then the active ingredient is added and the vehicle made up to volume.

Clarification

The BP has stringent requirements for the absence of particulate matter in eye drop solutions. Sintered glass filters or membrane filters of 0.45 – 1.2 µm pore sizes are suitable. The clarified solution is either filled directly into the final containers which are sealed prior to heat sterilization or filled into a suitable container prior to filtration sterilization. Clarified vehicle is used to prepare eye drop suspensions which are filled into final containers and sealed prior to sterilization.

Sterilization

This can take the form of:

- Autoclaving at 115°C for 30 minutes or 121°C for 15 minutes.
- Heating at 98 – 100°C for 30 minutes together with either benzalkonium chloride 0.01% w/v or chlorhexidine acetate 0.01% w/v or phenylmercuric acetate or nitrate 0.002% w/v or thiomersal 0.01% w/v. This method is described in the BP (1980) but is no longer a pharmacopoeial recommended method.
- Filtration through a membrane filter having a 0.22 µm pore size into sterile containers using strict aseptic technique. Filling should take place under Grade A laminar airflow conditions. A suitable filter holder for extemporaneous preparation. The filter assembly is sterilized by autoclaving before use.
- Dry heat sterilization at 160°C for 2 hours is employed for non-aqueous preparations such as liquid paraffin eye drops. Silicone rubber teats must be used.

Immediately following sterilization the eye drop containers must be converted with readily breakable seal, such as a viskring, to distinguish between opened and unopened containers.

Packaging

Containers: Eye drops should be packed in neutral glass containers or in suitable plastic containers. Traditionally, eye drops were stored in vertically fluted amber coloured glass bottles fitted with a bakelite cap carrying a dropper. The glass used in the formation of container must be passing the test of alkalinity, recently eye drops are packed in plastic container with applicators. Labelling for eye drops contain the direction for use (for external use only).

Labelling requirements are summarized in Tables 13.1 and 13.2.

Table 13.1: General labelling requirements for eye drop containers

Requirement	Include on label
Fully identify the product	Title; either name and concentration of active ingredients or reference to official monograph giving these details. If monograph allows more than one concentration then state the one used.
Specify storage conditions	"Store in a cool place" or "Protect from light".
State product expiry date	Month and year of expiry
Warning label	"Not to be taken"
Specify volume	e.g. 5ml
Ensure correct use	e.g. "Shake the bottle" for a suspension

Table 13.2: Additional labelling requirements for use in specific locations

All locations	Include concentration of active ingredient and name and concentration of any antimicrobial present.
Hospital	Patient's name. The eye to be treated. Date of opening of bottle and/or date to discard.
Wards	Single dose for once-only use. Marked with indication and concentration of active ingredient. No preservative.
Operating Theatres Clinics	Outer package fully labelled. Single dose or multidose used once only.
Domiciliary	"Avoid contamination of contents during use" Discard 4 weeks after opening" Keep out of reach of children. Plus instructions on how to use.

II. Preparation of Eye Lotions

The purpose of eye lotions is to assist in the cleaning of the external surfaces of the eye. This might be to help remove a non-impacted foreign body or to clean away conjunctival discharge. Eye lotions intended for use in surgical or first-aid procedures should not contain antimicrobial preservatives and should be in single-use containers. There is no intention to use an eye lotion to deliver any active ingredient to the eye but rather to remove unwanted gross contaminants from the eye. Thus, these preparations should be very simple and the most common eye lotion consists of sterile normal saline. This preparation typifies the requirements of an eye lotion, which are:

- Sterile and usually containing no preservative.
- Isotonic with lachrymal fluid.
- Neutral pH.
- Large volume but not greater than 200 ml.
- Non-irritant to ocular tissue.

Packaging

They are packed in amber coloured Screw capped fluted bottles.

Labelling

These should include:

- Title identifying the product and concentration of contents
- Sterile until opened
- Not to be taken
- Use once and discard remaining solution
- Expiry date

Preserved eye lotion would need the additional labelling:

- Avoid contamination of contents during use
- Discard remaining solutions not more than 4 weeks after first opening

The lotions should be supplied in coloured fluted bottles and sealed to exclude microorganisms.

III. Preparation of Eye Ointments

Eye ointments are popular and duplicate many of the therapeutic options offered by eye drops. Ointments have the disadvantage of temporarily interfering with vision, but have the advantage over liquids of providing greater total drug bioavailability. However, ointments take a longer time to reach peak absorption.

Eye ointments must be sterile and may contain suitable antimicrobial preservatives, antioxidants and stabilizers. USP ophthalmic ointments packaged in multi-dose containers are to contain an antimicrobial substance unless otherwise directed in the monograph or if the formulation itself is bacteriostatic. The most commonly used agents include the two mercurials, phenylmercuric nitrate and thiomersal, the parabens and chlorobutanol. It is necessary also those ointments are free from particulate matter that could be harmful to the tissues of the eye. The EP and BP have limits for the particle size of incorporated solids which will be met if all particles have been reduced to <25 µm.

The basic components of an eye ointment are given below:
- Liquid paraffin 1 part.
- Wool fat 1 part (to facilitate incorporation of water).
- Yellow soft paraffin 8 parts.
- Hard paraffin as required to produce required consistency in hot climates.

Preparation of Eye Ointments

Eye ointments are normally prepared using aseptic techniques to incorporate the finely powdered active ingredient or a sterilized concentrated solution of the medicament into the sterile eye ointment basis. Immediately after preparation the eye ointment is filled into the sterile containers which are then sealed so as to exclude microorganisms. The screw cap should be covered with a readily breakable seal. All apparatus used in the preparation of eye ointments must be scrupulously clean and sterile. Certain commercial eye ointments may be sterilized in their final containers using ionising radiation.

Preparation of Eye Ointment Basis

The paraffin and the wool fat are heated together and filtered, while molten, through a coarse filter paper in a heated funnel into a container which can withstand dry heat sterilization temperatures. The container is closed to exclude micro-organisms and together with contents is maintained at 160°C for 2 hours.

Containers for Eye Ointments

Eye ointments should be supplied in small sterilized collapsible tubes made of metal or in a suitable plastic. The tube should not contain more than 5 g of preparation and must be fitted or provided with a nozzle of a suitable shape to facilitate application to the eye and surrounds without allowing contamination of the contents. The tubes must be suitably sealed to prevent microbial contamination. Eye ointment may also be packed in suitably designed single-dose containers.

Labelling

This includes the following:
- The names and percentages of the active ingredients.
- The date after which the eye ointment is not intended to be used.
- The conditions under which the eye ointment should be stored — normally at a temperature not exceeding 25°C.
- The name and concentration of any antimicrobial preservative or other substance added to the preparation.
- A statement to the effect that the contents are sterile providing the container has not been opened.

13.9 SELECTION OF PACKAGING MATERIALS

Packaging for eye drops and other vision/ophthalmic products must protect, educate and impart the idea of purity.

When products help people see well, the packaging needs to look good. Packaging for vision/ophthalmic products such as eye drops, contact lenses and lens-care materials has to meet a unique set of demands. Like many over-the-counter (OTC) pharmaceuticals, they need to compete on the shelf and instruct consumers on their use-often with extremely limited surface area.

In addition, the concepts of purity and product protection are especially important for ophthalmic products. Both structurally and graphically, the best packaging for such products will reinforce the notion that it's safe to put this stuff in (or near) eye.

Eye drops are among the most common vision products sold OTC. One of their biggest packaging challenges is the tiny quantities involved. Eye drops are literally used a few drops at a time and it's common for them to be sold in small fractions of an ounce.

The most obvious packaging strategy for such products, and indeed the most common one, is to put a small plastic vial in a carded, peggable blister. But some marketers of vision products have moved beyond that concept. They're using packaging to improve the product's portability and ease of use.

Squeeze Play

A vial of high-density polyethylene (HDPE), the most common material used for eye drop containers, can be hard to use properly. Consumers often get too little or too much with each squeeze, and the amount of force needed varies as the vial empties.

One way to increase both portability and ease of use is to go to single-use containers. Several companies market eye drops in blow-fill-seal plastic vials, usually packaged a half-dozen or more to a paperboard carton. Single-use b-f-s vials, when filled under sterile conditions, have the additional advantage of enabling the product to be formulated without preservatives; most products in multi-use containers need preservatives to counteract the ingress of microorganisms after each use.

Preservative Bottle

When the consumer pushes on the bottle's base, the liquid compresses. The multiple valves and airless pump inside the bottle dispense a single drop, which passes over a silver coil in the bottle's tip. Because silver has antibacterial qualities, the coil helps maintain the product's sterility. After dispensing, the valves close, preventing air from entering the bottle and causing contamination.

"The priorities and imperatives for packaging are ensuring the integrity of the formula and making the product easy to use for a variety of consumers. Many of the containers used for eye drops and other ophthalmic products are fairly prosaic and utilitarian in appearance. They are round or slope-shouldered, and either white or translucent (a function of the HDPE or polypropylene used for the bottle). But Mentholatum distributes its flagship Rohto V eye drops in a striking, clear, flat oval container with a tinted top".

Lens Cleaners

This problem-solution orientation comes into play in a line of eye-care products where consumer education is an important part of the packaging. Nanofilm, wipes, sprays and other products designed to help consumers take care of their eyeglasses.

"Industries will easily reach for their clothing (to wipe their glasses) more often than not. So our (packaging) is a balance of something that's very attractive, but at the same time, if we can try to educate the consumer a little bit on that package, to make them understand why they really need to be cleaning their glasses with a professional product and not their clothing, that makes it even more of a win".

Nanofilm uses polyethylene terephthalate (PET) bottles for its Ultra Clarity lens cleaning fluid, with clear front and back labels. The back label, visible from the front through the bottle, completes a motif of a forest scene. "It ties into the calmness of being out in the forest, to clear the mind-that sense of clarity to it".

Nanofilm sells multi-component packages, which include sprays and pre-moistened towelettes. These packages give the company billboard space to educate consumers on the virtues of professional lens-cleaning products. "It's also to bring up the price point a little bit," Products need packaging that can suggest purity, dispense efficiently and educate consumers effectively.

13.10 PACKAGING OF AEROSOLS

Aerosol is a suspension of fine solid particles or liquid droplets in a gas. Examples are smoke, oceanic haze, air pollution and CS gas. In general conversation, aerosol usually refers to an aerosol spray can or the output of such a can. The word aerosol derives from the fact that matter "floating" in air is a suspension (a mixture in which solid or liquid or combined solid-liquid particles are suspended in a fluid). To differentiate suspensions from true solutions, the term sol evolved-originally meant to cover dispersions of tiny (sub-microscopic) particles in a liquid. With studies of dispersions in air, the term aerosol evolved and now embraces both liquid droplets, solid particles, and combinations of these.

I. The Packaging of Aerosol Technology

When a person spray any aerosol product, whether it is paint, mosquito repellent, or a disinfectant, they are all being delivered in the same way: aerosol container technology. The word "aerosol" refers to: "An integral ready-to-use package incorporating a valve and a product which is dispensed by pre-stored pressure in a controlled manner when the valve is operated".

But actually, the word aerosol can refer to any tiny particle or droplet suspended in a gas. This includes clouds, haze, and fog. The science that creates fog is recreated when we create an artificial mist with a spray can. The word "aerosol" gained stigma decades ago, when it was discovered that some of the chemicals used in spray cans were damaging our Earth's atmosphere and Ozone layer. Even though those chemicals, known as "CFCs" (chlorofluorocarbons), are no longer used to propel the contents out of the can, many people still falsely, believe that aerosol products are bad for the environment.

II. Component of Aerosols Package

Valve

At the top of the can is the valve. The valve is actually quite a complex little thingamajig. The valve or stem is attached to the dip tube, which grants access to the product inside. The valve can operate in two different ways, but its purpose is the same. Either press down on a button (actuator) to open the valve, or in the case of whipped cream, push a stem to the side. Either way, the purpose of the valve is to open up the can to release the pressure being asserted on the liquefied propellant/product solution. It is that change in pressure that reacts with the propellant and ultimately pushes the product out of the can. Now, inside the can, there is more than just paint. There is a delicate balance of pressurized gases.

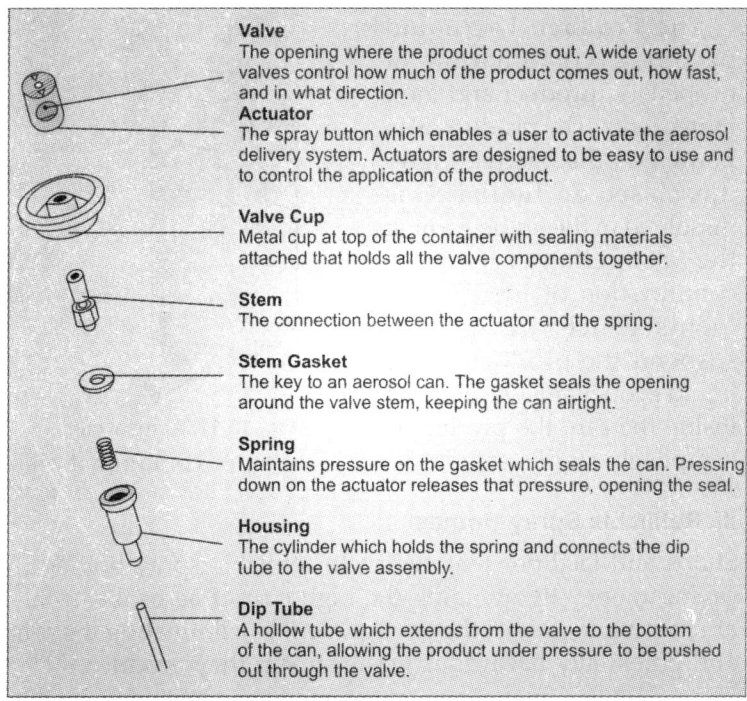

Valve
The opening where the product comes out. A wide variety of valves control how much of the product comes out, how fast, and in what direction.

Actuator
The spray button which enables a user to activate the aerosol delivery system. Actuators are designed to be easy to use and to control the application of the product.

Valve Cup
Metal cup at top of the container with sealing materials attached that holds all the valve components together.

Stem
The connection between the actuator and the spring.

Stem Gasket
The key to an aerosol can. The gasket seals the opening around the valve stem, keeping the can airtight.

Spring
Maintains pressure on the gasket which seals the can. Pressing down on the actuator releases that pressure, opening the seal.

Housing
The cylinder which holds the spring and connects the dip tube to the valve assembly.

Dip Tube
A hollow tube which extends from the valve to the bottom of the can, allowing the product under pressure to be pushed out through the valve.

The head space: When the can is filled, there is space left at the top to allow for some of the propellant to remain a gas.

The gaseous propellant: The same chemical propellant which is in liquid form mixed with the product, but at the top the propellant remains is gaseous form, which maintains a constant pressure inside the can.

Some propellants used today include propane, butane, which are naturally occurring hydrocarbons. Other propellants include compressed gasses such as nitrogen or carbon dioxide. Only a minuscule minority of modern aerosols uses CFC propellants, and this only because an appropriate substitute as not yet been found. These products, which are exempt from the EPAs ban, are primarily pharmaceutical products, which account for less than one percent of all aerosol products in consumer use. Soon, even these products will no longer use CFCs, once a proper alternative has been determined.

The Product: The liquid part is a combination of propellant, product and inert ingredients. The product, also known as the "active ingredient" see on the label, is dissolved in the liquid form of the propellant, using a combination of inert ingredients which are used to suspend the product in the liquid propellant. Once sealed inside the can, the product is completely sterile, safe from evaporation or contamination.

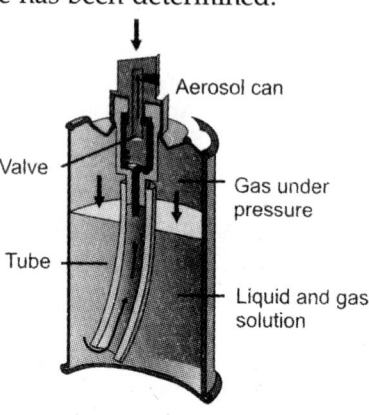

Fig. 13.11: Aerosol can

III. Refillable Spray Bottles

Shops and facilities that switch to refillable spray bottles are saving money by avoiding the high cost of aerosol cans and are helping to protect the environment by eliminating the solid and potentially hazardous waste stream they produce.

There are two basic types of refillable spray bottles:
1. Metal bottles that spray product using compressed air.
2. Plastic bottles that use a hand pump to spray product.

Refillable metal bottles more closely resemble aerosol cans in terms of their design and performance. These bottles are filled with product (for example, brake cleaner) from a bulk container and are pressurized with air at 80 to 200 pounds per square inch using a compressed-air hose. Plastic bottles are also filled from bulk containers but do not require compressed air. Instead, pumping a trigger to create a mist or stream of product operates them.

Construction material: Refillable spray bottles are available in different materials and with different finishes (aluminium, stainless-steel, brass, and steel) for use with different types of bulk product.

Nozzle type: 1-quart, refillable spray bottles come with standard spray and stream nozzles. A nozzle that can be adjusted from stream to spray is also available. Smaller bottles (16 and 8-fluid ounce) are available that closely resemble the size and shape of aerosol cans and have a spray pattern similar to an aerosol can spray.

Nozzle extensions: Nozzle extensions up to 12 inches long are available for spraying areas that are otherwise difficult or impossible to reach.

Advantages of Pharmaceutical Aerosols

 i. They are convenient and easy to use.
 ii. Medicament delivered directly to the affected area in the desired form and in high concentration.
 iii. Since application of the medicament is without manual contact with the skin irritation of painful areas avoided.
 iv. Dose of medicament can be removed without contamination of the remaining portion.
 v. Stability of air and moisture sensitive substances is enhanced.
 vi. The fine mist required for inhalation purposes can be easily formed.
 vii. Sterility of the product can be maintained if required.
 viii. For products requiring regulation of dose, a metered valve can be used.
 ix. Application of medicament is in thin layer giving immediate local action and reducing unnecessary losses. It is suitable for dispensing of medicaments in solid, semisolid or liquid form.

Along with the ability to adopt a wide range of appearances, from sleek to industrial, aerosols perform very well. Aerosol containers are clean and hygienic, and will not leak in bags during transport or in the bathroom. The containers are airtight, resulting in long product shelf life and 100% resistance to bacteria or dust contamination. The contents do not evaporate and the product's characteristics will not change over its lifetime. In terms of application, aerosols allow for controlled product dispensing, facilitating consumer use and the ability to reach some otherwise inaccessible spots.

Empty aerosol containers are recyclable, as they are made from tinplate steel or aluminium. They are also environmentally friendly, due to regulations that prohibit the use of chlorofluorocarbon (CFC) propellants in almost all aerosol products manufactured and sold around the world.

Disadvantages of Pharmaceutical Aerosols

i. A major disadvantage of aerosol formulation is its higher cost as compared to other conventional dosage form.
ii. Toxicity due to propellants may cause health problems specially in case of inhalation therapy.
iii. The cooling effect of highly volatile propellants may cause irritation and discomfort on injured skin.
iv. High pressure may develop on exposure to heat.

IV. Regulations

US EPA and many states may consider used aerosol cans that are not empty hazardous waste.

Required Paperwork

- *Purchasing:* Request a Material Safety Data Sheet (MSDS) for all aerosol products. Occupational Safety and Health Administration (OSHA) regulations require products. (Hazard information should also be provided in foreign languages for employees who may not understand English).
- *Storage:* Inspect all hazardous waste storage areas and document inspection results.
- *Shipping:* Keep shipping papers/manifests for a minimum of three years to show waste has been shipped properly.
- *Disposal:* Know where waste is going. Request proof that the waste has been received and disposed of or recycled properly. Keep records for a minimum of three years.

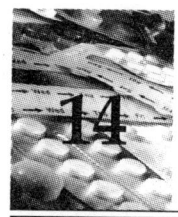

Defects in Packages

14.1 INTRODUCTION

Defects is the deviations from the specification, they are depends upon their effect on patient, product, pack or production operation. They require laboratory as well as possibly production and market application testing.

Category

Defects are classified in to following category:

Category 1 : Minor defect, high percentage AQL (Acceptable Quality Level).

Category 2 : Major defect medium percentage AQL.

Category 3 : Critical defect low percentage AQL.

Category 4 : Intolerable defect 0% AQL.

Minor defect: Minor defects are not likely to materially affected usability but are departures from normal commercial standards, i.e. damage the appearance but not the function of package.

Example: Stones, air bubbles in glass bottle, uneven or corrugated surface of bottle, dents and scratches on case, printing out of specification.

Major defects: They are likely to reduce the usability of the container or end product. It reduce the identity by virtue of graphic defects, to result in the product not meeting the require standard.

Example: Heat seal to narrow, rough weight edges, liner encoding specifications below weight.

Critical defects: Critical defects are likely to result in hazardous conditions for potential users or packaging operation. They cause hazards in handling or disposal.

Example: Cracks and penetrating, wrong copy size in levels, leakage on seal in metallic container.

General Example of Critical Defect

- Cracked and shipped bottle
- Fracture in the can end or body
- Missing liner in the closure
- Fracture in the pouch
- Unglued can flap

General Example of Minor Defect

- Split ring
- Split body: in any direction in the body
- Checked ring: anywhere on ring
- Crizzle ring: elsewhere on ring.

14.2 DEFECTS IN PACKAGING MATERIAL

Defects in package ultimately depend on the defect in packaging material including both primary and secondary packaging material.

- Glass defect
- Plastic defect
- Metal defect
- Rubber
- Closure defect
- Label defect
- Shipper defect
- Blister and strip package defect
- Paper board and corrugated material

I. Defects in Glass

Glass having some defects is given below:

1. Ring
   - *Bulged ring:* bulged out of shape and out of specification.
   - *Bent ring:* Tilted to one side.
   - *Dipped ring:* Severe dip in the sealing surface.
2. Neck and shoulder
   - *Bent neck:* Tilted neck

3. Body
  - *Sunk:* Body is sunk inwards.
  - *Bulged:* Body is bulged outside.
  - *Uneven distribution:* Vary in thickness of bottle wall.
  - *Corrugated:* Uneven surface.
4. Bottom
  - *Wedged bottom:* Glass is thicker at one side.
5. Thin corner
6. Rocky bottom
7. Spinner.

General Defects of Glass

- *Bird swing:* A thread of glass extends between two internal points of bottle or glass.
- *Stuck:* Lump of glass annealed with outside of container.
- *Stones:* Batch inclusion in glass.
- *Seed:* Small bubbles formed.
- *Blisters:* Bubbles forms in the body of glass.
- *Airline:* Single line in glass surface.
- *Wrinkle:* Wrinkles are formed on the surface of glass.
- *Spike:* Sharp projection on inside of container.
- *Glass inside:* Pieces of glass annealed inside of container
- *Flaking:* It is process of extraction of alkali from the surface of glass containers. Because of this formation of silica rich layer on the surface of glass. This sometimes gets detached or can be detected as shining flakes in the contents. This problem occurs at higher temperature storage condition. This is very harmful to the parenterals.
- *Weathering:* This is because moisture condensing on the surface of glass containers can be extracts some weakly bounded alkali leaving behind a white deposit this is loss of brilliance of glass.

II. Defect in Plastic/Drug-plastic Consideration

There problems or defect include:
1. Permeability of the container to atmosphere gases and moisture vapour.
2. Heating of the constituent of container into the internal content.

3. Sorption of drugs from the content to the container.
4. Transmission of light through the container.
5. Alteration of the container on storage.

1. Permeation of the container: Permeability is the process of saturation and diffusion with the penetrant initially dissolving in the plastic material on one side and diffusion through to the other side. Permeability is the function of several factors like nature of polymer, amount and type of plasticizer and fillers.

2. Leaching of the constituent of container into the internal content: Leached material whether dissolved into content or present in minute particles passes a health hazard to the patients.

Remedies: Soft walled container of PVC are frequently used to package various IV solution and blood for transfusion.

3. Sorption: Sorption include both the term adsorption and absorption. Sorption is a term used to indicate the binding the molecules to polymer materials. Sorption occurs though chemical or physical means with the phenomenon related to the chemical structure of the solute molecules and physical and chemical properties of the polymers. The process of sorption is depending upon the penetration or diffusion of a solute into the plastic. Sorption of drug components from a pharmaceutical solution reduces the concentration of that agent in the solution render the product unreliable as to potency and unacceptable for use. The sorption of following material may take place by the container, i.e.

- Sorption of antimicrobials and stabilizer.
- Sorption of colourants and flavours.
- Active ingredients, e.g. insulin.

Remedies: Use of soft plastic, plastic prepared by coextrusion using barrier layer and formed into sheets.

4. Transmission of light: Clear and uncoloured plastic container behave in much the same manner as clear and uncoloured glass container is allowing destructive light transmission.

Remedies: Agents termed UV absorber may be added to the plastic to decrease the transmission of there short UV rays and then may be used to protect light destructive drugs.

5. Alteration in container: The physical and chemical alteration of the packaging material by the drug product is called modification.

Phenomenon such as permeation, sorption, leaching play a role in altering the property of the plastic and may also leads to its degradation.

Example: Deformation in polyethylene container is alter caused by permeation of gases and vapours from the environment or by less of content through the container walls. Some solvent system are found to be responsible for change in mechanical properties of plastics.

Example: Oils have a softening effect on PE. Fluorinated hydrocarbons attack on PE and PVC.

SAA'S also causes changes in PE. In other case contents may extracts the plasticizer, antioxidants or stabilizers thus changing the flexibility of the package.

Remedies: Use of super plastic.

Some other Defects Terminology for Plastics

1. **Stress cracking:** Phenomena related to low density polyethylene and certain cracking agents as such as melting agents, detergents and volatile oils.
2. **Paneling or cavitations:** Containers shows inwards distortion or particle collapse achieving to absorption of gases form head space, absorption causing swelling of plastic.
3. **Crazing:** A surface reticulation which can occur particularly with polystyrene cause crazing.
4. **Poor key of print:** Certain plastics such as polyolefines need pre-treating before in with additive that migrates to the surface of plastics may cause printing problem.
5. **Poor impact resistance:** Both polystyrene and PVC have poor in resistance. This can be improved by inclusion of some modification.

III. Defects in Metals

Metals generally used are tin, plastic coated tin, tin coated lead, aluminium. Now in metals removal of metal particle is main problem. Nowaday generally coated metal are used but it has additional problem that coating is incompletely occurs the underlying materials so defects like, Cracking, solvent resistance can occur.

The metal in presence of some preparation may result in unwanted product, i.e.

- Aluminium react with fatty alcohol emulsion to form a while encrustation of such tube are unstable for mercury containing compounds.
- The cracking may occur at outside pH range of 6.5–8.0.
- *Corrosion:* Metal spontaneously undergo gradual destruction when exposed to the atmosphere in chemical terminology such as destruction is known as corrosion.

IV. Defects of Rubber

There are mainly two problems in rubber packaging.

1. Sorption of active ingredient, e.g. antibacterial, preservative or other material to the rubber. This may affect the stability of the preparation.
2. Extraction one or more components of rubber into vial solution. This may cause the toxicity and pyrogenicity of injectables preparation.

Remedies: An epoxy lining to rubber stopper may reduce amount of extractive leached form the stopper, but they is no effect on separation of preservative from solution.

Use of Teflon coated rubber stopper prevents sorption as well as leaching out of rubber closure.

V. Defects of Closures

Class A

These defects, which prevent the closure from performing there function of protection.

- A crack in metal anywhere on cap.
- Missing liner.
- No threads or shallow threads that do not engage to the glass threads.
- Missing colour or copy in lithography.
- Dimension outside of tolerable limits.

Class B

Defects which cause boarder line functionally.
- Liners loose and particularly having out.
- Copy illegible in lithography.
- Bulges in the center panel of the cap.

Class C

Defects, which impair appearance but not function.
- Blotchy lithography.
- Scratches on scruff marks on outside surface of cap.
- Rest spots on cap.

VI. Defects in Labels

- Wrong copy or size.
- Missing colour.
- Labels in stack, stack together.
- Severe curl.
- Tear of holes.
- Uneven stuck.
- Smeared or illegal copy.
- Rough cut edges.
- Scratches or below standard scuff resistance.
- Mattling
- Improper identification.

VII. Shipper Defects

Class A

Defects which prevent shipper from safety containing the primary package through national distribution by common carriers.
- Loose manufacturing points.
- Dimension outside of tolerance limits.
- Wrong colour graphics.
- Any tears, puncture, holes which loosely adhesing board particles.
- Bottom flaps.
- Turn on bent portions.

Class B

Which make function questionable and borderline.
- Incomplete printing.
- Bends other than on second line.
- Liner not completely glued to corrugated medium.
- Absence of howskid coating on top and bottom flaps.
- Moisture contents under 5% or 3%.

Class C

Which impair appearance but not function.
- Light or blotchy graphics.
- Uneven colour or stain on outer surface.

VIII. Defects in Blister Package

Class A

Faults, which compromise, package integrity.
- Cracks or holes anywhere on blister.
- Wall thickness.

Class B

Which reduce stability.
- Scratches and gets, waves.
- Discolouration
- Embedded foreign matters.
- Failure to meat scratch resistance test.

Class C
- Rough cut flanges.
- Mould marks on side of blister.

IX. Paperboard and Corrugated Fiberboard Defects

1. Cartons

Class A

Faults, which prevent the cartons from containing the detergent.
- Excessive opening or spring back force.
- Dimension out side of limits.
- Tears, holes or scuff.
- Missing colour.
- Misregistration of colour.

Class B

- Scuff surface.
- Inadequate surface for easy opening.

Class C

Faults affecting appearance only.
- Rough printed surface.
- Slight off colour match.

2. Corrugated Boxes

Class A

- Incomplete liner adhesive.
- Dimensions outside of tolerance.
- Weight below minimum.
- Loss manufacturing joints.

Class B

- Incomplete tape joint.
- Deep slots.
- Outer flaps not meeting by gap.
- Bad scores.
- Excessive high/low moisture contents in board.
- Treatment was not specified.

Class C

- Rough out-slots.
- Wash board appearance making for poor printing.
- Bad printing for any other reason.
- Cluster.

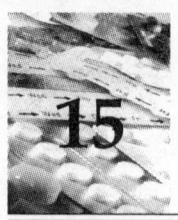

15

Labelling of Packages

15.1 INTRODUCTION

The oxford dictionary defines a label as "a slip of paper, card, liner, metal for attaching to an object and indicating its nature, owner, name, destination, etc". Labelling is the manual or electromechanical process of attaching the 'label' to the correct particular product or packaging or service.

From the simple manual operations of sticking the paper label to the container with animal glue, the labelling technology has progressed significantly, offering a variety of labelling materials, adhesives and machinery, tailored to suit particular labelling equipment. Sometimes, the function of the label is done by the container/package itself which is printed with all the information which the label normally carries.

15.2 FUNCTIONS OF LABELS

- To identify the product.
- Provide ingredients.
- Purpose/use of the products.
- Providing aesthetic appeal.
- Decoration as evidence.
- Child safety.
- Other information like maximum retail price (MRP), Batch No, Shelf-life/Best-before date, etc.

Information is required by all the links in the packaging chain, but the medium (i.e. the labels) used to carry that information represent only a minute part of the whole product. The quantum of information required has increased and is likely to do so again in the future; in particular, consumers, who influence the legislators, are demanding yet more information on products. Most parts of the production, storage and distribution systems are becoming more sophisticated in their use of barcodes and computers to track and record where goods are located, thereby requiring the design of specialist bar coding systems. Some or all of this information may have to be enshrined on the label.

Increased information on the labels is influenced by:
- *Health and safety issues:* More and detailed information is required on the product, from the point of view of human health, safety of the consumer and more comprehensive contents/ingredients listings.
- Better inventory control.
- Much more environmental pressure, particularly on packaging waste.
- National and international legislations.
- Growing internationalization of the label and labelling market leading to more languages being used.
- Increased problems with tampering, look-alikes and the counterfeiting of goods.

15.3 TYPES OF LABELS
- Non-adhesive label materials.
- Glue applied – Wet glue, hot-melt glue.
- Shrink/stretch sleeve – Formed into tube and shrunk on with heat.
- In mould – Placed in mould prior to injection or blow moulding.
- Pre-adhesive label materials.
- Gummed – Activate with water.
- Heat activated – Activate with heat.
- Pressure sensitive – Protective backing removed then applied with pressure.

15.4 COMMON APPLICATIONS
Common applications of varieties of labels:
- Back label – Used on back of containers.
- Band label – Partially wrapped around the container (does not cover the entire container).

- Can label – Used on cylindrically shaped tinplate container.
- Die-cut label – Label having special design.
- Embossed label – Label having portion raised giving a three dimensional effect.
- End label – Fixed at the end of carton or used for wrapper pack.
- Neck label – Used for neck of bottle.
- Over all wrap – Used for covering entire pack.
- Spot label – Used to cover a smaller portion of pack
- Tag: Generally fixed to the container with the help of string or wire
- Wrap around label – Generally covers sides and ends of the pack except top/bottom.

15.5 LABEL SUBSTRATE MATERIALS

The two major label substrate materials are plastic films and paper. They are rivals in many areas of label production and application although since 1993 films have tended to make more headway into the primarily paper dominated label areas. However, the paper label using the wet-glue application system remains firmly entrenched in many industries as one of the quickest systems and certainly the cheapest, so there seem to be plenty of good reasons for keeping that particular type of labelling system in operation. Having said that, the increase in shrink/stretch labelling techniques is brought about only by the peculiar properties of plastic film. Each material has its place, advantages and disadvantages.

Filmic Materials

Past few years have seen the use of filmic material in labels. Various plastic films and its combinations are used. PVC, BOPP, OPP, PP, PE and many other films are used. It is reported that a company in UK has introduced a novel way of reducing the costs of high-quality filmic (PP) labels by as much as 60% (as is reported), thereby reducing the cost to near that of paper labels as there is no need for pre-laminated labelstock. A narrow web label press is modified with two unwinds. Filmic facestock is printed on the underside, the second unwind being from ultraviolet silicone-printed filmic label liner, which is adhesive coated. After bonding and die cutting, matrix waste remains bonded to the liner.

BOPP

Biaxially Oriented Polypropylene (BOPP) is being a popular replacement of label face material to PVC. This versatile film has been used by two roll fed label stock manufacturers as the backing (carrier) layer for pressure-sensitive labels. This was used to eliminate the problem of paper dust (or lint). Secondly, it is reported that coatings are used on BOPP of 30 μm thickness to replace the traditional glassine backing paper, giving the advantage of using half the weight of material. The surface smoothness allows the adhesive on the label to smoothen out, thereby giving it a better chance of wetting the adhered surface. It is forecasted that 30 μm BOPP will become one of the most important filmic materials for pressure-sensitive labelling. BOPP is also the major material used for promotional labelling Roll-on Shrink-on (ROSO) technique. This is being introduced into Europe, having been successfully used in the USA.

OPP

Oriented Polypropylene (OPP) is reported as replacing paper and aluminium foil in some instances in food packaging particularly in identified butter and ice-cream wrappers and used in a metallised form for coffee pouches.

PP and PE

It is reported that the PE films in the range have improved their physical and mechanical properties, whilst the PP films are said to be of lower density, more moisture and chemical resistant and with greater tensile strength than the PE alternatives.

PVC

PVC labels are used as shrink labels and shrink sleeves on the neck of the bottles for tamper evidence. These labels are put on many of the packaged drinking water, drinks, etc.

PO

A recent introduction into the already very competitive pressure-sensitive film labelling market is a PO film that is carried on either a 67 µm or 80 µm glassine paper carrier with a range of both aqueous dispersion or solvent-based adhesives. It is thought that the combination of PO labels on to plastic containers should help alleviate the recycling problems of mixed plastics. Filmic materials used for labelling are said to be expanding their market at three times the rate of the paper label expansion.

15.6 BARCODES

Barcodes have become an important part of the pharma labelling industry, so much so that it is becoming very difficult today to find retail or warehouse labels that do not have barcodes printed upon them. The whole idea behind barcode symbols relies upon them being capable of being read accurately at the correct point in the industrial/retail system. Barcodes make easy purchasing in super markets, inventory control and keeping records. They are printed using inkjet printers using UV ink.

15.7 PRINTING PROCESSES

Printing is the soul of a label. Quality initiatives in the label printing industry are the improvements that have been noted in both the pre-press stages and actually on the printing machines themselves. Different techniques are used based on the priority, requirement, type of substrate and cost. Thermal transfer printing, inkjet printing, flexographic printing for the filmic materials, gravure printing, letterpress, screen, pad or tampon, waterless offset and digital printing are used for label printing. Novel decorating techniques are explained here.

Hot Foil Lamination

A UK based company has announced a novel method of using this printing technique. This system uses screen printing with a heat-activated ink, with heated rollers when the foil and labelstock meet. It is claimed that the powerful adhesive acts exactly like conventional screen ink. This helps in making the pack more attractive.

Metallising

There does not seem to be much progress in this field except, perhaps, in the area of vacuum deposition of metals to the surface of label stock, where better control of the vacuum and rate of coating has produced cost savings in the process. Metallised labels are used in high grade or high rate food products.

Holography

The type of holography that is used in labels and labelling may be divided into two distinct sectors by function. There is a hologram used for security purposes and the hologram that is used purely as a marketing tool.

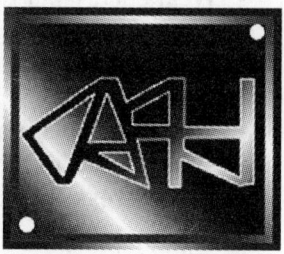

Sleeves

Shrink sleeves have overtaken other means of providing tamper-evident

Fig. 15.1: Hologram

food packages. Sleeving decoration is seen as maintaining perceived value differentials and enhancing pure design innovation on clear glass or PET containers. Nowadays thermochromic inks can be used for temperature colour changes and easy removal for promotional offers. These are tamper evident and require no adhesive. These are used for health drinks like malted milk food, juice bottles, carbonated beverage bottles, sauces, and many other products.

15.8 SECURITY DEVICES

There are several basic ways in which labels are used as security devices:

- To prevent tampering, e.g. tamper evident.
- To prevent pilferage and theft from retail, e.g. radio-frequency detectors for in-store security.

- To be used as anti-counterfeiting devices, either designed to deter or designed to identify (e.g. overt security hologram-identified labels to reassure the customer that the article is genuine, or one of the several covert devices designed to give the manufacturer positive proof that the article is of their manufacturing).

On-press label verification, online label verification, tamper evidence, anti counterfeiting, etc. help for security of the product.

For tamper evidence of pharma products various techniques are used:

- The use of 'fragile' materials that breach obviously when tampered with.
- Weakened label materials (e.g. perforations).
- Laminated materials with differential tear zones.
- Differential adhesives which may show 'VOID' if tampered with.
- 'Reactive' labels that change colour if tampered with.
- Labels with 'stripes' incorporated in their structure.
- Air ingress into sealed packs which creates a colour change.
- Overwrap the entire pack with a label or shrink or stretch film.

Anticounterfeiting worldwide is increasing. There are many ways of looking at anticounterfeiting techniques.

- Overt or showing a complicated, difficult to reproduce device or design that can be clearly seen and is aimed at deflecting the counterfeiter away from the product.
- Covert or including secret marks or information known only to the manufacturer, usually used for identification in the storage, distribution and retail systems.
- Security inks are also used. A new ink has been developed for the inkjet printers. This has been used in a multiple coding system designed to prevent empty used wine or spirit bottles being refilled and resold. Some of the codes are printed invisibly across joints, thereby making it more difficult to match them up.
- Holograms are used as one of the anti-counterfeiting techniques.

15.9 PROMOTIONAL OPPORTUNITIES

Use of promotional devices in packaging is on the increase. The advent of the shrink sleeve gave the marketers one type of surface upon which to practice their methods and others are the two sided printed and replaceable labels.

Label Leaflets

The basic concept of combining the basic labelling information with additional consumer information is expanding, e.g. on the pack of honey a leaflet is provided Security Device on the cap which says about different usage and positive side of the honey. Second example is of pickles pack which used to provide a tag on the neck of the bottle that mentioned the type of the pickle in that pack and one recipe which could be made with that pickle.

Decoration

A novel patented decoration technique, using gravure printing, has been developed in Europe. This is claimed to be an alternative to conventional aluminium coated labels. The process consists of printing with gravure offset, using a specialized ink containing very finely divided aluminium particles, which may also be coloured to give gold or metallised colour effects. The advantage over conventional techniques is that significantly less pollution is generated by the process, i.e. less inks and heavy metals and no solvents used. The technique is called AluPart and has been used as decoration on a beer brand.

Fragrance Labels

These are made by special kind of process. An introduction into this area is the micro-encapsulation process. The label gives the fragrance, when stretched.

15.10 FUTURE DEVELOPMENTS

Developments are likely to take place in variety of aspects.

Laminated labels: Labels are developed with different types of laminates, which increases the shelf-life of label, attraction and other aspects.

Security labelling: In the short term, the closer integration of the embossed hologram with the label manufacturer/ converter is becoming a reality. The newly-created photo-polymer holograms are starting to make an entry into the industry and are predicted to expand in the longer term. Usage of this kind of technique will help in tamper evidence.

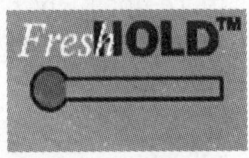

Fig. 15.2: Temperature labelling

Time/temperature labelling: This type of labels will be used more and more for common food products in India.

Sleeves: Sleeves are always likely to be required where there is a need for both a large surface area of decoration and the need for tamper evidence, particularly on regular-shaped containers. There are likely to be developments of a hybrid sleeve that contains some adhesive, which could be activated by some external means.

Barcodes: It appears that the barcode is here to stay. It has developed into data compression with 2D codes and it would not be surprising if this is continued and extended to 3D codes as well. There is talk of a 'watermark' invisible barcode system

Fig. 15.3: Barcode

that will help to solve the use of area on small labels more efficiently, since they would be underneath the printed decoration, be scannable but not affect the copy design. This might also be utilized as a covert security system.

15.11 LEGAL REQUIREMENTS OF LABELS

A. Prescription Label Requirements

Legal Requirements of the Prescription Label

(As dispensed to the patient upon a valid prescription order).

1. The name and address of the pharmacy.
2. The serial number of the prescription.
3. The date of the prescription (date of filling or refilling).
4. The name of the prescriber.
5. The name of the patient.

6. The directions for use, including precautions if indicated.
7. The name of the drug and strength, if any.
8. Caution: Federal Law Prohibits the Transfer of this drug to any other person than for whom it was prescribed. (Controlled Substance Rx's ONLY).

Not Required on the Rx Label but Common

1. The address of the patient.
2. The initials or name of the pharmacist.
3. The telephone number of the pharmacy.
4. The manufacturer's lot number.
5. The expiration date of the drug, if any.
6. The name of the manufacturer or distributor.
7. The quantity of the medication dispensed.
8. The number of refills left.

B. Labelling of Nonprescription Drugs

Drugs that may be safely used by the average person without medical supervision may be sold without a prescription and are called over the counter drugs. These drugs are usually referred to as OTC's. OTC's must bear a label containing specific information. While OTC labelling requirements are usually associated with the manufacturer, a pharmacist is subject to the same requirements if they remove the drug from its original package and convey it to an ultimate user. The labelling required on an OTC product includes:

1. The name of the product.
2. The name and address of the manufacturer, packer or distributor.
3. The net contents of the package.
4. The established name of all active ingredients and the quantity of other ingredients whether active or not.
5. The name of any habit-forming drug contained in the preparation.
6. Cautions and warnings that are needed for the protection of the user.
7. Adequate directions for safe and effective use.

C. Labelling of Commercial Containers of Legend Drugs

FDA Regulations require that the label of legend drugs (prescription drugs), as conveyed to the pharmacist, contain the following information:

1. The name and address of the manufacturer, packer or distributor.
2. Ingredient information.
3. A statement of identity-the generic and proprietary names.
4. The quantity in terms of weight or measure applicable to the drug.
5. The net quantity of the package contents (e.g. 100 tablets).
6. A statement of dosage or a reference to the package insert for dosage information.
7. The expiration date of the drug.
8. The lot number
9. The statement "Caution: Federal Law Prohibits Dispensing Without A Prescription".
10. The National Drug Code (NDC number) is requested by FDA and is usually included.

D. Prescription Labelling

Definition

The term "label" means a display of written, printed or graphic matter upon the immediate container of any article, any word, statement, or other information appearing on the label shall not be considered to be complied with unless the word, statement, or other information also appears on the outside container, or wrapper, if any there be, of the retail package of the article, or is easily legible through the outside container or wrapper.

The term "labelling" means all labels and other written, printed or graphic matter:

a. Upon an article or any of its containers or wrappers; or
b. Accompanying the article.

Label for Prescriptions – Exception

Every prescription dispensed by a pharmacist in this Commonwealth after July 1, 1972, shall bear upon the label the name of the medication in the container unless the practitioner indicates in the manner of his choice on the prescription "Do Not Label." (If the prescriber indicates "Do Not Label" on the Rx, you may not legally place the name of the drug on the label).

Labelling of Rx when Product Selection (Substitution) is Utilized-Board of Rx Ruling

The Kentucky Board of Pharmacy has addressed generic labelling and has come up with the alternatives when product selection is utilized. Alternatives the Board recognizes in lieu of using just the name of the drug dispensed on the label of the prescription container when product selection (substitution) is made are as follows:

1. Methyldopa "generic substitution made for" Aldomet.
2. Methyldopa "dispensed in place of" Aldomet.
3. Methyldopa "substituted for" Aldomet.
4. Methyldopa "generic for" Aldomet.
5. Methyldopa "dispensed for" Aldomet.
6. Methyldopa "generic as" Aldomet.

The label must refrain from wording such as "same as" or any inference that the substitution is the same as the trade name drug. Using only the trade name and the generic name on the label is not acceptable when denoting drug product selection. These alternatives were adopted by the Board to meet the requirement when the physician requests that both names appear on the label. This also should help those pharmacists supplying nursing homes and are required to have the name of the medication as it appears on the physician's order in the chart.

15.12 XML BASED SPL – FDA DRUG LABELLING STANDARD FOR PHARMAS MAKES FOR SAFER MEDICATION

The FDA's Structured Product Labelling (SPL) initiative promises greater safety and will help pharmaceutical companies better disseminate critical drug information. The FDA itself will be able to review label changes more quickly than it can now. Drug companies will be able to exchange label information more efficiently and health information providers will have access to the data in a computer-usable format. "All these (capabilities) are geared to benefiting the users of the labelling – including the prescriber, dispenser and patient – by promoting patient safety and by making the medication information more accessible," Levin adds.

Single Data Repository

The SPL format is now an approved ANSI standard. The effort was started in mid 2002 when the FDA approached Health Level Seven (HL7), a pharmaceutical organization, with the idea to develop a standard for drug product labelling based on another HL7 document standard – the Clinical Document Architecture (CDA). The FDA needed the standard to facilitate review of labelling and support the DailyMed initiative, which involves provision of up-to-date drug product labelling through a National Library of Medicine (NLM) database. Under this initiative, all the pharmaceutical label information will be stored at the NLM, providing a single, easily accessible repository of the data. Healthcare providers could then retrieve this data and make it available to patients. Despite the reprieve, pharmaceutical firms still face the challenge of converting existing labelling to SPL format. Most of the firms involved have their existing labelling in Microsoft Word, which is turned into PDF for submission. To comply with DailyMed they will need to convert Microsoft Word files to XML and then add the necessary meta-data associated with the format.

Master Labelling Document

While all this might take time to implement, there are benefits to be gained from the change over. Because SPL is based on XML, it means the content is separate from the formatting. Consequently manufacturers can create one format-independent XML master document, which includes all the labelling information for a given product. From that master document, all of the other labelling documents for that product can be generated and formatted automatically. In other words, the data is created once, but used many times throughout the organization.

Kris Spahr, of the SPL Working Group, believes there is a whole list of benefits to be gained from using XML to create labelling documents. "XML helps with eliminating redundant data collection used for other submissions," he says. "It also increases efficiency in internal label management, allowing the potential for more reusable product content across the enterprise. Plus it defines a consistent, predictable means of exchanging labelling content." As well as this, the FDA says SPL enables users to easily search all of its documents for keywords, something that could not readily be done with PDF files.

European Initiative

The European equivalent of the FDA – European Agency for the Evaluation of Medicinal Products (EMEA) – also got in on the act when it introduced its Product Information Management (PIM) standard, which is aimed at creating consistent labelling across the region. Like the SPL standard, PIM also relies on XML. Multinational companies, however, expect to incorporate both standards into their business processes. The FDA is becoming increasingly interested in introducing structured authoring into FDA submissions.

15.13 GMPs AND PHARMACEUTICAL LABELLING

Mislabeled drug products can pose a threat to public health and, according to FDA rulings, lead to costly product recalls with significant product liability. To help prevent mislabelling (and thereby protect consumers) manufacturers of pharmaceutical packaging components conform to good manufacturing processes (GMPs) designed to maintain product identity and ensure product quality. Requirements for label inspection and identity control have become increasingly stringent. Those same requirements have been passed on to packaging component suppliers. To maintain product identity when printing packaging components, manufacturers increasingly rely on electronic verification of the printed product.

Electronic Verification

Several methods of electronic verification are available to assure that the packaging component produced is exactly what the customer ordered. Most printed packaging components come in either sheets or rolls. Each method presents unique challenges for maintaining product integrity.

Sheet Items

For sheet items at the printer, packaging components - such as folding cartons, patient information literature, and cut labels are laid out so that the maximum sheet size is used. The goal is to get the most individual images of the same item on the press sheet. Putting multiple items on the same press sheet is strongly discouraged because it increases the risk of a product mix-up.

Bar Codes and IC Marks

Electronic detection devices can scan a number of different bar codes or identity control (IC) marks on individual sheets or pieces. Many components incorporate bar codes into the artwork, but codes and IC marks can be added in the waste area of the sheet when necessary. This unique form of identification is particularly helpful when common sheet sizes are used for similar items. After printing, the sheets are cut into individual pieces. Item-specific bar codes are then scanned on these pieces at the final folding or gluing operation for further identification and control. In addition, IC marks can be used for visual confirmation of the product identity. It is recommended that a unique item- or revision-specific bar code be used, rather than a universal product code (UPC) because the same UPC may be used on different revisions of the same packaging. That can cause the electronic scanner to fail to detect a mix-up of a different revision of the same item. To further assure compliance, bar codes and part numbers should be used (and recorded) for each product batch. Bar coding on both front and back sides allows a manufacturer to verify that a product is correct and that copy exists on both sides if necessary to comply with the product specifications. Bar code verification traditionally includes examining print contrasts, magnifications, bar heights, light margins and bar width. It can also give an assessment of overall print quality.

Roll products, such as labels and patient information literature, present different inspection and identity detection challenges. Like sheet producers, roll product producers maximize the capabilities of their equipment by putting as many images as possible on a press repeat. With the amount of information required on the label, sometimes there just isn't enough space for bar codes. This makes full electronic inspection using bar codes impossible. Although bar codes can be added to the outer edge of roll stock, that can get quite expensive, especially if producers have to special order a roll width just to accommodate the bar code. In addition, every label might not need scanning – just every repeated label.

Electronic inspection and detection of all the copy on a label is often accomplished with vision inspection equipment. Such equipment uses a camera that photographs the "truth copy" and compares it to the product's set specifications and guidelines. Although only a handful of companies use "100% vision inspection," it provides many advantages for compliance with various GMP interpretations. For example, copy-specific controls can be set to allow precise verification of key label components. In addition, suppliers and their customers can determine critical pieces, then check only those items, while still remaining in compliance.

High-level vision inspection equipment is a combination of inspection hardware and software that uses patented algorithms to view the labels in question. One hundred percent vision inspection systems allow standard print variations, yet can still identify critical defects. In contrast to other systems that view only a portion of each label, 100% vision inspection verifies everything on each label. In addition, a line-scan camera and pipeline vision are used to process the labels, even when labels are on a moving web at full production speeds. The process can also be used to identify marks and imperfections on the printing stock surface. Stricter enforcement by FDA has encouraged the adoption of vision inspection technology, and the increased emphasis drug companies place on quality and efficiency may increase its use by manufacturers of printed packaging components. Leaders in quality control use vision inspection equipment despite its higher cost. Several GMPs cover distribution and storage of pharmaceutical labels, and manufacturers have taken steps to promote the traceability of their products. Work-in-progress tags should indicate job, part, purchase order (PO), and lot numbers. Records with this level of detail allow traceability from packaged product back to the raw materials. FDA's pharmaceutical labelling requirements were enacted to reduce public health and safety risks stemming from drug labelling mix-ups. In response, printers and manufacturers of these products have enacted policies and purchased the equipment necessary to comply with the requirements—and defect-free labels are the intended end result.

15.14 PRINTING

Printing is a process for reproducing text and image, typically with ink on paper using a printing press. It is often carried out

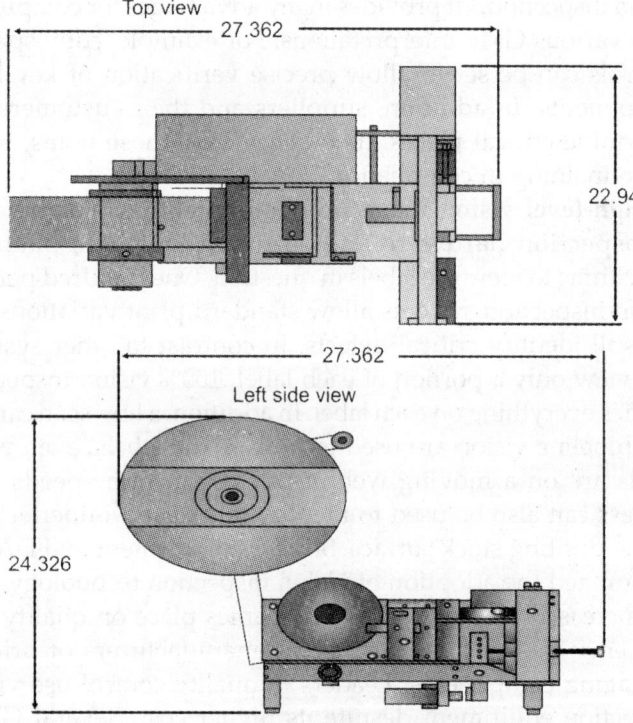

Fig. 15.4: Label printing machine

as a large-scale industrial process and is an essential part of publishing and transaction printing.

Modern Printing Technology

Across the world, over 45 trillion pages are printed annually. In 2006 there were approximately 30,700 printing companies in the United States, accounting for $112 billion, according to the 2006 US Industry and Market Outlook by Barnes Reports. Print jobs that move through the Internet made up 12.5% of the total US printing market last year, according to research firm InfoTrend/CAP Ventures.

Books and newspapers are printed today using the technique of offset lithography. Other common techniques include:

Flexography

Flexography (also called surface printing), often abbreviated to flexo, is a method of printing most commonly used for packaging (labels, tape, bags, boxes, banners, etc).

A flexo print is achieved by creating a mirrored master of the required image as a 3D relief in a rubber or polymer material. A measured amount of ink is deposited upon the surface of the printing plate (or printing cylinder) using an anilox roll. The print surface then rotates, contacting the print material which transfers the ink.

Originally flexo printing was basic in quality. Labels requiring high quality have generally been printed offset until recently. In the last few years great advances have been made to the quality of flexo printing presses.

The greatest advances though have been in the area of Photopolymer Printing Plates, including improvements to the plate material and the method of plate creation — usually photographic exposures followed by chemical etch, though also by direct laser engraving.

Digital Direct to Plate systems have dominated the industry recently with their incredible quality and ability to print four colour process as well as offset. Companies like Dupont in DE and PlateCrafters in Colmar, PA have pioneered the latest technologies with advances in FAST washout and the latest screening technology, even companies who make plates in house are going to trade shops to get these high quality plates.

Laser-etched anilox rolls also play a part in the improvement of print quality. Full colour picture printing now occurs, and some of the finer presses available today in combination with a skilled operator allow quality that rivals the lithographic process. One ongoing improvement has been the increasing ability to reproduce highlight tonal values, thereby providing a workaround for the very high dot gain associated with flexo print.

Flexo has an advantage over lithography in that it can use a wider range of inks and is good at printing on a variety of different materials. Flexo inks, like those used in gravure and unlike those used in lithography generally have low viscosity. This enables faster drying and, as a result, faster production; that means low cost. Printing press speeds of 450 meters per minute are regular with modern technology high end printers, like Windmoeller und Hollscher or Schiavi type. The main printing process worldwide for flexible packaging is rotogravure, for very large runs, and flexo for large and medium runs.

Typical products printed using flexography include brown corrugated boxes, flexible packaging including retail and shopping bags, food and hygiene bags and sacks, flexible plastics, self adhesive labels, and wallpaper. A number of newspapers now eschew the more common offset lithography process in favour of flexo.

Relief Print

A relief print is an image created by a printmaking process, such as woodcut, where the areas of the matrix (plate or block) that are to show printed black (typically) are on the original surface; the parts of the matrix that are to be blank (white) having been cut away, or otherwise removed. Printing the image is therefore a relatively simple matter of inking the face of the matrix and bringing it in firm contact with the paper; a printing-press may not be needed as the back of the paper can be rubbed or pressed by hand with a simple tool.

Screen Printing

Screen printing, silkscreening, or serigraphy is a printmaking technique that creates a sharp-edged image using a stencil. A screenprint or serigraph is an image created using this technique.

Rotogravure

Rotogravure is mainly used for magazines and packaging. It is a type of intaglio printing process, in that it involves engraving the image onto an image carrier. In gravure printing, the image is engraved onto a copper cylinder because, like offset and flexography, it uses a rotary printing press. The vast majority of gravure presses print on reels of paper, rather than sheets of paper (Sheetfed gravure is a small, specialty market.) Rotary gravure presses are the fastest and widest presses in operation, printing everything from narrow labels to 12-feet-wide rolls of vinyl flooring. Additional operations may be in-line with a gravure press, such as saddle stitching facilities for magazine/brochure work.

Inkjet

Inkjet is used typically to print a small number of books or packaging, and also to print a variety of materials from high quality papers simulate offset printing, to floor tiles. Inkjet is also used to apply mailing addresses to direct mail pieces. Inkjet printers are a type of computer printer that operates by propelling tiny droplets of liquid ink onto paper. They are the most common type of computer printer for the general consumer due to their low cost, high quality of output, capability of printing in vivid colour, and ease of use.

Dye Transfer

The dye transfer process is a continuous-tone colour photographic printing process, popularized by the Eastman Kodak Company in the 1940s. It is sometimes referred to by such generic names as wash-off relief printing and dye imbibition transfer printing. The process involves making three matrices for each colour, which absorb dye in proportion to the density of the relief. A colour print is formed, by transferring the dyed film matrices in physical contact onto a mordanted dye receiver paper. Eastman Kodak Company stopped making materials for this process in the mid 1990s. The dyes used in the process are very spectrally pure compared to normal coupler induced photographic dyes, with the exception of the Kodak cyan. Also the dyes have excellent light and dark fastness. The dye transfer process posses the largest color gamut and tonal scale than any other process, including inkjet. Another important characteristic of dye transfer is it allows the practitioner the highest degree of photographic control compared to any other photochemical colour print process.

Laser Printing

Laser printing is mainly used in offices and for transactional printing (bills, bank documents). Laser printing is commonly used by direct mail companies to create variable data letters or coupons, for example. A laser printer is a common type of computer printer that rapidly produces high quality text and graphics on plain paper. Like photocopiers, laser printers employ a xerographic printing process but differ from analog photocopiers in that the image is produced by the direct scanning of a laser beam across the printer's photoreceptor.

Pad Printing

Pad Printing for applying a flat image on a curved substrate. Pad Printing is sometimes also called "Tampo" or "Tampo Printing". Pad printing is used for decorating products in many industries including medical, automotive, promotional, apparel, electronics, appliances, sports equipment and toys. It can also be used to deposit functional materials such as conductive inks, adhesives, dyes and lubricants.

16 Package Testing and Testing of Containers and Closures

16.1 INTRODUCTION

Package testing or packaging testing involves the measurement of a characteristic involved with packaging. This includes packaging materials, packaging components, primary packages, shipping containers, and unit loads, as well as the associated processes.

Testing measures the effects and interactions of the levels of packaging, the package contents, external forces and end-use.

Testing can be a qualitative or quantitative procedure. Package testing is often a physical test. With some types of packaging such as food and pharmaceuticals, chemical tests are conducted to determine suitability of food contact materials. Testing programs range from simple tests with little replication to more thorough experimental designs.

Purposes

Packaging testing might have a variety of purposes, such as:
- Determine if, or verify that, the requirements of a specification, regulation, or contract are met.
- Decide if a new product development program is on track: Demonstrate proof of concept.
- Provide standard data for other scientific, engineering, and quality assurance functions.
- Validate suitability for end-use.
- Provide a basis for technical communication.
- Provide a technical means of comparison of several options.
- Provide evidence in legal proceedings: product liability, patents, product claims, etc.
- Help solve problems with current packaging.

- Help identify potential cost savings in packaging.
- Predict, in a laboratory, the performance of a package during distribution and the acceptance by customers.

Importance of Testing

For some types of products, package testing is mandated by regulations: food, pharmaceuticals, medical devices, dangerous goods, etc. This may cover both the design qualification, periodic retesting and control of the packaging processes. Processes may be controlled by a variety of quality management systems such as HACCP, statistical process control, validation protocols, ISO 9000, etc.

For unregulated products, the degree of package testing can be a business decision. Risk management may involve factors such as:

- Costs of packaging
- Costs of package testing
- Value of contents being shipped
- Value of customer's good will
- Product liability exposure
- Other potential costs of inadequate packaging

With distribution packaging, one vital packaging development consideration is to determine that a product will not be damaged throughout the entire process of getting to the customer from the manufacturer. A primary purpose of a package is to ensure the safety of a product during transportation and storage. If a product is damaged during this process, then the package has failed to accomplish its primary objective and the customer will either return the product or be unlikely to purchase the product altogether. Package testing is often a formal part of Project management programs. Packages are usually tested when there is a new packaging design, a revision to a current design, a change in packaging material, and various other reasons. Testing a new packaging design before full scale manufacturing can save time and money.

Laboratory Affiliation

Many suppliers or vendors offer limited material and package testing as a free service to customers. It is common for packagers to partner with reputable suppliers: Many suppliers have certified quality management systems such as ISO 9000 or allow customers to conduct technical and quality audits. Data from testing is commonly shared. There is sometimes a risk that supplier testing may tend to be self-serving and not completely impartial. Large companies often have their own packaging staff and a package testing and development laboratory. Corporate engineers know their products, manufacturing capabilities, logistics system, and their customers best. Cost reduction of existing products and cost avoidance for new products have been documented. Another option is to use paid consultants, Independent contractors, and third-party test laboratories. They are commonly chosen for specialized expertise, for access to certain test equipment, for surge projects, or where independent testing is otherwise required. Many have certifications and accreditations: ISO 9000, ISO/IEC 17025, and various governing agencies.

Procedures

Several standards organizations publish test methods for package testing. Included are:
- International Organization for Standardization, ISO
- ASTM International
- European Committee for Standardization
- TAPPI
- International Safe Transit Association, etc.

Governments and regulators publish some packaging test methods. There are also many corporate test standards in use. A review of technical literature and patents also provides good options to consider for test procedures. If a test is conducted with a deviation from a published test method, the test report must fully disclose that deviation.

Materials Testing

The basis of packaging design and performance is the component materials. The physical properties, and sometimes chemical properties, of the materials need to be communicated to packaging engineers to aid in the design process. Suppliers publish data sheets and other technical communications that include the typical or average relevant physical properties and the test method these are based upon. Sometimes these are adequate. Other times, additional material and component testing is required by the packager or supplier to better define certain characteristics. When a final package design is complete, the specifications for the component materials needs to be communicated to suppliers. Packaging materials testing is often needed to identify the critical material characteristics and engineering tolerances. These are used to prepare and enforce specifications. For example, shrink film data might include: tensile strength (MD and CD), elongation, Elastic modulus, surface energy, thickness, Moisture vapor transmission rate, Oxygen transmission rate, heat seal strength, heat sealing conditions, heat shrinking conditions, etc. Average and process capability are often provided. The chemical properties related for use as Food contact materials may be necessary.

Conditioning, Testing Atmosphere

The environmental conditions of testing are critical. The measured performance of many packages is affected by the conditioning and testing atmospheres. For example, paper based products are strongly affected by their moisture content: Relative humidity needs to be controlled. Plastic products are often strongly affected by temperature. Conditions of 23°C (73.4°F) and 50% relative humidity are common but other standard testing conditions are also published in material and package test standards. Engineering tolerances for the conditions are also specified. Often the package is conditioned to the specified environment and tested under those conditions. This can be in a conditioned room or in a chamber enclosing the test. With some testing, the package is conditioned to a specified environment, then is removed to ambient conditions and quickly tested. The test report needs to state the actual conditions used.

Thermal Testing

Many packages are used for products that are sensitive to temperature. The ability of insulated shipping containers to protect their contents from exposure to temperature fluctuations can be measured in a laboratory. Ovens, freezers, and environmental chambers are commonly used for this and other types of packaging. Exposure to high temperatures is also for shelf life testing of products: temperature (and other factors such as relative humidity) can accelerate the degradation of many products. The ability of packaging to control product degradation is frequently a subject of laboratory and field evaluations. Temperature is also one of the factors that can accelerate the natural aging of packaging. Accelerated aging of packaging can be based on time and the exposure to temperature, relative humidity, light, the contents of the package, and several other environmental factors. An Arrhenius equation is often used to correlate chemical reactions at different temperatures, based on the proper choice of Q10 (temperature coefficient). Digital data loggers are used to measure temperatures experienced in different distribution systems. This data is sometimes used to develop unique test methods for that distribution system.

Vacuum Testing

Vacuum chambers are used to test the ability of a package to withstand low pressures which might be encountered during distribution. They are also used to stress the package to test the strength of seals and the tendency for leakage.

Barrier Properties

Moisture vapor transmission rate, oxygen transmission rate, and carbon dioxide transmission rate.

The ability of a package to control the permeation and penetration of gasses is vital for many types of products. Tests are often conducted on the packaging materials but also on the completed packages, sometimes after being subjected to flexing, handling, vibration, or temperature.

Shock and Impact

Instrumented drop test of cushioned package to measure the transmitted shock.

Both primary (consumer) packages and shipping containers have a risk of being dropped or being impacted by other items. Package integrity and product protection are important packaging functions. Tests are conducted to measure the effectiveness of package cushioning to isolate fragile products from shock.

Vibration

Vibration tester to simulate vibration frequencies at which packaged products are subjected during shipments. Vibration is encountered during shipping (vehicle vibration, rough roads, etc) and movement on conveyors. The ability of a package to withstand these vibrations and to protect the contents can be measured by several laboratory test procedures. Some allow searching for the particular frequencies of vibration that have potential for damage. Others use specified bands of random vibration to better represent vibrations measured in field studies of distribution environments.

Compression

Compression testing relates to stacking or crushing of packages, particularly shipping containers. It usually measures of the force required to crush a package, stack of packages, or a unit load. Packages can be empty or filled as for shipment. A force-deflection curve used to obtain the peak load or other desired points. Other tests use a constant load and measure the time to failure or to a critical deflection.

Large Loads

Large pallet loads, bulk boxes, wooden boxes, and crates can be evaluated by many of the other test procedures previously listed. In addition, some special test methods are available for these larger loads.

Dangerous Goods

Hazardous materials, dangerous goods are highly regulated. There are some material and construction requirements but also Performance testing is required. The testing is based on the packing group (hazard level) of the contents, the quantity of material, and the type of container.

Medical Packaging

Medical packaging is highly regulated. Often medical devices and products are sterilized in the package. The sterility must be maintained throughout distribution to allow immediate use by physicians. A series of special packaging tests is used to measure the ability of the package to maintain sterility.

Test Protocols for Shipping Containers

Shipping containers are often subjected to sequential tests involving a combination of individual test methods. A variety of standard test schedules or protocols are available for evaluating transport packaging. They are used to help determine the ability of complete and filled shipping containers to various types of logistics systems. Some test the general ruggedness of the shipping container while others have been shown to reproduce the types of damage encountered in distribution. Some base the type and severity of testing on formal studies of the distribution environment: instrumentation, data loggers, and observation. Test cycles with these documented elements better simulate parts of certain logistics shipping environments.

16.2 TESTING OF CONTAINERS AND CLOSURES

A. Glass Containers for Injectable Preparation

Containers intended for injectable preparation may be ampoules, vials or bottles hydrolytic resistance test is used.

Hydrolytic resistance test (IP): Three types of containers (Type I, Type II and Type III) are suitable for use. The types are distinguished by resistance to water attack of new containers the degree of attack being determined by the amount of alkali released from the glass under the conditions specified.

Test: For test no. containers to be examined and volume of test solution to be used in Table 16.1.

Table 16.1

Nominal capacity of container (ml)	No. of containers to be used	Volume of test solution to be use for titration (ml)
05 or less	At least 10	50.0
06-30	At least 5	50.0
>30	At least 3	100

Rinse each container with water at least twice at room temperature

↓

Just before the test, rinse each container with freshly prepared distilled water

↓

Empty, determined average overflow volume

↓

Fill container to 90% of their calculated overflow volume

↓

Cover with borosilicate glass previously rinsed with freshly prepared distilled water

↓

Place the container in an autoclave

↓

Close autoclave

↓

Displace the air by passage of stream for 10 minute

↓

Rise the temperature from 100 to 121°C over 20 minute

↓

Maintain temperature at 121°C for 60 minute

↓

Reduce the temperature from 121 to100°C over 40 minute

↓

Remove the container from autoclave

↓

Cool containers in a bath of running tape water

↓

Carry out following titration within 1 hour of removing the containers from autoclave

↓

Combine the liquids from containers being examined

↓

Measure the volume of test solution specified in table into a conical flask

↓

Add 0.15 ml of Methyl red solution for each 50 ml of liquid

↓

Titrate with 0.01M HCl

↓

End point is colour obtained by repeating the operation using the same volume of freshly prepared distilled water

↓

The difference between the titrations = Volume of 0.01M HCl required for each 100 ml of test solution

The result should not be greater than stated in Table 16.2.

Table 16.2

Capacity of container (ml)	Volume of 0.01M HCl/100ml test solution Type I or II	Type III glass (ml)
<1	2	20.0
1–2	1.8	17.6
2–5	1.3	13.2
5–10	1.0	10.2
10–20	0.80	8.1
20–50	0.60	6.1
50–100	0.50	4.8
100–200	0.40	3.8
200–500	0.30	2.9
>500	0.20	2.2

Distinguish between Type I and Type II Glass

Rinse the containers with water

↓

Fill completely with 4% v/v solution of HCl

↓

Allow to stand at room temperature for 10 minute

$\downarrow$

Empty the container

$\downarrow$

Rinse 5 times with water

$\downarrow$

Carry out the procedure of hydrolytic resistance

$\downarrow$

Compare the results with Table 16.2.

Type I glass: Values obtained are similar to those for type I or type II.

Type II glass: Values exceed for type I or II and are similar to those given for type III glass.

Arsenic: Carry out the test on ampoules the inner and outer surfaces of which are washed 5 times with freshly distilled water.

Prepare a test solution as that for hydrolytic resistance for adequate no. ampoules to produce 50 ml

$\downarrow$

Pipette out 10 ml of solution from the combined contents of all ampoules into a flask

$\downarrow$

Add 10 ml of HNO_3

$\downarrow$

Evaporate to dryness on a water bath

$\downarrow$

Dry the residue in an oven at 130°C for 30 minute.

$\downarrow$

Cool and add 10 ml of hydrazine-molybdate reagent

$\downarrow$

Swirl to dissolve

$\downarrow$

Heat under reflux on water bath for 30 minute

$\downarrow$

Cool to room temperature

$\downarrow$

Determine absorbance of resultant solution at 840 nm

$\downarrow$

Abs-test solution should not exceed absorbance of 0.1 ml of arsenic standard solution (10 ppm arsenic)

B. Metal Containers for Eye Ointments

Select a sample of 50 tubes from the lot to be tested
↓
Fill the tube with molten eye ointment base
↓
Close the open end of each tube through double folds
↓
Allow filled tubes to cool over night at temperature 15–20°C.
↓
Assembled a metal bacteriological filter with a paper supported on a suitable perforated plate to a temperature above the melting point of base
↓
Remove caps from cooled tubes
↓
Apply uniform pressure to closed end of each tube in a manner that the time taken to express as much as possible through each nozzle is not less than 20 sec
↓
Collect extruded base from each tube
↓
Apply suction to stem of filter. When all melted mass has been remove wash the wall of filter
↓
Expose the filter paper to three successive quantities each of 30 ml of $CHCl_3$
↓
Allow filter paper to dry
↓
Examine the filter paper oblique light with the aid of magnifying glass with graticule of 1mm^2 (1 is subdivided into 0.2 mm^2).

Note

1. No. of metal particle 1 mm in length and longs   50
2. No.in the range 0.5–1 mm   10

3. No. in the range of 0.2–0.5 mm   02
4. No. in the rang of <0.2 mm   Nil

Carry out two further examinations with different positions. Calculate average no. of metal particle in range of specified.

Tubes pass the test if total score is <100, tubes does not pass the test if total score is >150, the total score is 100–150 test is repeated.

Lot passes the test if sum of total scores is <150.

C. Plastic Containers

1. Testing of Thermoplastics

Tensile tests: ISO 527 –1/–2 and ASTM D 638 set out the standardized test methods. These standards are technically equivalent. However, they are not fully comparable because of the difference in testing speeds. The modulus determination requires a high accuracy of ± 1 micrometer for the dilatometer.

Flexural tests: 3-points flexural tests are among the most common and classic methods for semi rigid and rigid plastics.

Pendulum impact tests: Impact tests are used to measure the behaviour of materials at higher deformation speeds. Pendulum impact testers are used to determine the energy required to break a standardized specimen by measuring the height to which the pendulum hammer rises after impacting the test piece.

2. For Non-injectable Preparation

Leakage Test

Fill ten containers with water

↓

Fit closer

↓

Keep inverted at room temperature for 24 hour

↓

There should be no sign of leakage from any container

3. Collapsibility Test for Collapsible Tube

A container, by collapsing inward during use should yield at least 90% of its contents at the required rate of flow.

4. For Oral Liquids

a. Clarity of Aqueous Extract

Select unlabelled, unmarked and non-laminated portion
from suitable containers

↓

Cut these portions into strips none of which should have
total area greater than 20 cm²

↓

Wash the strip by shaking them with at least two portions
distilled water for about 30 second

↓

Drain off the water

↓

Select washed portions of sample with a total surface area of
125 cm²

↓

Transfer to a flask previously cleaned with chromic acid
mixture and rinsed with several portions of distilled water

↓

Add 250 ml of distilled water

↓

Cover the flask with a beaker, autoclave at 121°C
for 30 minutes

↓

Carry out blank determination using 250 ml distilled water

↓

Cool and examine the extract, it should be colourless and
free from turbidity

b. Non-volatile Residue

Evaporate 100 ml of extract obtained in test for clarity
of aqueous extract

↓

Dry to constant weight at 105°C

↓

Residue weight should not be more than 12.5 mg.

5. Plastic Container for Injectable Preparation

Characteristics

1. Container should be transparent.
2. If a filled container should be sterlizable by heat or any other method, without shrinkage, distortion, discolour-lation loss of transparency, cracking, tackiness.
3. Container should be of such design that is desire, any attachment is possible.

D. Test on Container: Leakage Test, Collapsibility Test

1. Transparency Test

Reagents: Standard suspension- 1 gm of hydrazine sulphate + sufficient water to produce 100 ml. set a side for 6 hr.

↓

25 ml of above sol. + 25 ml of 10%w/v hexamine

↓

Mix. allow to stand for 24 hr.

15 ml → dilute to 100 ml → standard suspension

Prepare a 16 fold dilution of standard suspension so as to give an absorbance at about 640 nm of 0.37 to 0.43 Fill five empty containers with diluted suspension

↓

Compare cloudiness with container of same type filled with water

2. Water Vapour Permeability

Fill five containers with nominal volume of water

↓

Heat seal the bottle with an aluminium foil – polyethylene laminate

↓

Weigh accurately each container

↓

Allow to stand for 14 days at RH of 60 ± 5 % and temperature between 20–25°C

↓

Reweigh the containers

The loss in weight in each container should not be more than 0.2%

E. Test on Container Material

1. Barelium

Moisten 2 gm material with HCl

↓

Ignite in Petri dish

↓

Dissolve residue in 10 ml of 1M HCl and filter

↓

Filtrate + 1 ml of 1M H_2SO_4

Carry out same procedure with a mixture of 10 ml of Ba standard sol. (10 ppm Ba) and 10 ml of 1M HCl. Turbidity should not be greater in sample solution

2. Heavy Metals

Take 2.5 gm of material in round bottom flask and add 20 ml H_2SO_4

↓

Char for 10 minute and add H_2O_2 sol. Drop wise to hot solution until it become colourless

↓

Heat between each addition until white fumes are evolved and cool

↓

Transfer to a Petri dish with the add of 10 ml water and evaporate to dryness

↓

Dissolve the residue in 10 ml of 1M HCl filter if necessary

↓

Add water to produce 25 ml–solution A

10 ml of solution A + 2 ml of acetate buffer of pH 3.5 + 1.2 ml of thioacetamide reagent and mix, allow to stand for 20 minute

↓

Yellow colour

a. It should not be more instance than yellow colour obtain by repeating the operation using 10 ml of standard Cd solution (10 ppm Cd) in place of solution A.

b. Any brown colour should not be more instance than colour obtained by repeating the operation using a mixture of 5 ml Pb standard solution (10 ppm Pb) and 5 ml of water in place of solution A.

3. Tin

10 ml of sol. A + 5 ml H_2SO_4 (20%) + 1 ml of 1% w/v sol. of sodium dodecyl sulphate + 1 ml of Zn dithiol reagent

↓

Heat on water bath for 1 minute and cool

↓

Allow to stand for ½ hr.

↓

Red colour

It should not be more instance than colour obtained by repeating operation using 10 ml of tin standard sol (5 ppm Sn) in place of sol A.

4. Zinc

One ml of solution A + water → to produce 100 ml

↓

10 ml of resulting solution A + 5 ml acetate buffer solution (pH 4.4) + 1 ml of 0.1M sodium thiosulphate + 5 ml of 0.001% w/v solution of dithizone in $CHCl_3$

↓

Shake and allow to stand for 2 minute

↓

Violet colour in CHCl3 layer

Colour should not be more instance than colour obtains by repeating the operation. Using a mixture of 2 ml of Zn standard solution (10 ppm Zn) and 8 ml of water in place of test solution. Carry out blank determination using 10 ml of water. Test is not valid until the $CHCl_3$ layer in blank determination is colourless.

F. Test on Extracts

1. Physicochemical Tests

From a homogeneous sample of plastic material, use a portion for each 20 ml of extracting medium equivalent to 120 cm^2 total surface areas (both sides combined)

↓
Subdivide into strips (5 cm long and 0.3 cm wide) and transfer subdivided sample to glass stoppered 250 ml graduated cylinder of Type I glass

↓
Add 150 ml of purified water and agitate for 30 second

↓
Drain of the liquid and repeat the operation

↓
Transfer to an extraction flask a quantity of prepared sample + 200 ml purified water

↓
Extract by heating in a water bath at 70°C for 24 hour

↓
Heat in an autoclave 121°C for 30 minute

↓
Cool (not below 20°C)

Appearance: Extract should be colourless and clear.

Light absorption: Using water as a blank light absorption is not more than 0.03 in the range of 220–240 nm and not more than 0.05 in the range of 240–360 nm.

pH: 20 ml extract + 0.1% w/v solution of $KClO_3$ → pH. Same process is applied for blank.

Difference in pH of two solutions is not greater than 15.

2. Non-volatile Matter

50 ml of extract in crucible and evaporate on water bath

↓
Dry the residue at 105°C for one hour

↓
Repeat the operation with blank

The difference between the residue obtained a from extract and blank should not be more than 15 mg.

3. Heavy Metals

Transfer 20 ml of extract into one of two nessler cylinder

↓
Adjust pH (3–4) with 1M CH_3COOH or 5M NH_3 dilute to water to about 35 ml and mix. Nessler cylinder II –2 ml lead

standard solution (1ppm Pb) + 20 ml blank and adjust
pH 3–4 with 1M CH_3COOH or 5M NH_3
↓
Dilute with water to about 35 ml and mix. To each cylinder
at 10 ml freshly prepared H_2S solution and dilute to 50 ml
with water
↓
Brown colour should not be more instance than obtained by
lead standard solution

4. Buffering Capacity

20 ml extract titrate with 0.01M HCl or 0.01M NaOH
to a pH of 7
↓
End point potentiometrically measured

Repeat the operation with 20 ml blank. If same titrant is used
difference in amount of titrant between extract and blank
should not be greater than 10 ml if different titrant are used,
total volume should not be greater than 10 ml.

5. Oxidisable Substances

20 ml of extract into glass-stoppered flask + 20 ml 0.002M
$KMnO_4$ +1 ml dilute H_2SO_4
↓
Boil for 3 minute, cool, add 0.1 gm of KI
↓
Shake and allow to stand in dark for 10 minute
↓
Titrate with 0.01M sodium thiosulphate using 0.25 ml starch
solution
↓
Repeat the operation with blank
↓
Difference between titration should not be more than 1 ml

G. Biological Tests

A sample is defined as an extract prepared from specimen.
Blank consists of same quantity of same extracting medium
that is used for specimen under test.

Systemic injection test: This test is design to evaluate systematic responses to extract the material under test, following injection into mice.

Test animals: Healthy, not previously used albino mice weighing between 17 and 23.

Apparatus: ......

Autoclave: Use autoclave that can maintain the temperature 121°C ± 2°C.

Oven: Maintain temperature 50–70°C ± 2°C.

Extraction containers: Ampoules of Type I glass or screw cap test-tube.

Preparation of apparatus: Clean all equipment with chromic acid mixture or with hot HNO_3.

Extracting Media

a. **NaCl injection:** A sterile and pyrogen free solution of NaCl in waters for injection it contains 0.9% w/v of NaCl.

b. 5% v/v solution of ethanol in NaCl injection.

c. PEG 400

d. Vegetable oil

Table 16.3

Form of plastic	Thickness	Amount of sample for each 20 ml of extracting medium	Subdivided into
Film or sheet	Less than 0.5 mm	Equivalent of 120 cm² total surface area	Strip of about 5 × 0.3 cm
	0.5 to1mm	Equivalent to 60 cm² total surface area	
Tubing	<0.5 mm	Length 120 cm² sum of ID and OD	Section of about 5 × 0.3 cm
	0.5–1 mm	Length 60 cm² sum of ID and OD	
Slabs, tubing and moulded items	>1 mm	Equivalent of 60 cm² total surface area	Pieces up to about 5 × 0.3 cm

Preparation of Sample

Select and subdivided the sample into portion as shown in
Table 16.3
Sample in 100 ml graduated cylinder of
Type I glass
↓
70 ml WFI agitate for 30 second and drain water
↓
Dry the pieces prepared for extraction with vegetable oil in
oven at <50°C

Preparation of Extracts

Sample in extraction containers + 20 ml extracting medium
Apply the same for blank
Extract by heating in an autoclave at 121°C for 2 hour in an
oven at 70°C for 24 hour or at 50°C for 72 hour
↓
Cool to room temperature and shake
↓
Decant each extract into dry, sterile vessel
↓
Store in temperature between 20–30°C

Procedure

Inject each of the five mice in a test with sample or blank.

Table 16.4

Extract or blank	Number of sites/animal	Dose/site (µl)
Sample	5	200
Blank	5	20

Table 16.5

Extract or blank	Dose/kg	Route	Injection rate(µl/sec)
NaCl injection	50 ml	IV	100
5% v/v solution of	50 ml	IV	100
PEG 400	10 gm	IP	
Vegetable oil	50 ml	IP	

Dilute each gm of extract of sample with PEG 400 and corresponding blank solution with NaCl injection obtained a concentration of 200 mg of PEG/ml.

Observe animal: Immediately after 4 hour, 24, 48 and 72 hr

Compare: If during the observation period none of the animal treated with extract so greater biological activity than blank sample passes the test.

H. Test for Rubber

1. Fragmentation Test

Place a volume of water corresponding to nominal volume minus 4ml in each of 12 clean vials

↓

Close vials with closure and secure caps for 16 hr.

↓

Pierce the closure with 21 SWG hypodermic needle (by angle of 10° to 14°) and inject 1 ml water and remove same quantity of air

↓

Repeat the above operation 4 times for each closure (use new needle for each closure)

↓

Count the number of fragments visible to the naked eye

↓

Total number of fragments should not be more then 10 except butyl rubber where the fragment not exceed 15

2. Self-sealability Test (for multi-dose container)

Fill 10 vials with water to nominal volume and close the vials with closure, secure cap.

↓

Pierce the cap 10 times at different sites with 21 SWG hypodermic needle.

↓

Immerse the vials in 0.1% w/v solution of methylene blue under reduced external pressure (27 K pa) for 10 minutes

↓

Restore the normal pressure and keep the container immersed for 30 minute

↓

Wash the vials. None of the vials should contain trace of coloured solution.

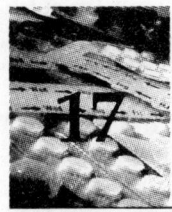

Stability of Packages

17.1 INTRODUCTION

The classic definition of stability is "difficult to move or change". Although stability may be a good thing, stability in package design is not. This is because a stable package, according to the definition, is difficult to change. Why is it bad if we cannot easily change a package? Because a change in any package might impact or break so many other packages that are package dependent on upon it. For example, imagine in your application, if you have the following package dependencies depicted in (Fig. 17.1).

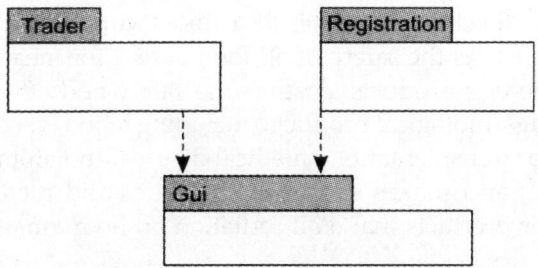

Fig. 17.1: The stable package syndrome

In this case, any change in package "gui" is likely to impact package "trader" and "registration" packages and similarly any other package that depends on "gui" package. This makes the "gui" package hard to change. In this scenario, the "gui" package is called "stable".

17.2 LEGISLATION

The Food and Drugs Act of 1906 was the first of more than 200 laws that constitute one of the world's most comprehensive and effective networks of public health and consumer protections. Here are a few of the congressional milestones:

- The Federal Food, Drug and Cosmetic Act of 1938 were passed after a legally marketed toxic elixir killed 107 people, including many children. The FD and C Act completely overhauled the public health system. Among other provisions, the law authorized the FDA to demand evidence of safety for new drugs, issue standards for food, and conduct factory inspections.

- The Kefauver-Harris Amendments of 1962, which were inspired by the thalidomide tragedy in Europe (and the FDA's vigilance that prevented the drug's marketing in the United States), strengthened the rules for drug safety and required manufacturers to prove their drugs' effectiveness.

- The Medical Device Amendments of 1976 followed a US Senate finding that faulty medical devices had caused 10,000 injuries, including 731 deaths. The law applied safety and effectiveness safeguards to new devices.

Today, the FDA regulates $1 trillion worth of products a year. It ensures the safety of all food except for meat, poultry and some egg products; ensures the safety and effectiveness of all drugs, biological products (including blood, vaccines and tissues for transplantation), medical devices, and animal drugs and feed; and makes sure that cosmetics and medical and consumer products that emit radiation do no harm.

17.3 REGULATION

The Food and Drug Administration (FDA) has issued two guidance documents and a Notice of Proposed Rulemaking (NPRM) on what information the Agency needs to review drug product applications, including information needed about packaging materials used with such products. One of the guidance documents explains the type of information FDA would like to see in drug master files (or in the drug company's application) on container closure systems for various types of drug products. The other guidance document (in draft) and the accompanying rulemaking, details the types of changes to packaging materials that require prior review and approval by the Agency and those that require notification prior to marketing.

Guidance for Container Closure Systems

Although FDA has not modified its guidance document on drug master files (DMFs), it has published a new guidance document for the drug industry which is also pertinent to packaging material suppliers.

Entitled "Container Closure Systems for Packaging Human Drugs and Biologics: Chemistry, Manufacturing and Controls Documentation," this document recommends how to submit information to FDA on materials used in packaging for drugs and biologics. It also provides guidance on qualifications and quality control on packaging components used for injection and ophthalmic drug products, liquid-based oral and topical drug products and topical delivery systems, solid oral dosage forms and powders for reconstitution and other dosage forms.

FDA published a draft of this guidance document in July of 1997, which was criticized by industry for several internal inconsistent statements concerning the applicability of the food additive regulations to drug packaging materials, among other things. In the final document FDA has clarified many of these matters, although in some instances, it is still overly restrictive in the information being requested and the substantive requirements for the packaging materials.

In its draft, FDA made inconsistent remarks about whether substances used to produce drug packaging materials need to be the subject of the food-additive regulations. However, in the final guidance document, FDA indicates that food-additive clearances are usually sufficient to support the safety of packaging materials for solid oral dosage forms and liquid oral dosage forms intended for short-term administration. But the Agency intimates that such clearances may not be acceptable for the evaluation of packaging materials for liquid oral dosage forms for chronic use. FDA's logic on this last point is, of course, entirely misplaced.

Food additives are cleared by FDA on the basis that exposure will occur over a life time involving a significant portion of the diet. Exposure estimates for materials used in packaging food are much greater than that related to medications, even if taken on a daily basis. This fact will be brought to the Agency's attention again; hopefully, FDA will provide clarification. Overall, the Agency now seems to much better recognize the relevance of food-additive clearances for packaging materials intended to be used with drug products. Several other statements in the guidance document still need further clarification by the Agency. For example, the Agency suggests that packaging manufacturers should report any formulation changes both to drug company customers and to the appropriate DMF. However, significant modifications to the DMF only require notification to customers that the DMF has been amended, as opposed to providing an update to the customer on the formulation change itself.

The guidance document also suggests that the DMF should contain the names of raw material suppliers and manufacturing process information. In our experience, such details are typically of no relevance to the Agency. Except in a few isolated instances, we strongly advise against providing such specific information to the Agency because of the continuing modifications that might have to be made to the DMF whenever even insignificant changes are made.

Regrind and Virgin Resins

On another matter – following work undertaken by the Society of the Plastics Industry (SPI) that compares the properties of polyethylene containers made with virgin materials and internal regrind – FDA has modified the final guidance document so that it makes no distinction between the use of virgin resin and regrind. FDA previously expressed concerns with the use of regrind in the production of packaging materials and suggested that only virgin polymers and resins be used. FDA's guidance continues to state that post-consumer recycled material should not be used to manufacture drug packaging components.

Easing Notification Requirements

In its other guidance document, entitled "Changes to an Approved NDA or ANDA," and in its proposed rulemaking, FDA deals with the question of equivalency considerations for changes to container closure systems. This issue has long plagued drug manufacturers both regarding packaging materials and other modifications that may be made to a drug product.

The current regulations specify that some modifications to a packaging material, such as a change from one container closure system to another, require submission of a supplemental application to the Agency for pre-market review and approval. Other modifications only require submission of a supplement to FDA, but do not require FDA approval. Still other changes (for example, a change from one polyethylene to another based upon a showing of equivalency in accordance with an official compendium) require only description of the change in the drug company's annual report.

In essence, the proposal would allow FDA a bit more latitude in easing these notification requirements by way of a guidance document, accomplished here with the draft guidance issued concurrently with the rulemaking. The draft guidance states in detail the types of modifications that the Agency sees as requiring submission of a prior approval supplement. The guidance document also sets out modifications that may require submission of a supplemental notice 30 days prior to marketing, although FDA prior approval, strictly speaking, is not required. In addition, the draft sets out modifications to the label that require prior approval from the Agency, as well as those that do not. Both guidance documents are available from FDA's website at www.fda.gov/cdr/guidance/index.htm. The proposed rule can be found in the Federal Register at 64 Fed. Reg. 34608 (June 28, 1999).

17.4 PHARMACEUTICAL STABILITY TESTING IN CLIMATIC CABINETS

Stability testing for pharmaceutical products has now been harmonized globally. All pharmaceutical products must undergo defined specific testing conditions in accordance to local climatic conditions. With the ICH guideline Q1A (R2) for stability, tests which was finalised in August 2003, and revised in 2005 (withdrawal of the chapter Q1F, which defines additional stress testing conditions in zones III and IV) new changes have taken place. With the withdrawal of chapter Q1F, the 10 member ASEAN countries have introduced their independent technical dossier related to the ICH guidelines and have adapted the testing conditions to suit their own climatic conditions. The enforcement of the ASEAN ICH guidelines into the ASEAN countries is currently in progress.

Climatic Stability Testing for Pharmaceutical Goods

The example of the ASEAN countries clearly demonstrates that the testing standard will become more intensive and specific. Individual advances from various countries to look into testing protocols under varying climatic conditions or more toughened testing conditions are in discussion. Once again the pharmaceutical industry sets new quality standards for the stability testing of pharmaceutical goods. It is a challenge for pharmaceutical companies but also a challenge to suppliers of testing equipment, to be prepared for the demands of tomorrow. After the latest revision and implementation for ICH stability testing the actual conditions are as now regulated in chapter Q1A (R2) for climatic stability testing and in chapter Q1B for photo stability testing (unchanged). The introduction of the ASEAN ICH guidelines which are defined as zone IVb created new regional testing conditions for the long term stability tests to be carried out in the 10 ASEAN (Association of South East Asian Nations). This leaves now following climatic zones (Grimm, 1980). It is now up to individual countries located in zone IV to decide whether they wish to join the newly created climatic zone IVb or to follow the testing conditions of zone IV defined by WHO / ICH.

- *Zone I:* Temperate zone
- *Zone II:* Mediterranean/subtropical zone
- *Zone III:* Hot dry zone
- *Zone IV:* Hot humid/tropical zone
- *Zone IVb:* ASEAN testing conditions hot/higher humidity

17.5 PHARMACEUTICAL STABILITY TESTING CONDITIONS

Chapter Q1A (R2) regulates the stability testing for long term testing at ambient, refrigerated and frozen storage conditions of pharmaceutical products. The testing conditions are displayed in Table 17.1.

Table 17.1: Long-term testing conditions

Climatic zone	Temperature	Humidity	Min. duration
Zone I	21°C ± 2°C	45% RH ± 5% RH	12 months
Zone II	25°C ± 2°C	60% RH ± 5% RH	12 months
Zone III	30°C ± 2°C	35% RH ± 5% RH	12 months
Zone IV	30°C ± 2°C	65% RH ± 5% RH	12 months
Zone IVb	30°C ± 2°C	75% RH ± 5% RH	12 months
Refrigerated	5°C ± 3°C	No humidity	12 months
Frozen	– 15°C ± 5°C	No humidity	12 months

Besides long term stability testing of various storage conditions, the ICH guidelines also requires accelerated testing conditions for all storage conditions (frozen, refrigerated and ambient) and an intermediate testing when the accelerated testing shows unacceptable deterioration (Table 17.2).

Table 17.2: Accelerated and Intermediate testing conditions

Climatic zone	Temperature	Humidity	Min. duration
Accelerated ambient	40°C ± 2°C	75% RH ± 5% RH	6 months
Accelerated refrigerated	25°C ± 2°C	60% RH ± 5% RH	6 months
Accelerated frozen	5°C ± 3°C	No humidity	6 months
Intermediate	30°C ± 2°C	65% RH ± 5% RH	6 months

Zone II Testing Only when Accelerated Testing Fails

While the exposure to climatic conditions in various climatic zones is undisputed and well accepted and carried out the photo stability testing in accordance to chapter Q1B is often not carried out or only sparsely performed. However, the chapter describes the stability testing procedures for new

substances and products which include generic pharmaceuticals as well. The chapter Q1B describes two options of
light sources. Option 1 is a light mix of D65/ID65 daylight mix,
xenon or metal halide light sources containing UV and daylight.
However, the UVB part needs to be removed and appropriate
filters need to be installed.

Option 2 is a two component light of UVA and visible light.
These light sources are usually specifically designed for UVA
(ICH compliant) and visible light. Filters are not necessary. The
use of option 1 and option 2 light sources depends on the
application. In a R and D, where a big number of substances
need to be tested in a short time, the use of xenon lights are
advantageous (short exposure time), while to test final products
the use of option 2 light sources are better suited to simulate
actual storage conditions, without additional heat impact.
Testing with option 2 is preferably to be carried out in climatic
chambers as the unwanted effect of heating (caused by
intensive light sources such as xenon) is eliminated and results
give real data about light impacts and storage precautions for
pharmaceuticals. The exposure times are defined by the
guidelines with a minimum of 1.2 Mio. Lux hours for visible
light and $200Wh/m^2$ for UVA light. It is important that the
light intensities of samples are determined at the sample
location. A recordable measurement at sample location will
provide the necessary information about effective intensities
and therefore required duration.

Stability Testing in Climatic Cabinets

What is the purpose of stability tests in constant climate
cabinets? and what role does the functionality of the chamber
play in this? The idea is that stability tests should reliably
indicate how and in what time the composition of a substance
or packaged product changes under environmental conditions.
This is done for the purpose of correctly determining and
declaring the shelf life of substances, products and medications.
In order to ensure that the process of making these
determinations is carried out by uniform criteria worldwide,
guidelines were developed, to be adhered to with regards to.

Temperature, humidity, light and carried out in an identical manner. The existence of various climatic zones on the globe makes this uniformity a little complicated – as already explained. To meet today's demands, a climate cabinet should, where possible, be constructed to "replicate" all climatic zones. This is of particular importance for manufacturers of pharmaceutical products who export into various climatic zones. For these manufacturers, chambers such as the ones manufactured by BINDER are of interest, since they are able to "replicate" all climatic zones—and meet all international standards required for this purpose: they are in agreement with the pharmaceutical ICH guidelines and beyond this, the FDA, GLP/GMP, etc.

17.6 BINDER CLIMATIC CHAMBERS

More Performance Reserves Needed

The climatic chambers from the BINDER KBF series are already prepared for future demands today. Their test spectrum permits not only the 30°C at 70% RH (Relative Humidity) required thus far, but also offers considerable performance reserves with options of 10°C at 90% RH They are open to all new standards, guidelines and changes. Therefore, those who are investing in a new climatic chamber today should look to the future. If testing must take place under other guidelines tomorrow, the chamber should be ready for it today.

Open to all Demands

Every user should check how open his products are to the demands of today and the near future. Manufacturers such as BINDER GmbH have thought about this well in advance and already have products on the market which meet all requirements. Chambers of the BINDER KBF series were constructed especially for the precise simulation of all climatic conditions with a constant climate, in accordance with the standards. This includes long-term storage and shelf life tests as per the pharmaceutical ICH guidelines and international standards. The KBF series guarantees high process security with tests which last for months under constant conditions, and precise, reproducible and constant humidity values in the entire work space. The humidity precision over time equals +/– 1.5% r.H. Adherence to the ICH guidelines and international standards applies to all climatic zones — and this will remain true in the future as well.

System Solutions are in Demand – Right Through to SMS Messaging

Even today, BINDER offers a spectrum, which reaches far beyond the normal range. It is important that BINDER offers not only a climatic chamber, but a complete solution — the climatic chamber, software, documentation, calibration/ validation and service. Everything is possible — right through to automatic SMS messaging to the user in the event of an alarm. High operating comfort and flexibility are provided by a colour screen programme controller which shows the actual and set point values of all process figures at a glance and permits up to 25-programme processes to be saved. A built-in monitoring controller, numerous alarm functions and an integrated line recorder round up the offer.

17.7 PHOTOSTABILITY TESTING

New Highlight for Photostability Tests (Q1B)

Proof that the products do not or not significantly change within a certain period of use must, among other things, be provided through the photostability test with light. For this purpose, BINDER offers the complete solution on the market– the KBF with standard equipment of ICH-conforming lighting. The special international ICH guideline Q1B was created for proving photostability. Since the fulfilment of this guideline must now mandatorily be documented by the authorities without exception, pharmaceutical companies are faced by new challenges in this regard in their test practices. For the new photostability tests, samples must be exposed to a light amount of 1.2 million Lux hours, as well as UV radiation of 200 Watt hours/m^2, in climatic chambers with ICH lighting.

But what is the most objective method of proving these light values? The fundamental prerequisite for reliable recording is the integration and display of the light values on the regulator, as in the BINDER KBF series with ICH lighting. This includes the automatic shutoff of the lamps (VIS and UV separately) when the freely selectable dosage values are reached. Reliable recording of the light amounts is provided at BINDER with Light Quantum Control, two spherical light sensors which, due to their direction-independent characteristics, function more precisely than planar sensors. However, the following should be decisive for the testing authorities: BINDER chambers possess APT-COM™ Data Control System software and therefore, excellent options for documenting the test conditions in every phase. The information from the light sensors flows into this system, providing optimal proof.

17.8 REVIEW OF PHARMACEUTICAL PRODUCT STABILITY, PACKAGING AND THE ICH GUIDELINES

The majority of pharmaceutical products show good stability over a wide range of climate conditions. A minority however display instability, which may be related to a wide range of challenges or a multiplicity of challenges such as variations in temperature, exposure to oxygen, light, moisture, etc. These challenges may be combated by storage under defined conditions (e.g., below x°C, in a refrigerator, etc.) or in packs which act as an effective barrier to the critical deterioration factor(s). The cause and route of this is normally determined for the Drug Substance and the product Dosage Form, early in the research and development stages, hence it should be relatively easy to find suitable storage conditions and a suitable form of protective packaging. However, the full role of the pack extends beyond that of basic protection as there are factors associated with overall quality, compatibility, assembly with particular emphasis on an effective closure system, economics, etc. right through to ultimate use and final disposal.

A pack product must therefore be seen as an effective marriage between the product and the pack, since the pack makes a major contribution to overall performance and to the declared shelf life. The importance of the pack must therefore not be under dated.

Having provided this short introduction with due emphasis on the role of the pack, it is now possible to consider the most likely impact of the International Conference on Harmonization (ICH) guidelines on the future of the pack and packaging in general, and vice versa. In the case of a new chemical entity (NCE, a molecule that is the product of drug discovery focused on a specific therapeutic area) which is then developed into a product dosage form, there is inevitably an assumption that sufficient testing has been carried out to establish, both in the research and development phases, that there will be no surprises when a formal stability programme is initiated. This later stage is often equated with a worst situation or theory both in the chosen testing conditions and the selection of the lower line in regression analysis as representative of the product shelf life. Variations within and between packs can also contribute to this situation by lack of effective evaluation and analysis within a stability programme. An example of this can arise where a pack on test is removed from a hot storage condition and is allowed to cool prior to chemical analysis being carried out. At the higher temperature of storage the closure fit could be loose or looser and then tighten up as it cools, hence giving the false impression of effectiveness if only checked prior to analysis. To cover this type of situation requires cap forces and physical appearance to be checked as follows:

(a) On immediate removal of products from the storage conditions.

(b) After cooling to the laboratory condition.

(c) Plus a possible further examination after product removal.

Tests (a) and (b) have to be carried out on separate samples. This also makes an assumption that such work has not been evaluated during development investigational stages. With such a background any resulting variations in analysis, then have a better chance of being coupled to possible pack variations or defects.

It should be noted that there could be an assumption that there is significant data on plastic screw caps on plastic screw threaded bottles. This can often be untrue as the plastic used on both cap and bottle may vary in addition to any dimensional detail. Experimentation is also complex as it needs to cover a range of torques (maximum, mean, minimum), immediate torques after removal from the storage condition, and torques after cooling or warming up, (packs can also be stored at colder temperatures). This work needs to be supported by full dimensional details as the tolerances allowed within the specification may also contribute. Since it is a destructive type of test, i.e. a cap can only be removed once, a full statistically designed experiment, can involve thousands of samples. What happens if the cap is reapplied and further stored and removed is yet another experiment.

The storage condition chosen under the ICH guidelines, 40°C, 75% RH, can be a very severe environment for a pack (try sitting in it for one hour and see how you like it?). An indication of its severity can be given by reference to a typical crisp biscuit like rich tea, where shelflife is related to its direct pickup of moisture, i.e. it looses the crispness, becomes soft and less palatable. Under a typical storage condition of 15°C to 20°C with an RH of 40%, storage at 40°C, 75% RH is likely to represent an acceleration factor of 32 times or more to such a biscuit, bearing in mind the accuracy of this calculation becomes more suspect once the factor exceeds 8 times. However, if moisture loss was a critical factor, under another set of circumstances, 40°C, 75% RH, can be a near equilibrium condition, should a product have an aqueous base containing dissolved salts in a permeable pack, hence little moisture loss might occur.

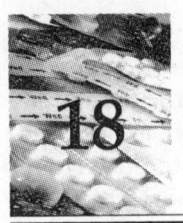 **Packaging Regulations and Legal Requirements**

18.1 INTRODUCTION

This guide is intended to assist both those involved in the placing of packaged goods on the market and the enforcement authorities to understand the application of the regulations. It aims to explain the regulations as interpreted by the DTI. The regulations themselves should always be read and understood, as they constitute the law, in contrast with the Guide, which is informative but has no legal authority. The regulations may be changed from time to time, so users should take care to keep themselves informed. The regulations are likely to be amended within the next 18 months. In this regard, information may be obtained from the DTI's Recycling Policy Unit.

18.2 THE REGULATIONS — IN BRIEF

The Packaging (essential requirements) regulations 2003 (S.I. 2003 No 1941) ("the Regulations") replace the packaging (essential requirements) regulations 1998 (SI 1998 No. 1165) ("the 1998 Regulations").

The regulations implement provisions of the European Parliament and Council Directive on Packaging and Packaging Waste (94/62/EC) ("the Directive") relating to the essential requirements to be satisfied by packaging in order to circulate freely on the single market.

The 2003 Regulations include the addition of derogations from the heavy metals limits in respect of certain glass packaging and plastic pallets and crates as set out in Commission Decisions 1999/177/EC and 2001/171/EC and the introduction of a set timeframe for producing proof of compliance of 28 days.

The definition of "packaging" in the Directive will be amended with the publication of the revised Directive in early 2004. This amendment will introduce an indicative list containing examples of what constitutes "packaging", in order to provide clarity for the purposes of producers and other interested parties. The definition of packaging in the regulations is due to be amended within 18 months of the publication of the new Directive.

These regulations do not affect the application of existing quality requirements for packaging, including those regarding safety, the protection of health and hygiene of the packed products, existing transport requirements or provisions on hazardous waste. In other words, existing legislation on these matters must also be complied with.

The Indian Pharmaceutical Industry today is in the front rank of India's science-based industries with wide ranging capabilities in the complex field of drug manufacture and technology. It ranks very high in the third world, in terms of technology, quality and range of medicines manufactured. From simple headache pills to sophisticated antibiotics and complex cardiac compounds, almost every type of medicines is now made in India.

Along with the complexity of the growing market the requirements of the packaging materials are also becoming complex. Glass as the preferred packaging material in the earlier days, being inert, did not pose any problem and in as much as it was properly closed the pack was safe for any pharmaceutical packaging. However, with the advent of plastics and other polymeric materials for packaging the situation has changed, as the problem of interaction with the product by the packaging material is a major concern to the users. Newer materials both for packaging and the product have thrown open newer challenges to the packaging technologists as it has to comply with the strict and stringent regulations applicable to the pharma industry.

18.3 REGULATION IN PACKAGING

The pharmaceutical industry is one of the most highly regulated industries in the world. Specific laws and directives govern each step from the product development and manufacture to the packaging and disposal.

In India there are two major government agencies responsible for drug regulation and control:

1. The Drugs Controller General of India (DCGI) and
2. The State Food and Drug Administrations (FDAs).

State FDAs monitor the drug manufacture, sale and testing by companies including packaging in their jurisdiction. The guidelines for packaging generally defines the type of container to be used, dividing into parenteral (glass or plastic) and non-parenteral (glass, plastic or metal) along with pressurised containers and bulk containers. Closure types are also listed including tamper evident and child resistant caps. Liners are also given prominence with inner seals and elastomers when used as closures.

The guidelines generally give the suitability of the packaging components in term of the physical, chemical and biological characteristics, specification and tests to be applied, stability and compatibility considerations and the involvement of adhesive and inks.

The ingredients added to the plastics such as plasticisers, pigments, etc. sometimes leach from the plastics into the product. Also certain ingredients of the product bind or get absorbed into the plastics. These are required to be tested with the extractive testing. The pharmacopoeia of different countries also provides lists of plastics that are permitted for use for pharmaceutical containers. If a material is not listed in the pharmacopoeia then generally reference is made to further directives dealing with plastic materials in contact with pharmaceutical product.

1. Labelling

Just as the container cannot be separated from the product in regulatory or technical terms, the label and leaflet are also intimately connected and in pharmaceuticals the term labelling generally includes both labels and leaflets. The function of a label and a leaflet is to inform the patient, the pharmacist, wholesalers to control the product in terms of its distribution and medical aspects and to reduce the risk of product liability claims. The patient has the label on the primary container and the packaging insert, the wholesalers has the carton and pallet labels, and the pharmacist has the immediate container label, carton label, packaging insert and possibly the summary of product characteristics (SPC). The doctor looks at the SPC or any such information.

All the information supplied should be accurate and consistent both scientifically and legally.

General labelling requirements for the primary pack of pharmaceutical products are:

- Product name.
- Active ingredients.
- Pharmaceutical form and contents.
- List of excipients (all for ophthalmic or parenteral) (any with recognizable effect).
- Method and route of administration.
- Special warnings.
- Expiry date.
- Special precautions.
- Name and address of authorisation holder.
- Authorisation number.
- Manufacturing batch number.
- Instructions for use for self-medication product.

Some smaller packs such as blister packs are sometime exempted from full labelling.

- Product name
- Authorisation holder's name
- Expiry date
- Batch number leaflet

All products must contain a patient leaflet unless all the information can be conveyed on the outer packaging label. The content of the leaflet and order of presentation must be as follows.

1. Identification of product.
2. Name of product, statement of active ingredients, pharmaceutical form, pharmacotherapeutic group, name and address of authorisation holder.

3. Therapeutic indications.
4. Information needed for taking the product.
5. Contraindications, precautions for use, interactions, special warnings, including use in pregnancy, elderly, effect on ability to drive vehicles and details of any excipients which may be important for safe and effective use of the product.
6. Instructions for use.
7. Dosage, method and route of administration, frequency of administration, duration of treatment where limited, action to be taken in the case of an overdose or lack of dosing and risk of withdrawal effects where possible.
8. Undesirable effects.
9. Effects that can occur under normal use of the product and action to be taken.
10. Expiry date.
11. Warning against use of the product after the date, appropriate storage precautions and warning against visible signs of deterioration.
12. Date on which package leaflet was last revised.

The leaflet must be written in clear understandable terms and has to be in the official language of the country. Package and environment of particular concern is the amount of packaging used and how it is disposed off. The concerns of packaging with respect to the environment are waste disposal, Ozone depletion and transport of harmful substances. As regards the waste disposal problems are concerned the approach has been to:

– Reduce the quantities of packaging material and therefore the waste.
– Reduction in harmfulness of waste.
– Promotion of reuse of packaging.
– Recycling and recovery of packaging waste.

Many countries have set targets of waste recovery thus necessitating the need for an efficient return collection and recovery system. Also it is necessary in many countries that the nature of the plastic to be identified by proper marking.

Pressurised aerosol plays a major part in pharmaceuticals and in many cases are perfect package efficiently protecting the product and dispensing an accurate dosage of the contents. A mixture of chlorofluorocarbons (CFCs) was used as propellant in such pack systems. This was causing depletion of the ozone layer. As a result their productions have been stopped in many countries. Alternative propellants are being developed and are being introduced in the market each day.

2. Hazardous Products

If the pharmaceutical products are hazardous in nature special regulations with respect to shipping of this either by air or by sea are in vogue. The packs for these hazardous products should comply with shipping regulations (IMDG or IAATA)

3. Barcodes

Bar codes are generally used as a product identification tool for use in the retail chains or for in-house applications like inventory management, sales tracking, etc.

Though EAN 13 is the most popular barcode for retail marketing special barcodes are developed for the pharmaceutical industries. EAN-13 is used worldwide for marking retail goods. The symbol encodes 13 characters: the first two or three are a country code which identify the country in which the manufacturer is registered (not necessarily where the product is actually made). The country code is followed by 9 or 10 data digits (depending on the length of the country code) and a single digit checksum.

Code 128 provides excellent density for all-numeric data and good density for alphanumeric data. It is often selected over Code 39 in new applications because of its density and because it offers a much larger selection of characters. The Code 128 standard is maintained by AIM (Automatic Identification Manufacturers).

Code 128 is generally used on the shipping container for coding additional informations such as batch number; lot number, etc. The pharmaceutical industry also uses some variations of the general codes for specific end uses in the industry. Some of them are: The Pharma Code is used for quality control and product identification for pharmaceutical products. Often one or more of the bars have different colour. The colours can be used to display extra information about the product each company can use different colouring for the bars, for example, a blue bar may mean the product may be taken orally.

The other main pharmaceutical barcode types are IKS, a variation of EAN 13, PZN (Pharma Zentralle Numer), MSI and IMH, used by the Italian health Ministry The bars encode a number which is not usually displayed.

Other pharmaceutical barcodes are often variations of standard labelling symbologies. Care should be taken, as sometimes the displayed number is not the number encoded in the bars.

The pharma industry the world over is a highly controlled industry. The regulations with respect to packaging are very stringent as the product is meant for such applications such as direct injections, intravenous fluids that are directly injected into the bloodstream.

A little mishap due to negligent or incompatible package will cause huge damage to the company by way of claims. The mandatory labelling requirements for safe use and dosage of the product is a must on the entire product. Various countries have different formats but the basic requirements remain the same - make the user aware of the safe usage of the product.

4. Entry into Force

The 1998 regulations came into effect on 31 May 1998. There was an exclusion from the requirements of the 1998 regulations for packaging manufactured before 31 December 1994 and lawfully placed on the market before 31 December 1999. The revised 2003 regulations came into effect on 25 August 2003.

18.4 REQUIREMENTS

The main requirement is that no person who is responsible for packing or filling products into packaging or importing packed or filled packaging into the United Kingdom may place that packaging on the market unless that packaging fulfils the essential requirements and is within the heavy metal concentration limits.

1. Legal/Essential Requirements

The essential requirements are:
- Packaging volume and weight must be the minimum amount to maintain necessary levels of safety, hygiene and acceptance for the packed product and for the consumer.
- Packaging must be recoverable in accordance with specific requirements.
- Noxious or hazardous substances in packaging must be minimised in emissions, ash or leachate from incineration or landfill.

2. Heavy Metal Limits

Aggregate heavy metal limits apply to cadmium, mercury, lead and hexavalent chromium in packaging or packaging components. The total by weight of such metals should not exceed:

600 ppm on or after 30 June 1998
250 ppm on or after 30 June 1999
100 ppm on or after 30 June 2001

Enforcement

Trading Drug Authorities Standards Officers may assess the compliance of any packaging by requesting technical documentation on both the essential requirements and the heavy metal limits. This documentation must be produced within 28 days of the request being made.

3. Packaging and the Single Market

Achieving the free movement of goods, in this case packaging, lies at the heart of the drive to create the single European market. In May 1985, European Community Ministers agreed on a 'New Approach to Technical Harmonisation and Standards' to fulfil this objective.

'New Approach' EC Directives set out the essential requirements (on products), usually written in general terms, which must be met before products may be sold in the United Kingdom or anywhere else in the European Community. Mandated European harmonised standards in respect of a product provide detailed characteristics and tests which, if met, provide a presumption of conformity with the essential requirements, with the result that the product should enjoy free movement anywhere within the community.

In this case, a series of seven standards were published by the European Committee for Standardization (CEN) in 2000 and have been in use in the UK for demonstrating compliance (*see* Annex A). References for two of the standards, EN13428:2000 on prevention by source reduction and EN13432:2000 on organic recovery, were published in the Official Journal and can now be used to presume compliance with those aspects of the essential requirements across the EC (except in relation to noxious and other hazardous substances).

Showing conformity with the non-harmonised standards is accepted by the UK as evidence of compliance. Until their references are published in the Official Journal, Member States are not obliged to grant market access to packaging meeting the standards. The standards have been through a revision process and are still in draft form, with a vote due at CEN in spring 2004. When the remaining standards are adopted, which will be late 2004 at the earliest, conformity with the standards must be taken as compliance with the essential requirements.

18.5 PACKAGING (ESSENTIAL REQUIREMENTS) REGULATIONS

These regulations apply to all packaging placed on the market in the United Kingdom as packed or filled packaging. Packaging is defined as "all products made of any material of any nature used for the containment, protection, handling, delivery and presentation of goods, from raw materials to processed goods, from the producer to the user or the consumer, but only where the products are sales or primary packaging; grouped or secondary packaging or transport or tertiary packaging". The full definition is in the regulations and further guidance as to the interpretation of packaging has been published by the Environment Agencies. However, anything recognized as packaging and in use as packaging would in general be likely to be covered by these regulations.

"Placing on the market" is not defined in the regulations, but is generally taken to refer to the first occasion on which the assembled (i.e. packed/filled) packaging is transferred with the intention of distribution on the EEA market. Whether the particular packaging product has been placed on the EEA market for the first time in the UK would need to be examined by reference to the particular circumstances of the case. Further guidance on this matter is available from the Local Authorities Co-ordinating Office on Regulatory Services (LACORS).

The reuse of packaging, for the same purpose for which it was conceived, is not considered to be a further placing on the market and therefore such reused packaging already in circulation is not covered by these regulations. Reusable packaging must fulfil the essential requirements and other requirements in the regulations on its first placing on the market. Where packaging has been reconditioned, remanufactured, repainted or altered for a different use, for example, it will be considered to be covered by the regulations when again placed on the market and the provisions of the regulations must be met.

The regulations do not apply:

a. To packaging used for a given product (that is, the packaging has been packed or filled) prior to 31 December 1994.

b. To packaging manufactured on or before 31 December 1994 and lawfully placed on the market on or before 31 December 1999.

c. To packaging manufactured, packed or filled for export without being placed on the market in the United Kingdom.

In all cases, packaging refers to the individual product, rather than the packaging design.

These regulations do not affect the application of existing quality or labelling requirements for packaging, including those regarding safety, the protection of health and hygiene of the packed products, existing transport requirements or the provisions of Council Directive 91/689/EEC on hazardous waste. In other words, existing legislation on these matters must be complied with.

Obligation

The obligation to ensure that these regulations are complied with lies with the packer/filler or importer of packed or filled packaging, and must be fulfilled when the packaged goods are placed on the market. In circumstances where the packaged product is marked with a brand or trade mark or other distinctive mark, the person so identified would normally be considered the packer/filler. It follows that, for an own-label product where the brand owner is not the packer/filler, the obligation to demonstrate compliance would fall upon the brand owner rather than the packer/filler.

The responsible person is obliged to ensure that all packaging (covered by these regulations) complies with the essential requirements and heavy metal limits, in addition to the other provisions of the regulations.

A. Legal/Essential Requirements

The essential requirements are:

1. Requirements Specific to the Manufacturing and Composition of Packaging

All packaging subject to these regulations must satisfy the following requirements:

a. "Packaging shall be so manufactured that the packaging volume and weight be limited to the minimum adequate amount to maintain the necessary level of safety, hygiene and acceptance for the packed product and for the consumer". This is not considered to indicate a preference between material types (e.g. glass versus plastics) or packaging systems (e.g. single trip versus reusable), although consideration of the overall environmental impact of the packaging system used would be encouraged.

b. "Packaging shall be designed, produced and commercialized in such a way as to permit its ... recovery, including recycling, and to minimize its impact on the environment when packaging waste or residues from packaging waste management operations are disposed of".

c. "Packaging shall be so manufactured that the presence of noxious and other hazardous substances and materials as constituents of the packaging material or of any of the packaging components is minimized with regard to their presence in emissions, ash or leachate when packaging or residues from management operations or packaging waste are incinerated or landfilled".

2. Requirements Specific to Reusable Packaging

Reuse is considered to be reuse for the same purpose for which the packaging was originally conceived. Packaging reused according to this definition need not comply with the regulations after first use. The following requirements must simultaneously be satisfied if packaging is declared as reusable:

a. The physical properties and characteristics of the packaging shall enable a number of trips or rotations in normally predictable conditions of use.

b. It must be possible to process the used packaging without contravening existing health and safety requirements for the workforce.

c. The requirements specific to recoverable packaging when the packaging is no longer reused and thus becomes waste must be met.

Reuse is not the same as reworking or reconditioning used packaging. Enforcement authorities may wish to see appropriate technical documentation to establish that reuse does not involve alterations which might impact upon compliance.

3. Requirements Specific to the Recoverable Nature of Packaging

All packaging, including reusable packaging, must fulfill at least one of the following:

(I) Packaging Recoverable Through Material Recycling

Packaging must be manufactured in such a way as to enable the recycling of a certain percentage by weight of the materials used into the manufacture of marketable products, in compliance with current standards in the Community. The establishment of this percentage may vary, depending on the type of material of which the packaging is composed. The revised standard on packaging reuse provides guidance on a "certain percentage". This is taken to mean that the packaging must make a positive contribution to the output of the material recycling process for which it is considered suitable. In other words, if packaging is considered suitable for a metal recycling process, it must be possible to extract metal from the packaging in the recycling process.

(II) Packaging Recoverable Through Energy Recovery

Packaging waste processed for the purpose of energy recovery shall have a minimum inferior calorific value (also known as 'minimum net calorific value') to allow optimisation of energy recovery. In the absence of harmonised standards, this is taken to mean that the packaging will make a positive contribution to the energy recovered in a waste incinerator.

(III) Packaging Recoverable Through Composting

Packaging waste processed for the purpose of composting shall be of such a nature that it should not hinder the separate collection and the composting process or activity into which it is introduced.

(IV) Biodegradable Packaging

Biodegradable packaging waste shall be of such a nature that it is capable of undergoing physical, chemical, thermal or biological decomposition such that most of the finished compost ultimately decomposes into carbon dioxide, biomass and water.

B. Heavy Metal Limits

The heavy metal limits refer to the sum of concentration levels of cadmium, mercury, lead and hexavalent chromium. The content of the specified heavy metals in packaging or any of its components must not exceed the following limits:

600 ppm by weight on or after 30 June 1998.
250 ppm by weight on or after 30 June 1999.
100 ppm by weight on or after 30 June 2001.

A packaging component is defined as any part of the packaging that can be separated by hand or by simple mechanical means. An example would be a bottle top. This does not include permanent coatings or pigments which would be regarded as a constituent of the packaging (or of the packaging component) and would thus be part of any calculation, but not required to meet the heavy metal limits independently. As an example, if a steel drum was coated in lead chromate based paint, it would only exceed the limit if the lead chromate was greater than the limit in relation to the mass of the drum and the paint taken together.

Testing is not specifically required nor defined in the regulations but note the section on 'Compliance' below. Compliance with the heavy metal limits is further addressed in Annex B.

The heavy metal limits do not apply to packaging which consists entirely of lead crystal glass.

There are two derogations from the heavy metals limits, which have been formally agreed at European level, and which have now been included in the regulations. These cover the placing on the market of plastic pallets and crates and enamelled glass and glass that may have been contaminated with lead by old glass in the recycling process.

C. Derogation for Plastic Pallets and Crates

Commission Decision 1999/177/EC of 8th February 1999 established the conditions for a derogation for plastic crates and plastic pallets in relation to the heavy metals concentration limits in the Directive and hence for the purposes of these regulations. This derogation came into force in UK legislation on 25th August 2003.

Until 4th March 2009, the Derogation allows plastic pallets and crates with heavy metals concentrations greater than those permitted by the regulations to be placed on the market if they fulfil a number of conditions, namely:

The plastic pallet or crate concerned must have been manufactured in a controlled recycling process, involving a maximum of 20% virgin material, and for which the remaining feedstock was other plastic pallets and crates. None of the identified heavy metals are intentionally added during the production process. The plastic pallet or crate may only exceed the heavy metal limits as a result of the addition of recycled materials.

Further to this, the crates and pallets must be introduced in a controlled distribution and reuse system in which:

New plastic pallets and crates containing the regulated metals are marked in a permanent and visible way.

A system of inventory and record-keeping is established.

The return rate of the pallets and crates over their lifetime is not less than 90%.

An annual declaration of conformity is drawn up by the responsible party, which must be made available on request for 4 years.

D. Derogation for Glass Packaging

Commission Decision 2001/171/EC of 19th February 2001 established the conditions for a derogation in relation to the heavy metals concentration limits in the Directive, and hence for the purposes of these regulations. This derogation came into force in UK legislation on 25th August 2003.

Until 30th June 2006, the derogation allows glass packaging heavy metals concentration limits greater than those permitted by the regulations to be placed on the market if they fulfil a number of conditions, namely:

No regulated metals have been intentionally introduced during the manufacturing process of glass packaging.

The limits are exceeded only as a result of the addition of recycled materials containing heavy metals.

That the responsible person placing the product on the market must submit a report to the enforcement authority verifying that the average heavy metals concentration levels of each glass furnace does not exceed a 200 ppm limit.

18.6 COMPLIANCE

The responsible person for the purposes of these regulations should demonstrate compliance with the regulations by providing the enforcement authorities on request with the necessary technical documentation. The responsible person must be able to supply technical documentation for a period of up to four years from the date on which the packaging is placed on the market. How and when such documentation is generated is not specified and is left to the person concerned; implicitly it could be compiled when a request is made by the enforcement authorities, although this would not be recommended as good practice. A request may be made at any time by the enforcement authorities, but reasonable notice would normally be given to allow the documentation to be supplied. The documentation must be produced within a maximum of 28 days of the enforcement authority making the request. This time limit was not defined in the 1998 regulations and came into effect on 25th August 2003.

One approach which may help businesses to meet a request from enforcement authorities would be if the responsible person had regard to the likely documentation required when designing new packaging. Until the remaining CEN standards have been published in the Official Journal, it will be the responsibility of the responsible person to ensure that information which shows that the packaging complies with the requirements is presented. In the interim period the illustrative compliance procedures in Annex A are offered for consideration, although they should not be regarded as definitive.

It is expected that the remaining CEN standards, covering the essential requirements, will be adopted, and can be applied and used to demonstrate compliance. The use of and demonstration of conformity with the CEN standards will carry with it the presumption of conformity of the packaging with the essential requirements in all Member States. In other words, if the standards are used, the product will be considered to meet the essential requirements unless there are grounds for suspecting otherwise. These standards are currently in draft awaiting a vote by CEN in Spring 2004 and are available from British Standards Institute (BSI). The final standards are not expected to be harmonised before late 2004. It should be noted that the standards represent only one means of demonstrating conformity with the essential requirements, and that other means may be acceptable. The procedures presented in Annex A are based on the draft standards and these may aid companies in considering their arrangements, but the similarity and relationship to the final standards cannot be guaranteed.

It may be appropriate for the responsible person to refer to their suppliers for relevant information, such as test results or technical information, or to specify requirements as part of the supply arrangements. However, it should be noted that such suppliers would normally only be able to provide information concerning those aspects of the essential requirements which are directly under their control and that legal responsibility remains with the responsible person. The umbrella standard (EN13427:2000) recommends the level in the supply chain at which the various assessments for conformity should be carried out.

Trade associations and materials organisations are encouraged to organise conformity testing or other supporting information covering their sectors to aid their members in assessing compliance. Where it is considered desirable to have an enforcement input into this, an approach can be made to LACORS.

18.7 ENFORCEMENT

It is the statutory duty of the following organisations to enforce the regulations within their area:

  a. In England and Wales, weights and measures authorities (the trading standards departments of local authorities); and

  b. In Northern Ireland, the Department of Enterprise, Trade and Investment.

  c. In Scotland, weights and measures authorities (the trading standards departments of local authorities); prosecutions against infringement of the regulations are brought by the procurator fiscal or lord advocate.

The enforcement authorities have available to them various powers based on the consumer protection Act 1987, including:

- Issuing suspension notices prohibiting the supply of packaging which is considered to breach the regulations.
- Making test purchases.
- Entering premises at any reasonable time.
- Requesting compliance documentation, inspecting processes and performing tests.

Enforcement practice will be based around the Home Authority Principle developed by LACORS. This means that any guidance given to a business by a 'home authority' (usually the one covering the area where the headquarters of the business is based) will be recognised by all Trading Standards Departments.

The principle is designed to consistency and common sense. The four express aims of the Home Authority Principle are to:

Encourage authorities to place special emphasis on goods and services originating within their area.

Provide businesses with a home authority source of guidance and advice.

Support efficient liaison between local authorities; and Provide a system for the resolution of problems and disputes.

18.8 OFFENCES AND PENALTIES

These regulations introduce the following offences:

1. Contravening or failing to comply with the essential requirements and heavy metal limits, penalised by a fine up to level 5 on the standard scale (currently £5000) on summary conviction or an unlimited fine on conviction on indictment.
2. Failing to submit compliance documentation at the request of the enforcement authorities, penalised by a fine up to level 5 on the standard scale.

These regulations refer to the following offences:

3. Contravening a suspension notice, penalised by up to 3 months imprisonment or a fine up to level 5.
4. Intentionally obstructing the enforcement authorities, penalised by a fine up to level 5.

5. Knowingly or recklessly making a false statement of compliance, penalised by a fine up to the statutory maximum on summary conviction (currently £5000) or an unlimited fine on conviction on indictment.

The defence of 'due diligence' applies to offences 1, 4 and 5. This means that a claim that a person took all reasonable steps and exercised all due diligence to avoid committing the offence may be made in defence. This may include reference to an act or default or information given by a third party, in which case it must be accompanied by information identifying the third party, or that information in possession of the person making the claim. In this case the provision in the regulations of 'liability of persons other than the principal offender' allows the third party to be prosecuted as though they had committed the offence.

Where an offence by a corporate body is shown to have been committed with the consent, connivance or through neglect of any director, manager or similar officer of the corporate body, they shall be regarded as having committed the offence as well as the corporate body.

- Contact points for further information.
- Enquiries should be addressed, in the first instance, to your local authority Trading Standards department (or 'home authority').
- Contact details of your local Trading Standards Office can be found by entering your postcode at: http://www.tradingstandards.gov.uk/
- 'The Agencies' Interpretation of Packaging booklet is available from these addresses or your regional environment agency office.
- Enquiries regarding the producer responsibility Obligations (packaging waste) regulations 1997 should also be referred to the Environment Agency (SEPA in Scotland, Environment and Heritage Service in NI).

18.9 ENVIRONMENTAL HELPLINE

The helpline is a government telephone enquiry service providing a comprehensive information and signposting service for firms seeking advice on a wide range of environmental issues that may affect their business. Case studies and guides to help with various packaging issues are available.

The Responsible Packaging Code of Practice, developed by INCPEN and endorsed by DTI, DEFRA and LACORS is available, priced at £5.00, from:

INCPEN (the Industry Council for Packaging and the Environment)

The following Draft Standards are available from BSI and contain greater detail than presented in the Annexes:

Title	Current Standard Number	Draft Standard Number (for public comment)
Packaging: Requirements for packaging recoverable by material recycling	EN 13430:2000	03/101363 DC
Packaging: Requirements for packaging recoverable through composting and biodegradation—Test scheme and evaluation criteria for the final acceptance of packaging	EN 13432:2000	N/A
Packaging: Requirements for packaging recoverable in the form of energy, including specification of minimum inferior calorific value	EN 13431:2000	03/101364 DC
Packaging: Requirements specific to manufacturing and composition-Prevention by source reduction	EN 13428:2000	03/101361 DC
Packaging: Reuse	EN 13429:2000	03/101362 DC
Packaging and the environment: Requirements for the use of European Standards in the field of packaging and packaging waste	EN 13427:2000	03/101360 DC

Contd...

Contd...

Packaging: Requirements for measuring and verifying the four heavy metals and other dangerous substances present in packaging and their release into the environment.		
Part 1: Requirements for measuring and verifying the four heavy metals present in packaging.	CEN/CR 13695-1:2000	*N/A*
Part 2: Requirements for measuring and verifying dangerous substances present in packaging, and their relese into the environment.	CEN/CR 13695-2:2002	*PrCEN/TR 13695-2 03/101404 DC*

ANNEX A

Illustrative Compliance Procedures

Design and Review Processes

Wherever possible, it is recommended that the concerns represented by the essential requirements and heavy metals limits are integrated into existing packaging design and review processes, particularly where formal quality or environmental management systems are in use.

Existing Packaging Lines

Although existing packaging portfolios may not refer to these concerns directly, other evidence of suitability for recovery processes may be found through primary evidence that such recovery does occur. In the case of other issues such as minimisation, supporting evidence as to the required strength of the packaging may be available through monitoring transit damage and similar parameters.

Overall

The following recommended procedures are written from the point of view of the design process. They can equally be applied to a review of an existing package.

In the procedures, packaging is considered as a packaging system made up of different functional units. Each functional unit is may be a single packaging unit or made up of several packaging components, which in turn are made of packaging constituents or packaging materials. An example would be a packaging system for the transport of beverages. This could be a cardboard carton used to transport filled bottles. The cardboard carton and the filled bottles would be functional units, interacting within the system but separable without affecting the product. The bottle would be made up of components: the empty bottle, the bottle top and the label, for example. The packaging constituents would be the cardboard of the crate, the glass of the bottle, any inks or pigments used and the materials of the bottle top and the label.

The compliance procedure should be applied to a packaging system as follows:

1. The packaging system should be minimised by weight and volume to take account of the system chosen and interaction between functional units where, for instance, a thinner bottle may require a stronger carton.
2. All packaging components should comply with the heavy metal limits currently in force (*see* Annex B).
3. All packaging components should comply with the requirement that the presence of noxious and other hazardous substances be minimised as constituents of the packaging material with regard to their presence in ash, emissions or leachate.
4. Any reusable functional unit should comply with the reuse requirement, particularly if designing for reuse affects the criteria for minimisation by weight and volume.
5. Each functional unit should comply with at least one recovery process, although different functional packaging in a packaging system may comply with different recovery processes.

Minimisation

It should be noted that the choice of system and material does not fall within the compliance procedure. Once the system is chosen and materials specified, they should be the minimum required for the design criteria.

These design criteria should establish the minimum adequate volume and weight usable for the packaging without compromising its performance.

A list of the relevant performance criteria should be produced in order to identify which criterion (called the critical area) prevents a further reduction in the quantity of material used. If it is not possible to identify a criterion preventing further reduction, then there is scope for further reduction until one of the criteria becomes the critical area.

The performance criteria identified in the draft standard are:

Product protection: Examples include protection against vibration, compression, humidity, light, oxygen, microbiological contamination.

Packaging manufacturing process: Examples include container shape, thickness tolerances, size, tooling, specifications minimising production waste.

Packing/filling process: Examples include impact and stress resistance, mechanical strength, packing line speed and efficiency, stability, heat resistance, closing, minimum headspace, hygiene.

Logistics (including transport, warehousing and handling) Examples include any handling requirement, space utilisation, palleting systems, damage resistance.

Product presentation and marketing Examples include product identity, brand recognition, labelling, retail display system requirements, pilfer resistance.

Consumer acceptance: Examples include unit size, ergonomics, tamper evidence, shelf life, dispensing methods, attractive presentation.

Information: Examples include product information, instructions, bar codes, expiry dates.

Safety: Examples include safe handling requirements, child resistance, hazard warnings, pressure release closures.

Legislation: Any requirements from national or international legislation or standardisation.

Other issues: Other economic, social or environmental implication not considered above relevant to weight or volume of packaging.

Noxious and Hazardous Substances

Noxious and hazardous substances must be minimised with regard to their presence in emissions, ash or leachate when packaging or residues from management operations or packaging waste are incinerated or landfilled. This implies that any noxious or hazardous substances should be reduced to the minimum level required for the effective functioning of the packaging. Where the presence of noxious or hazardous substances is included by design, the same procedure as presented for minimisation can be applied. This should be done by applying the procedure to the material containing the noxious or hazardous substance, although allowance should be made for the possible substitution, in part or full, of the noxious or hazardous substance by an alternative.

If the presence of noxious or hazardous substances is due to impurities then it may be appropriate to regard this as a quality control issue rather than a functional criterion.

As the regulations do not define noxious or hazardous substances, it is taken to mean any substance described as such in national or international law.

Reuse

Packaging must conform to the reuse requirement only when design criteria for other requirements, particularly minimisation, are developed with the intention of reuse. In other words, where packaging has been designed for reuse, and is therefore stronger and uses more material than single trip packaging, it must comply with the reuse requirement.

The requirements for reuse are fulfilled if:

1. The physical properties of the packaging are such that it can be reused. That is, it must be capable of being unpacked and then repacked (with or without reconditioning).
2. A reuse system is in place enabling the packaging to be reused.

The recognised reuse systems are closed loop, open loop or hybrid systems. They are defined below.

A closed loop reuse system is one where reusable packaging is circulated by a company or an organised group of companies.

An open loop reuse system is one in which reusable packaging circulates amongst unspecified companies.

A hybrid system consists of a reusable packaging item which stays with the end user with no redistribution, and one way packaging used to transport the contents to the reusable packaging, (this must fulfil the essential requirements in its own right). An example of such a system would be detergent pouches used to refill a reusable container that stays in the home.

3. Reusable packaging is subject to the same requirement of recoverability as set out below.

Recovery

Each recovery option (i.e. material recycling, energy recovery, composting and biodegradation) has its own requirements and design issues. Packaging must be designed to comply with at least one recovery option in full.

Material Recycling

To be considered to comply with this recovery process the packaging and its associated life cycle must be compatible with at least one specified recycling process. As such it depends on the criteria of the recycling process specified. The following is a general list of considerations common to recycling processes.

The considerations are:

* That raw materials in the combination used as packaging constituents should allow a positive contribution to the material reclaimed; that is, the packaging must contribute to the output of the recycling process.

* That effective emptying or residue removal is possible, to the extent that any remaining traces of product adhering to the packaging have no negative effect on the recycling process.

- That materials are separable if they may be required to undergo separate recycling processes (e.g. mixed plastics).
- That further aids or improvements to collection, sorting or recycling processes may be incorporated, (e.g. material identification markings, reduction in undesired materials).

Energy Recovery

Packaging composed of >50% by weight organic materials (e.g. wood, cardboard, paper and other organic fibres and plastics) shall be considered to comply. Thin gauge aluminium foil up to 50 μm thick shall be considered to comply.

If packaging does not fall into the above description, it may still comply by the application of the methods below:

1. Any packaging which has a calculated net calorific gain which is positive shall be considered to comply (described below).
2. Any packaging which has a positive net calorific gain determined experimentally, e.g. by ISO/DIS 1928 or ISO/5660: Part 1, shall be considered to comply.

The net calorific gain is defined as:

$$Q_{net} = Q - H_a$$

This must be positive for the packaging to be considered to comply.

Where:

Q is the energy released on combustion.

H_a is the energy required to adiabatically heat the post-combustion residues of a material from ambient temperature to the final combustion temperature. In this case the ambient temperature is defined as 25°C and final temperature as 850°C.

Composting and Biodegradation

The conditions for composting and biodegradation are fulfilled when the packaging complies with the following: Packaging should be largely combustible solids; that is, the residue after incineration should be less than 50% of the packaging. This figure is taken as indicating the organic content. The organic materials should be inherently and ultimately biodegradable materials that are break down to carbon dioxide, mineral salts, biomass and water or methane. Chemically unmodified materials of natural origin such as wood, wood fibre, paper pulp and jute are accepted as biodegradable for these requirements. The packaging should disintegrate in the waste treatment process. The packaging should not retard or adversely affect the waste treatment process. The packaging should not degrade the quality of the resulting compost. Packaging material demonstrated to be organically recoverable in a particular form shall be accepted as organically recoverable in any other form having a smaller mass to surface ratio or wall thickness.

ANNEX B

Comments on Heavy Metals in Packaging

Although it is recognised that heavy metals are rarely intentionally added to packaging, there are some known uses that may occur. In particular: Glass (undecorated). Glass containers may contain lead due to its unintentional introduction to recycled glass. This may be from lead containing glass or old wine bottle capsules. Levels of lead over 600 ppm have been detected in some European glass containers, and as there is no known environmental or health risk through heavy metals in glass, a derogation has been agreed at european level. The regulations were amended to reflect this in 2003. Glass (decorated). Enamels used to decorate or print on glass may contain lead oxide as a basic component and cadmium may be used in bright red and yellow enamels. A number of major producers signed a voluntary agreement aiming to phase out the use of heavy metals in enamels in enamelled glass. In the interim, a derogation has been agreed at European level. The regulations were amended to reflect this in 2003.

Non food grade plastics. Pigments containing cadmium are occasionally still found, as is the use of lead chromate for yellow, orange and red pigments. A derogation from the heavy metal limits has been agreed at european level for plastic pallets and crates manufactured by recycling old plastic pallets and crates in closed loop schemes. The regulations were amended to reflect this in 2003. Drums lead chromate or other hexavalent chromium compounds may be used in some colours of coatings for metal drums. Non-food metal containers. Rarely, lead solder may be used in metal container construction.

Pigments and inks. May in a few cases be based on lead, cadmium or hexavalent chromium compounds. More generally, the specified heavy metals will occur in small levels in most materials and some level of compliance monitoring should be performed.

Compliance

It is recommended that, wherever possible, an upper limit of the heavy metal concentration is calculated on the basis of data from the constituent materials. If testing is considered to be required, any suitable test for a given material or packaging may be used. If such testing is carried out, particular care should be taken to ensure that a sample is representative of all the constituent materials and the proportion in which they are used. For example, a sample taken from a drum could be seriously affected if the drum had a red stripe which contained lead chromate, yet the rest of the coating did not. *Some potentially useful standards and documents exist*: 'Survey of the content of heavy metals in packaging on the Danish market' H Andreasen, N Bernth, I Christensen, PH Jensen (Danish DTI). This document describes sampling and testing methods used in the survey, in particular the use of wavelength dispersive X-ray fluorescence (WDXRF) and microwave assisted acid digestion followed by inductively coupled plasma atomic emission and mass spectrometry (ICP – AES and ICP - MS). *United States Environment Protection Agency Methods*: US EPA Method 3050: Acid digestion of sediments, sludges and soils and other matrices. This method is used for the CONEG regulations, which are similar to the heavy metal limits in these regulations, and uses ICP – AES, ICP – MS, graphite furnace atomic absorption spectroscopy (GFAA) and flame atomic absorption spectroscopy (FLAA).

US EPA Method 3052: Microwave assisted acid digestion of siliceous and organically based matrices. A total digestion method for glass similar to the Danish DTI method. It is a microwave assisted nitric and hydrofluoric acid digestion method. US EPA Method 3060: This is an alkaline digestion method for extracting hexavalent chromium from soluble, absorbed and precipitated forms of chromium compounds in soils, sludges, sediments and similar waste. It is included as the other methods do not distinguish between trivalent and hexavalent chromium. This method can be followed by US EPA method 7196 or 7199 (colorimetrically by UV spectrophotometry or ion chromatography respectively).

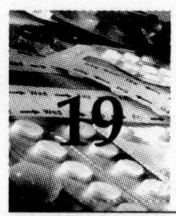

The Package Line and Packaging Functions

19.1 INTRODUCTION

The packaging function essentially comprises of the following packaging systems, such as:

Primary Packaging System

Such package components as well as subcomponents which actually come into contact with the product, or those that may have a direct effect on the product shelf-life.

Secondary Packaging System

These emphatically include such items as: cartons, corrugated shippers and pallets. Historically, the pharmaceutical packaging actually consists of the following aspects, namely:

- Effective containment of pharmaceutical dosage forms so that at any material line before the stipulated expiry date of the drug product – one may enjoy the availability of a safe and efficacious dosage form.
- Based upon the intensive stability studies there should be no interaction between product and package.

Present scenario: A virtual revolution has taken place in the recent past very much within the preview of the ever – growing domain of pharmaceutical technology due to the emerging intricacy and complexity prevailing both in dosage form and in packaging forms.

The tremendous developments in pharmaceutical industry across the globe have become so interwined that virtually the drug product should need to be defined in terms of both packaging and formulation.

Typical examples:

1. Prefilled syringes
2. Transdermal patches
3. Metered dose inhalers/nasal sprays

Contemporary definition of pharmaceutical packaging may be stated as that – combination of components necessary to contain, preserve, protect and deliver a safe, efficacious drug product. However, the previously mentioned definition is very much restricted to the primary package components, i.e. the components, and sub-components that come into direct contact with the product during storage and delivery.

19.2 PACKAGING FUNCTIONS

Nevertheless, the packaging of pharmaceuticals essentially involves containment as well as protection from potentially damaging environmental factors, for instance: moisture, oxygen, temperature and light.

Transport: The packaging system must also safely transport the product via distribution channels either to the pharmacist or to the physician.

Deliver: The overall packaging system may deliver the drug product to the end- user (i.e. patient). In this specific instance, the package essentially constituents an integral part of the dosage form because ultimately the package actually controls or affects the amount of the drug delivered, i.e. the dosage intended.

In short, a modern-day pharmacist should be critically aware of:

- A broad spectrum of packaging issues related directly to the stability and acceptability of the dosage form.
- During the process of development – this array of relationship of container material and their respective properties should be understood, and managed to optimize shelf life, whereas at the other end of the development chain, the retail pharmacist must not compromise that shelf life via improper or under packaging.

19.3 PACKAGE LINE

1. Practical requirements of operating pharmaceutical packaging lines

The cardinal objectives of any pharmaceutical packaging line may be broadly described as:

- Filling
- Closing
- Identification and
- Protecting

The finished product safely to be predetermined specification, besides considering closely an economic cost involved. Unfortunately, the design as well as operational functions seems to be more complicated in nature than usually expected.

Evidently, the lost of other requirements are:

- High steady output.
- Zero dour time due to stoppages.
- No wastage or rejects.
- Superb consistent quality.
- Low maintenance, labour, services costs.
- No risk of any possible mix-ups.
- Excellent hygienic environment.
- Minimum depreciation.
- Minimum wear and tear.
- Regular and effective maintenance.
- Effective operation and operating staff training.
- Provision of adequate safety for staff.

2. A typical pharmaceutical packaging line essentially needs only

  i. **Materials:** Product and packaging materials carefully supplied to predetermined and agreed specifications.
 ii. **Services:** e.g. electricity, compressed air, water, low-pressure steam to predetermined standards.
iii. **Personnel:** Properly and effectively trained operators, engineers, quality control and other supportive staff.

3. Split-up various activities of a typical packaging line

The following activities of a typical packaging line are as stated under:

- Bringing the materials (both product and packaging) on to the line.
- Packaging line services needed absolutely to make the line operate duly.
- Filling the product right into the prime container.
- Closing the prime container.
- Labelling the prime container.
- Addition of leaflet.
- Cartoning, i.e. secondary packaging.
- Collation, casing and palletisation for warehousing and distribution.
- On line testing.
- Provision of motivated trained production support staff.

Interestingly, the filling and packaging operations may be accomplished on one either single machinery or be split across several machines, such as:

i. **Fill and seal (single machines):** For example, blister packs-where the product gets duly filled-closed-labelled.
ii. **Bottle filling (multiple machines):** For example, (a) unscrambling-cleaning-rinsing, (b) Filling-closing-labelling are two distinct separate operations to reach the same state of completion.

4. Speed of packaging line

It is one of the most vital and critical considerations that may be justifiably expressed as below:

i. **Design speed,** i.e. the speed of the line running under no load and optimum parameters.
ii. **Capacity,** i.e. the upper sustainable limit of acceptable product passing a point on the line prior to warehousing.
iii. **Running speed:** The instaneous operating rate.
iv. **Output,** i.e. the exact quantity of acceptable quality product that passes from the line under load conditions to warehouse in a standard time.

5. Packaging–line operations

In fact, a typical complex packaging line, the most observed critical operation invariability comprise of the following cardinal factors, include:

- Operators at almost the stipulated (recommended) output speed, i.e. the filling operation.

- Other machines meant for upstream and downstream must be designed in such a manner so as to have a bare minimum queuing of unfinished packaging as practically possible to accomplish, which may be clearly seen from the following Table 19.1.

Table 19.1

Funning speed (containers per minutes)	Machine function	
113	Unloaded packaging materials	up stream
110	Unscrambled containers	"
105	Clean containers	"
100	Filling product into prime container	"
105	Closing prime container	downstream
108	Labelling prime container	"
110	Cartoning and leaflet addition	"
115	Collation of a stand. quantity of prime containers	"
117	Casing of a stand. number of collations	"
120	Palletisation to preset stack pattern of cases	"

6. Packaging – line services

Certainly, the packaging-line services cannot function in isolation. It essentially needs several most critically required services, such as:

Clean-dry-oil free air -electricity -gases (N_2 and O_2) cooling water -vaccum -removal of waste materials -and finally removal of finished packs.

However, one may classify the packaging -line services into three convenient heads and therefore, must be taken into consideration before building the line:

1. Atmosphere, sterility level of cleanliness, environment, removal of waste materials.
2. Line -layouts -operators -loading points.
3. Specifications -maintenance -planning -inventory control - testing off line — and QA/QC support.

Solutions to cleanliness problems: These are as follows:

1. Must isolate the filling and closing operation in a GMP - classified zone (European class A or B; FDA class 100). Here, all materials entering an aseptic area should be perfectly sterile.
2. For non-sterile situations necessary to build up a floor to ceiling, partition bet the filling/closing equipment and the secondary packaging operations and must restrict the movement of fibre-shedding materials.
3. Strip off all fibre-shedding packaging materials to the line in plastic containers and using an aluminium pallet.
4. Keep the fibre-shedding materials away from the close/ immediate viccinity of product contact materials.
5. To provide special closed containers for solid wastes like: Cases, cleaning cloths, plastic coverings, etc.
6. Special instructions for recovery/reworking of reject packs produced on the line to substantially reduce contamination.

Planning and inventory control: Do have the important task of ensuring that for any given order:

1. Services in the production building will all be available for the time needed for the order completion like: heating-ventilation -AC -power.
2. Requisite QC -passed materials available for job.
3. Requisite man power available including scheduling of on line changeover -engineering support -QC, etc. presence is available promptly.
4. Internal transport, warehouse space, etc. available for the finished packed goods.

Index

Reader's Notes

Reader's Notes